# 500 Best Quinoa Recipes

## 100% Gluten-Free
## Super-Easy Superfood

## Camilla V. Saulsbury

Robert ROSE

500 Best Quinoa Recipes
Text copyright © 2012 Camilla V. Saulsbury
Photographs copyright © 2012 Robert Rose Inc.
Cover and text design copyright © 2012 Robert Rose Inc.

*For complete cataloguing information, see page 528.*

**Disclaimer**
The recipes in this book have been carefully tested by our kitchen and our tasters. To the best of our knowledge, they are safe and nutritious for ordinary use and users. For those people with food or other allergies, or who have special food requirements or health issues, please read the suggested contents of each recipe carefully and determine whether or not they may create a problem for you. All recipes are used at the risk of the consumer.

We cannot be responsible for any hazards, loss or damage that may occur as a result of any recipe use.

For those with special needs, allergies, requirements or health problems, in the event of any doubt, please contact your medical adviser prior to the use of any recipe.

Design and Production: Kevin Cockburn/PageWave Graphics Inc.
Editor: Sue Sumeraj
Recipe Editor: Jennifer MacKenzie
Proofreader: Sheila Wawanash
Indexer: Gillian Watts

Cover and interior photos (pages 12–15 of color inserts): Colin Erricson
Associate Photographer: Matt Johannsson
Food Stylist: Kathryn Robertson
Prop Stylist: Charlene Erricson

Interior photos (pages 2–11 and 18–31 of color inserts) by Tango Photography
Food Stylist: Solène Thouin
Prop Stylist: Jacques Faucher

Other photographs: © iStockphoto.com/Sayarikuna (page 1 of color inserts),
© iStockphoto.com/Marek Uliasz (page 16 of color inserts),
© iStockphoto.com/Cat London (page 17 of color inserts),
© iStockphoto.com/Debbi Smirnoff (page 32 of color inserts)

Cover image: Herbed Chicken and Pomegranate Salad (page 200)

We acknowledge the financial support of the Government of Canada through the Book Publishing Industry Development Program (BPIDP) for our publishing activities.

Published by Robert Rose Inc.
120 Eglinton Avenue East, Suite 800, Toronto, Ontario, Canada M4P 1E2
Tel: (416) 322-6552 Fax: (416) 322-6936
www.robertrose.ca

Printed and bound in Canada

2 3 4 5 6 7 8 9 IMG 20 19 18 17 16 15 14 13 12

FSC
www.fsc.org
MIX
Paper from responsible sources
FSC® C103567

# Contents

# Keen on Quinoa

Francisco Pizarro may have been a master conquistador, but he would have made a rotten dietitian. Following his invasion of the Incan empire in the early 16th century, he returned to Spain with two New World crops — potatoes and corn, which were destined to change European cuisine — while nearly obliterating a third crop in his wake. Little did he realize that third crop, first cultivated by the Incas thousands of years earlier, would one day be lauded as one of the world's most nutritious foods.

The crop? Quinoa.

Although cooked and eaten like a grain, quinoa (pronounced *KEEN-wah*) is technically a seed, classified as a "pseudocereal." Quinoa seeds are harvested from a broadleaf plant that belongs to the goosefoot (*Chenopodium*) family, which is closely related to spinach, beets and chard. Quinoa plants can grow upwards of 7 feet (2.1 m) and have brilliantly colored, flowering seed heads in shades ranging from orange, yellow and pink to red, purple and black. Once the seed head is dried, the small quinoa seeds are simply shaken out. The edible seeds are typically white or pale golden, but can be pink, red, orange, purple or black. They are coated in saponin, a bitter, resin-like substance that protects the plant from insects and birds.

## A Nutrition Superstar

Quinoa has now been classified a superfood by nutritionists and a "super-crop" by the United Nations. The reason is clear: quinoa has a near-perfect balance of protein, carbohydrates and dietary fiber. Further, it is rich in vitamins and minerals, namely thiamine, riboflavin, vitamin $B_6$, folate, magnesium and vitamin E, and is a good source of iron, calcium, phosphorus and zinc. Of all whole grains, quinoa is also highest in potassium, a mineral that is essential for optimal brain function, blood sugar regulation, muscle function and sound mental health.

Quinoa's protein content has garnered considerable attention because it includes all of the essential amino acids humans need. The National Academy of Sciences calls quinoa "one of the best sources of protein in the vegetable kingdom" and the World Health Organization rates the protein in quinoa as comparable to milk protein (casein), a position supported by extensive nutritional research. Quinoa is an especially good source of the amino acid lysine (linoleic acid), a member of the omega-6 group of essential fatty acids. Rarely found in plants, lysine assists in the building of muscle protein and is important in the production of antibodies, hormones and enzymes, collagen formation and tissue repair.

Thanks to its hardiness and high yield, quinoa is being hailed as a food of the future and as a possible relief crop for battling famine and malnutrition. Unlike most grains, which require massive irrigation and infrastructure to grow, quinoa can flourish almost anywhere, under relatively harsh conditions. Further, the seed head from a single quinoa plant typically contains enough seeds to plant a quarter of an acre. So quinoa requires fewer resources to grow, while simultaneously providing outstanding nutrition.

## Quinoa Nutrition Profile

| 1 cup (250 mL) Uncooked Quinoa | | 1 cup (250 mL) Cooked Quinoa | |
|---|---|---|---|
| Calories | 626 | Calories | 222 |
| Fat (total) | 10 g | Fat (total) | 3.5 g |
| Saturated fat | 1 g | Saturated fat | 0 g |
| Trans fat | 0 g | Trans fat | 0 g |
| Cholesterol | 0 mg | Cholesterol | 0 mg |
| Sodium | 8 mg | Sodium | 13 mg |
| Carbohydrates | 109 g | Carbohydrates | 40 g |
| Dietary fiber | 12 g | Dietary fiber | 5 g |
| Protein | 24 g | Protein | 8 g |

*Source:* Nutrient Data Laboratory. Retrieved January 29, 2012, from the USDA National Nutrient Database: http://www.nal.usda.gov/fnic/foodcomp/search/index.html.

# A Gluten-Free Option

Another of quinoa's appealing attributes is that it is naturally gluten-free, so it's safe for anyone with celiac disease or gluten or wheat sensitivities. Quinoa can be particularly valuable for those with celiac disease, who are often deficient in calcium and magnesium. Quinoa is a good source of calcium, and its lysine content assists in the absorption and storage of calcium. Quinoa also offers a good source of magnesium: 1 cup (250 mL) of cooked quinoa provides about 30% of the daily requirement.

Quinoa flour rivals wheat flour for versatility, making it possible to create myriad gluten-free baked goods that bake up quickly and easily, with excellent flavor and texture.

# A Culinary Triple-Threat

Beyond its phenomenal nutritional profile, quinoa is a rare culinary triple-threat: it's delicious, easy to prepare and ultra-versatile. In other words, quinoa is a home cook's best friend.

## Seeds in Space

Because of their high nutrient content and infinite culinary possibilities, quinoa seeds are currently being considered by NASA as a possible long-term renewable food source for astronauts going into space on multi-year missions.

## What Is Gluten?

Gluten is the elastic protein in wheat, rye, barley, durum, einkorn, graham, semolina, bulgur, spelt, farro, Kamut and triticale. Its elasticity is what holds breads together, makes cupcakes peak and makes biscuits as light as air. Think of gluten as the glue ("gluten" comes the same Latin root as "glue") in wheat, rye and barley.

The easiest way to prepare quinoa is to cook it like rice (see page 11). A quick simmer on the stovetop and it's done. Once cooked, quinoa has a light, fluffy texture and a delicate crunch. It looks similar to couscous, but is semi-translucent, with a white band or tail. It works beautifully in everything from salads to soups to breakfast porridge, and in just about any main dish imaginable. Quinoa's delicate, nutty flavor imparts distinction to any dish, savory or sweet.

And that is merely the tip of the iceberg. Quinoa seeds can be lightly toasted until golden and crunchy, then used in much the same way as toasted nuts. Or they can be sprouted for an über-nutritious addition to sandwiches and wraps. They can be steamed and rolled into flakes (called quinoa flakes) akin to rolled oats and used in recipes much the same way. Or they can be ground into flour for use in a wide variety of gluten-free baked goods and to make pasta.

# The History of Quinoa

Thousands of years before its present-day popularity, the Incas recognized and celebrated the superfood qualities of quinoa.

Quinoa is native to the Andean mountains of Peru, Bolivia and Chile, but it was the Incas who cultivated it and used it to feed an empire. They gave it the name *la chisiya mama* ("the mother grain") because of its ever-bearing and nourishing properties, and it remains the staple food of the Quechua and Aymara peoples, descendants of the Incas who still inhabit the rural Andean areas of Peru, Boliva, Ecuador and Chile.

The Incas were geniuses of plant domestication, and quinoa was arguably their most sacred crop. Each year, the Inca emperor broke the soil with a golden implement and sowed the first seeds. Religious festivals included an offering of quinoa in a fountain of gold to the sun god, Inti, and in ancient Cuzco, Incas worshipped entombed quinoa seeds as the progenitors of the city. Quinoa was eaten daily as porridge, in soups and stews, ground into flour for flatbreads, and fermented into a drink (one of the many types of South American *chichi*) that was considered the "drink of the Incas." Inca warriors are believed to have carried small balls of cooked quinoa and animal fat (called "war balls") into battle for stamina, energy and strength.

When Spanish conquerors, led by explorer Francisco Pizarro, arrived in the Andes in 1532, the quinoa landscape was altered both literally and figuratively for centuries to follow. Wary of how quinoa was revered in Incan culture, the conquistadors deemed it a threat to Christianity and thus heretical. They destroyed the intricately cultivated quinoa fields, replacing them with traditional European crops such as wheat, barley, carrots and broad beans. Moreover, they marginalized quinoa, stigmatizing it as a "trash" food better suited for animal feed than human consumption. It was only in the remotest areas of the Andes that small groups of indigenous people continued to eat quinoa.

Despite its obscurity, quinoa gained some notice in the modern era. Traveling through Colombia in the early 19th century, Alexander von Humboldt, a German naturalist who explored many regions of Latin America, observed that quinoa was to the region what "wine was to the Greeks, wheat to the Romans, cotton to the Arabs." He was excited by the crop because, at that time, starvation was rampant all over the world, and he had gone to South America looking for new foods to combat it.

Quinoa also received periodic attention in Western books and magazines. Articles about it appeared in *Popular Science Monthly* in 1893, *National Geographic* in 1916, *Encyclopedia of Gardening* in 1931 and *The Farm* quarterly in 1950. A 1918 *Bulletin of the Pan American Union*, published by the U.S. government, featured a lengthy article on the wondrous but little-known crop called quinoa. Along with in-depth descriptions of how quinoa was prepared and eaten by indigenous peoples, the author marveled at how such a remarkable crop could have been overlooked in the West and urged correction of the oversight.

But the spark that ignited the sensational rediscovery of quinoa did not occur until many decades later, and it did not originate from a government entity but rather from two Americans, Stephen Gorad and Don McKinley, who had learned about the wonders of quinoa while studying in South America under Oscar Ichazo, a Bolivian spiritual leader who encouraged his followers to eat quinoa to help them reach higher plains of spirituality while meditating. The two men returned to the U.S. and eventually founded the Quinoa Corporation in Boulder, Colorado, in 1983, initiating the first significant cultivation of quinoa since the Incas were wiped out. Agricultural research focusing on the remarkable crop soon followed at major universities, and by the mid-1980s, quinoa was making regular appearances in health food and specialty stores in North America and Europe.

Since then, quinoa has grown steadily in popularity and has found a new life as a replacement for rice and other grains, while gaining a reputation as a potent functional food, prized for its delicious taste as much as for its nutritional benefits. While most quinoa is still grown in South America, it is also cultivated in the U.S. (in Colorado and California), Canada, China, Europe and India. It is also being cultivated experimentally in Finland and the UK.

# Quinoa 101

Cooking with quinoa is easy, quick and convenient, and quinoa can be incorporated into countless meals and recipes. Consider this your quinoa primer, a comprehensive, instructive guide to purchasing, preparing, eating, storing and savoring this versatile supergrain. You'll find that integrating quinoa into your daily menu — whether for breakfast or lunch, at snack time or dinnertime, or even as a sweet treat — is a cinch.

## Forms of Quinoa

Quinoa comes in dozens of colors, making it as beautiful as it is delicious. It can be steamed and rolled into delicate flakes that can be used like quick oats, or ground into a fine-textured flour that is naturally gluten-free and can be used to make baked goods and gluten-free pasta. This section identifies the primary quinoa products available on the market and explains how they are used and how to store them.

### Quinoa Seeds

When most people speak of quinoa, they are referring to quinoa seeds. At first glance, the uncooked seeds resemble couscous or millet. Upon closer inspection, they have two flat surfaces and rounded sides, like tiny aspirin tablets. Although quinoa seeds come in many colors, the most commonly available varieties are white (or pale golden), followed by red and black. Any color of quinoa seeds can be used in any of the recipes in this collection; when I call for a particular color, it is primarily for a dramatic appearance.

To keep quinoa seeds as fresh as possible, store them in an airtight container in the refrigerator for up to 6 months or in the freezer for up to 1 year.

### Quinoa Flour

Quinoa flour is made by grinding quinoa seeds to a fine consistency. It looks and feels like all-purpose wheat flour and is easily adapted to a broad range of baking recipes, from desserts to muffins to breads (with the exception of yeast breads). Quinoa flour can also be added directly to soups and stews as a thickening agent, or used like a protein powder in smoothies and shakes.

Unlike other gluten-free flours or flour blends, there is no need to add gums (such as xanthan gum or guar gum) to make quinoa flour "work" in baking recipes, a feature that is particularly appealing to home bakers interested in gluten-free

---

**Quinoa Leaves**

Although quinoa seeds receive all the attention, the leaves of quinoa plants — which resemble large spinach or chard leaves — are among the most nutritious greens. They can be enjoyed raw in salads or gently cooked in sautés, soups or stews.

baking, incorporating nutritious non-wheat flours into their diets or creating baked goods that fit into a high-protein/low-carbohydrate diet. Most importantly, quinoa flour, with its naturally nutty and slightly sweet flavor, appeals to anyone interested in delicious baked goods.

Because quinoa flour has a distinctive earthy, nutty flavor, you may want to begin with recipes that feature other bold flavors, such as dark molasses, cocoa powder or a mix of strong spices. The more familiar you become with quinoa flour, the more you will love the unique flavor it imparts to recipes.

When baking with quinoa flour, keep in mind that it tends to absorb more liquid than traditional wheat flour. Recipes for quick breads and muffins tend to benefit from the addition of an extra egg. Because quinoa flour does not contain gluten, baked goods may taste and feel slightly heavier; an additional egg and a small increase in leavening can make all the difference in producing a delicious, pleasing result. Follow the recipes in this collection for guidelines, then have fun experimenting with your own recipes and variations.

Quinoa flour, like whole wheat flour and many other gluten-free flours, is higher in fat than all-purpose flour, so it can spoil easily. For the best flavor and freshness, always check the expiration date on the package, and store it in an airtight container in the refrigerator or freezer to prolong freshness. Let the cold flour return to room temperature before using it.

> ### If Cooking Gluten-Free, Avoid the Bulk Foods Section
>
> If you are following a gluten-free diet, avoid buying quinoa products from the bulk foods section. The lower prices are appealing, but the chances of cross-contamination with gluten-containing products is high. Someone may have used the same scoop for quinoa and for bulgur!

## Make Your Own Quinoa Flour

While quinoa flour is readily available in many supermarkets — typically in the health food section — and natural food stores, you can also make your own at home, using a grain mill or a clean coffee or spice grinder. This is a great way to experiment with quinoa flour without buying an entire package of it; it is less expensive to grind your own.

Place 1/4 cup (60 mL) of quinoa seeds in the grinder (adding any more will overload the grinder and prevent the seeds from being ground to a fine consistency). Using on/off pulses, process, shaking the grinder every few pulses to ensure an even grind, until the seeds are finely and evenly ground. Repeat with more seeds until you have the desired amount of flour. Note that 3/4 cup (175 mL) of whole quinoa seeds yields about 1 cup (250 mL) of fine quinoa flour.

## Quinoa Flakes

Quinoa flakes are made by steaming and flattening the seeds with huge rollers (much like the process to create rolled oats). The resulting flakes can be prepared into a quick-cooking porridge akin to oatmeal. Quinoa flakes can be used as a substitute for oats in most recipes, from granola to cookies to cake. They can also be used to thicken soups and stews and to add protein to smoothies.

As with quinoa flour, it is best to store quinoa flakes in an airtight container in the refrigerator or freezer to prolong freshness.

## Quinoa Pasta

Quinoa pasta is made from a nutritious blend of quinoa flour and corn, and is available in several shapes and sizes. It is gluten-free, and its flavor, texture and appearance are very close to those of regular pasta.

I do not focus on quinoa pasta in this collection because swapping quinoa pasta for regular pasta is so straightforward: simply use it in place of traditional pasta in your favorite recipes. So long as the other ingredients in the pasta or soup recipe are gluten-free, it is a quick and easy way to make a pasta dish gluten-free.

# Preparing Quinoa

A significant part of quinoa's appeal is its ease of preparation. It can be cooked several different ways to produce a tender, fluffy grain, or it can be toasted (dry or in a bit of oil or butter), yielding crisp, crunchy quinoa that can be used as you would chopped nuts. One constant, no matter how you plan to cook quinoa, though, is a quick rinse to remove any residual saponin coating.

## Before You Cook: Removing Saponin

Virtually all quinoa that reaches consumers in North America and Europe has already had the saponin removed (this includes quinoa flour and quinoa flakes). Nevertheless, it is important to give quinoa seeds a brief rinse before use, to remove any saponin residue that may remain after processing. Place the quinoa in a fine-mesh strainer and rinse thoroughly under cold water for 30 to 60 seconds. This ensures that the cooked quinoa will have a delicately sweet, pleasant flavor.

If you are uncertain whether the quinoa you purchased has had the saponin removed (for example, if you bought quinoa from a bulk foods container), soak it more thoroughly: submerge the quinoa in enough cold water to cover it by 1 inch (2.5 cm). Let stand, stirring once or twice, for at least 5 minutes or as much as 2 hours. Drain the quinoa through a fine-mesh sieve and rinse thoroughly under cold water for 30 to 60 seconds.

## Quinoa Cooking Methods

To cook quinoa for a side dish or breakfast porridge, or for use in a recipe that calls for cooked quinoa, you can use the simmer method, the pasta method or the rice cooker method. All yield equally good results.

### Ancient Quinoa

Archaeological evidence relating to the consumption of quinoa in ancient Andean societies has been found in a prehistoric tomb in Chile and among the contents of a mummy's possessions in Peru. According to findings in northern Chile, archaeologists believe quinoa was in use prior to 3000 BC. Further evidence from the Ayacucho area places the domestication of quinoa before 5000 BC.

## The Simmer Method

Simmering is the most common way to prepare quinoa, and the process is very similar to cooking rice: simmer one part quinoa with two parts water until the liquid is absorbed. However, it takes less time from start to finish than rice (a boon for busy cooks), and it is, I would contend, easier to produce consistent results.

To prepare 3 cups (750 mL) of cooked quinoa, combine 1 cup (250 mL) quinoa and 2 cups (500 mL) water in a medium saucepan (see chart below for other amounts of quinoa and water and their corresponding yields). Bring to a boil over medium-high heat. Reduce heat to low, cover and simmer for 12 to 15 minutes or until liquid is just barely absorbed. Remove from heat. Cover and let stand — 2 to 3 minutes for an al dente texture, ideal for salads; 5 to 6 minutes for a light, fluffy texture, ideal for side dishes; or 8 to 10 minutes for a softer texture best suited to desserts, breakfasts and incorporation into baked goods. Fluff with a fork.

Darker quinoa seeds — particularly red and black seeds — use the same quinoa-to-water ratio as the more common white quinoa. However, they do not always absorb all of the water in the designated cooking time. If excess liquid remains at the end of the cooking time, simply drain it off.

## Cooked Quinoa Yields

| Uncooked Quinoa | Water | Cooked Quinoa |
| --- | --- | --- |
| 2 tbsp (30 mL) | ¼ cup (60 mL) | ⅓ cup (75 mL) |
| ¼ cup (60 mL) | ½ cup (125 mL | ¾ cup (175 mL) |
| ⅓ cup (75 mL) | ⅔ cup (150 mL) | 1 cup (250 mL) |
| ½ cup (125 mL) | 1 cup (250 mL) | 1½ cups (375 mL) |
| ⅔ cup (150 mL) | 1⅓ cups (325 mL) | 2 cups (500 mL) |
| ¾ cup (175 mL) | 1½ cups (375 mL) | 2¼ cups (550 mL) |
| 1 cup (250 mL) | 2 cups (500 mL) | 3 cups (750 mL) |
| 1⅓ cups (325 mL) | 2⅔ cups (650 mL) | 4 cups (1 L) |

*Note:* The pasta method and the rice cooker method produce the same yield ratios for uncooked and cooked quinoa as the simmer method.

## Are Nutrients Lost with the Pasta Method?

The moisture-bound nutrients in quinoa and other whole grains are found in the oils in the outer, protein-rich layer of the endosperm (the aleurone layer) and within the endosperm, both of which are dense enough that the nutrients cannot seep out to the outer layer of the grain. Hence, nutrient loss from boiling and draining quinoa (the pasta method) is negligible.

## The Pasta Method

The easiest way to cook quinoa is to boil it like pasta. This method is particularly good for individuals who detect residual bitterness from the quinoa saponins. It is not necessary to rinse the quinoa before using this method.

Fill a large pot with water, add salt if desired and bring to a boil. Add the desired amount of quinoa and cook for 10 to 13 minutes or until tender. Drain the quinoa through a fine-mesh sieve. Return the quinoa to the still-warm pan (off the heat), cover and let stand for 2 to 3 minutes. The moisture in the cooked quinoa will steam it slightly, producing a light and fluffy texture.

If using this method to prepare quinoa for a salad, do not return the drained quinoa to the pan. Instead, rinse it under cold water until cooled. Shake the sieve to remove as much water as possible, then transfer the quinoa to a bowl and fluff with a fork.

### The Rice Cooker Method

Prepare the quinoa in a rice cooker using one part quinoa to two parts water. Follow the manufacturer's instructions for cooking white rice. When the cooking cycle is complete, fluff the quinoa with a fork.

### The Thermos Method

Quinoa (and almost any other grain) can be prepared with ease using this little-known method. Place 1 cup (250 mL) quinoa in a 4-cup (1 L) Thermos. Add 2 cups (500 mL) boiling water. Tightly close the Thermos and turn it upside down several times to combine the quinoa and water. Let stand for 6 to 8 hours. Remove lid, shake quinoa into a medium bowl and fluff with a fork. This method yields 3 cups (750 mL) cooked quinoa. You can use the quinoa immediately (it will still be warm) as a side dish or as part of a main dish. If prepared overnight, it is also a perfect way to have ready-to-eat quinoa for breakfast: simply drizzle the quinoa with milk or non-dairy milk and sprinkle with your favorite toppings. Alternatively, let the quinoa cool and refrigerate or freeze it for future use.

## Toasting Quinoa

Dry-toasting quinoa deepens the nutty sesame flavor of the seeds. Dry-toasted seeds can be used like chopped nuts in baked goods such as muffins, quick breads and cookies. You can also dry-toast quinoa before cooking it (using any method) or before grinding the seeds into flour.

Toasting the seeds in a bit of butter or oil makes them crisp and crunchy, perfect for sprinkling on salad or yogurt, or adding to trail mix. Dried herbs, ground spices or fine sea salt can be added to the quinoa mixture before toasting for additional flavor and variety.

### Dry-Toasting

Rinse quinoa, drain, then transfer to a clean, dry dish towel to remove remaining moisture. Heat a large skillet over medium-high heat. Adding no more than $1/4$ cup (60 mL) quinoa at a time, toast quinoa, stirring occasionally, for 3 to 4 minutes or until golden brown and just beginning to pop. Transfer to a large bowl and let cool. Store in an airtight container in the refrigerator for 6 to 8 weeks.

## Toasting in Butter or Oil

Rinse quinoa, drain, then transfer to a clean, dry dish towel to remove remaining moisture. Preheat oven to 350°F (180°C). In a small bowl, combine quinoa and melted butter or oil (such as vegetable oil, olive oil, toasted sesame oil or warmed coconut oil), using 1 tbsp (15 mL) butter or oil for every $1/2$ cup (125 mL) quinoa. Spread the mixture in a single layer on a large rimmed baking sheet. Bake for 9 to 12 minutes, stirring once or twice, until fragrant. Transfer to a large bowl and let cool. Store in an airtight container in the refrigerator for 6 to 8 weeks.

# Sprouting Quinoa

Quinoa sprouts are delicious, easy to make and a wonderful way to enjoy quinoa raw. Sprouting activates the natural enzymes in the seeds, boosting their vitamin content and softening them so that they can be added directly to salads, sandwiches and other recipes without being cooked.

Sprouting does not require any special equipment, but you will need to allow 2 to 3 days for the sprouts to appear and grow long enough to eat. Keep in mind that the quality of the sprouts will depend on the quality and age of the seeds. For the best results, use organic seeds that are well within the expiration date on the package.

In a medium glass bowl or an 8- or 9-inch (20 or 23 cm) square glass baking dish, combine $1/2$ cup (125 mL) quinoa and 2 cups (500 mL) filtered, reverse osmosis or distilled cold water. Stir to completely immerse all of the seeds, then loosely cover with a clean dish towel or cheesecloth. Let stand at room temperature for 1 hour. Drain the seeds in a fine-mesh sieve and rinse with cold water. Return the quinoa to the bowl and loosely cover with the dish towel. Let stand at room temperature for 8 to 10 hours. Rinse and let stand for 8 to 10 hours two to three more times, until the sprouts have emerged from the seeds (they are very small and short). Shorter sprouts will keep in the refrigerator for up to 5 days; longer sprouts should be kept in the refrigerator and used within 24 hours.

### Quinoa and Kon-Tiki

Having read about its high nutritive value, Thor Heyerdahl took quinoa on the raft Kon-Tiki to sustain himself and his crew on their long journey.

# Stocking the Quinoa Pantry

This ingredient guide will ensure that all of the quinoa dishes you prepare from this collection are healthful and delicious. Those following a gluten-free diet should use gluten-free versions of the following ingredients:

- Cornmeal
- Oats
- Baking powder
- Chocolate
- Vanilla extract
- Almond extract
- Soy sauce
- Tamari
- Miso
- Broth

## Grains

As tasty as it is on its own, quinoa also works in harmony with a variety of other grains, most notably in baked goods. In this collection, quinoa is combined with cornmeal and oats in a variety of recipes, to delicious effect.

## Cornmeal

Cornmeal is simply ground dried corn kernels. There are two methods of grinding cornmeal. The first is the modern method, in which milling is done by huge steel rollers, which remove the husk and germ almost entirely; this creates the most common variety of cornmeal found in supermarkets. The second is the stone-ground method, in which some of the hull and germ of the corn is retained; this type of cornmeal is available at health food stores and in the health food sections of most supermarkets. The two varieties can be used interchangeably in most of the recipes in this collection, but I recommend sticking with the stone-ground variety where specified, as it has a much deeper corn flavor and is far more nutritious.

## Rolled Oats

Two types of rolled oats are called for in these recipes: large-flake (old-fashioned) rolled oats are oat groats (hulled and cleaned whole oats) that have been steamed and flattened with huge rollers; quick-cooking rolled oats are groats that have been cut into several pieces before being steamed and rolled into thinner flakes. For the best results, it is important to use the type of rolled oats specified in the recipe.

---

### Gluten-Free Cornmeal

Although cornmeal is naturally gluten-free, cross-contamination from wheat and barley during the milling process makes many brands unusable in gluten-free baking. However, there are many brands of gluten-free cornmeal, so if you are following a gluten-free diet, check the packaging (and phone the manufacturer) to make sure the cornmeal is gluten-free before using it.

### A Note about Oat Tolerance

A small percentage of people with celiac disease may not tolerate oats at all. If you are unsure about your tolerance, consult your doctor.

If you're following a gluten-free diet, it is imperative to buy oats that are certified gluten-free, as oats can easily be contaminated with wheat during harvest, storage or other stages of processing. Gluten-free oats are available in large-flake (old-fashioned) and quick-cooking.

# Frozen Fruits and Vegetables

Keeping a selection of frozen fruits and vegetables in the freezer is a great way to make quick and simple quinoa dishes in an instant, whether for quick soups or for morning smoothies.

In addition to its convenience, frozen produce can sometimes be more nutritious than fresh. When fresh fruits and vegetables are shipped long distances, they rapidly lose vitamins and minerals thanks to exposure to heat and light; by contrast, frozen fruits and vegetables are frozen immediately after being picked, ensuring that all of the vitamins and minerals are preserved.

Whenever possible, choose organic frozen fruits and vegetables. Some varieties to keep on hand include:

- Winter squash purée (typically a blend of acorn and butternut squash)
- Petite peas
- Chopped greens (e.g., spinach, Swiss chard, mustard greens)
- Chopped onions
- Vegetable stir-fry blends
- Broccoli florets
- Shelled edamame
- Corn
- Lima beans
- Berries (blueberries, blackberries, raspberries, strawberries)
- Diced mangos
- Diced pineapples
- Sliced peaches

## Hidden Gluten

Gluten is found in many obvious places (breads and bread products), but it is also hidden in thousands of products you would never think to suspect, from meats to flavorings to Popsicles. Reading labels is critically important, as is becoming familiar with the names of potential gluten ingredients. Celiac organizations such as the National Foundation for Celiac Awareness, Celiac.com, the Center for Celiac Research and the Celiac Disease Center offer information about hidden gluten ingredients on their websites.

# Interpreting Organic Labels

Understanding the various organic labels can be a challenge. Here's what the four most common labels and claims mean:

| | |
|---|---|
| **"100% Organic"** <br> USDA ORGANIC | For a food product to be labeled "100% organic" and be able to bear the USDA organic seal, it must be made with 100% organic ingredients. The product must also have an ingredient list and list the name of the certifying agency. |
| **"Organic"** <br> USDA ORGANIC | For a food product to be labeled "organic" and be able to bear the USDA organic seal, it must be made with 95% organic ingredients. The product must also list the name of the certifying agency and have an ingredient statement on the label in which organic ingredients are identified as organic. |
| **"Made with Organic Ingredients"** | To make this claim, a food product must be made with at least 70% organic ingredients. The product must also list the name of the certifying agency and have an ingredient statement on the label in which organic ingredients are identified as organic. |
| **"Some Organic Ingredients"** | Food products with less than 70% organic ingredients cannot bear the USDA seal nor have information about a certifying agency or any reference to organic content. |

# Shelf-Stable Tomato Products

Choose organic tomato products whenever possible, as they tend to be lower in sodium and residual chemicals.

## Diced Tomatoes

Canned diced tomatoes can replace diced fresh tomatoes in most recipes, especially soups and stews. Stock up on diced fire-roasted tomatoes, too, as they add a subtle smoky flavor to dishes.

## Crushed Tomatoes

Canned crushed tomatoes (sometimes called ground tomatoes) are a convenient way to add fresh tomato flavor to soups, stews and pastas without the separate step of puréeing.

## Tomato Sauce

Tomato sauce can be used to make delicious sauces, stews and soups when you want to give them a distinct tomato flavor. For true tomato flavor with minimal processing, be sure to select a variety of tomato sauce that is low in sodium and has no added seasonings.

## Tomato Paste

Tomato paste is made from tomatoes that have been cooked for several hours, then strained and reduced to a deep red, richly flavored concentrate. It is available in both cans and convenient squeeze tubes. Just a tablespoon or two (15 or 30 mL) can greatly enrich a wide variety of dishes, adding acidity, depth and a hint of sweetness. Select a brand that is low in sodium and has no added seasonings.

## Sun-Dried Tomatoes

Sun-dried tomatoes are a flavorful and nutritious way to add an extra bit of zest to quinoa recipes. Look for organic sun-dried tomatoes, which are often processed at a lower temperature than most commercial varieties, preserving some of the nutrients.

## Marinara Sauce

Jarred marinara sauce — a highly seasoned Italian tomato sauce made with onions, garlic, basil and oregano — is typically used on pasta and meat, but it is also a great pantry staple for creating a range of quinoa meals in minutes. For the best tomato flavor and the most versatility, choose a variety with minimal ingredients and low sodium. The majority of marinara sauces on the market are gluten-free, but check the label to be certain.

## Chunky Tomato Salsa

Like marinara sauce, ready-made chunky salsa — rich with tomatoes, peppers, onions and spices but low in calories — packs tremendous flavor into quinoa recipes in an instant. For the best flavor and nutrition, select a brand that is low in sodium and has a short list of easily identifiable ingredients.

| Gluten-Free Tomato Paste |
|---|
| If you're following a gluten-free diet, choose a tomato paste that is clearly labeled "gluten-free." A small number of brands use wheat-based additives as thickening agents. |

# Dried Fruit

A variety of dried fruit is essential for adding depth of flavor and sweetness to quinoa recipes. Whenever possible, opt for organic dried fruit. The following are top picks:

- Raisins (both dark and golden)
- Dried currants (sometimes labeled Zante currants)
- Dried cranberries (preferably sweetened with fruit juice)
- Dried cherries
- Dried apricots
- Dried apples
- Dried figs
- Prunes (dried plums)

# Legumes

Legumes are nutritional powerhouses, very low in cost and easy to prepare for use in a wide variety of quinoa recipes. In this collection, legumes are used in a wide variety of forms, from canned beans to dried split peas and lentils to tofu and tempeh.

## Canned Beans

With their high protein content, wide availability, low cost and convenience, canned beans are ideal in combination with quinoa for quick, healthy meals. For the best flavor and versatility, select varieties that are low in sodium and have no added seasonings. The following varieties are great choices to keep on hand for everything from dips to entrées:

• Black beans
• White beans (e.g., cannellini and white navy beans)
• Pinto beans
• Red kidney beans
• Chickpeas

## Dried Split Peas (Green and Yellow)

A variety of yellow and green peas are grown specifically for drying. These peas are dried and split along a natural seam (hence, "split peas"). Split peas are very inexpensive and are loaded with good nutrition, including a significant amount of protein. They are available packaged in supermarkets and in bulk in health food stores. Unlike dried beans, they do not require presoaking.

## Dried Lentils

Lentils are inexpensive, require no presoaking, cook in about 30 to 45 minutes and are very high in nutrients (soybeans are the only legume with more protein). Lentils come in a variety of sizes and colors: common brown lentils and French green lentils can be found in supermarkets, and increasingly, so can red and black lentils.

## Soybean Products

Just a short while back, soybean products — tofu, soy milk, tempeh, soy cheese and soy yogurt — were considered health food oddities. Now, most of these items have gone mainstream and are usually available in well-stocked grocery stores.

### Tofu

All of the recipes in this collection were tested with refrigerated tofu. While shelf-stable tofu is convenient, the flavor and texture are markedly inferior. Tofu, or bean curd, is made from soybeans that have been cooked, made into milk and then coagulated. The soy milk curdles when heated, and the curds are skimmed off and pressed into blocks. Tofu can be found in extra-firm, firm and soft varieties in the refrigerated section of the supermarket. Be sure to use the variety specified in the recipe for optimal results.

### Tempeh

Tempeh (pronounced *TEM-pay*) is a traditional Indonesian food. It is made from fully cooked soybeans that have been fermented with a mold called rhizopus and formed into cakes. Some varieties have whole grains added to the mix, creating a particularly meaty, satisfying texture. Tempeh, like tofu, takes on the flavor of whatever it is marinated with, and also needs to be stored in the refrigerator.

# Nuts, Seeds and Nut/Seed Butters

Nuts and seeds — including natural nut and seed butters — are very nutritious and are a perfect complement to the naturally nutty, sesame-like flavor of quinoa. In addition to being excellent sources of protein, nuts and seeds contain vitamins, minerals, fiber and essential fatty acids (such as omega-3 and omega-6).

## Nuts

A wide variety of nuts are used in this collection, including walnuts, cashews, pecans, almonds, peanuts, hazelnuts and pistachios. Many of the recipes call for the nuts to be toasted before they are used. Toasting nuts deepens their flavor and makes them crisp. To toast whole nuts, spread the amount needed for the recipe on a rimmed baking sheet. Bake in a preheated 350°F (180°C) oven for 8 to 10 minutes or until golden and fragrant. Alternatively, toast the nuts in a dry skillet over low heat, stirring constantly for 2 to 4 minutes or until golden and fragrant. Transfer the toasted nuts to a plate and let them cool before chopping.

## Ground Flax Seeds (Flaxseed Meal)

Flax seeds are highly nutritious, tiny seeds from the flax plant. They have gained tremendous popularity in recent years thanks to their high levels of omega-3 fatty acids. But to reap the most benefits from the seeds, they must be ground into meal. Look for packages of ready-ground flax seeds, which may be labeled "flaxseed meal," or use a clean spice or coffee grinder to grind whole flax seeds to a very fine meal. The meal adds a warm, nutty flavor to a wide range of recipes. Store ground flax seeds in an airtight container in the refrigerator for up to 5 months or in the freezer for up to 8 months.

### Green Pumpkin Seeds (Pepitas)

Pepitas are pumpkin seeds with the white hull removed, leaving the flat, dark green inner seed. They are subtly sweet and nutty, with a slightly chewy texture when raw and a crisp, crunchy texture when toasted or roasted. They can be used much as nuts are used — sprinkled atop salads, soups and entrées for a pleasant, contrasting crunch, or added to muffins, cookies or breads.

### Shelled Sunflower Seeds

Sunflower seeds are highly nutritious and have a mild, nutty flavor and texture. The recipes in this collection call for seeds that have been removed from their shells. They can be used in place of nuts in both sweet and savory dishes.

### Sesame Seeds

Tiny and delicate, the flavor of sesame seeds increases exponentially when they are toasted. Used as a flavoring in many Asian preparations, sesame seeds are also delicious in sweet and savory baked goods.

### Nut and Seed Butters

Delicious, nutritious, ultra-convenient nut and seed butters are a boon for any meal of the day, as well as for snacks, desserts and quick breads. They can also impart instant richness to a wide range of sauces and dressing.

A wide variety of all-natural, unsalted nut and seed butters is increasingly available at well-stocked supermarkets, co-ops and natural food stores. Seed butters, such as tahini and sunflower seed butter, are an excellent substitution for nut butters for those with tree nut allergies or sensitivities.

Below are some of the butters used in this collection. They may be used interchangeably in any recipe calling for nut butter, unless otherwise specified. Store opened jars in the refrigerator.

- Unsweetened natural peanut butter
- Unsweetened natural almond butter
- Unsweetened natural cashew butter
- Tahini (sesame seed butter)
- Sunflower seed butter

# Eggs, Dairy and Non-Dairy Milks

Eggs, dairy products and non-dairy milks are essential ingredients in any healthy pantry, helping you prepare everything from short-order breakfasts and dinners to countless baked goods.

## Eggs

All of the recipes in this book were tested with large eggs. Select clean, fresh eggs that have been handled properly and refrigerated. Do not use dirty, cracked or leaking eggs, or eggs that have a bad odor or unnatural color when cracked open; they may have become contaminated with harmful bacteria, such as salmonella.

## Decoding Egg Labels

These days, egg cartons are covered in labels ranging from "organic" to "cage-free" to "animal welfare approved." It's confusing, to say the least. Here's a quick guide to the terms you need to know, according to USDA guidelines:

- *Organic:* Chickens must be cage-free with some outdoor access (amount not defined), cannot be given antibiotics, and must be fed organic, vegetarian food. The USDA organic seal is the only official egg label claim that's backed by federal regulations.
- *Free Range:* Chickens are out of cages, and can roam freely around a farmyard for at least part of the day, but there is no regulation in the U.S. about the amount or quality of outdoor access. There are no restrictions on what the birds can be fed.
- *Cage-Free:* Chickens have continuous access to food and water and are out of cages, but do not necessarily have access to the outdoors. They may be tightly packed into a shed, with no access to a farmyard.
- *Certified Humane:* Chickens are out of cages inside barns or warehouses, but may not have access to the outdoors. There are regulations to ensure that the chickens can perform natural behaviors and to limit the density of birds. More information is available at www.certifiedhumane.com.
- *Animal Welfare Approved:* This term is given to independent family farmers with flocks of up to 500 chickens that are free to spend unlimited time outside on pesticide-free pasture and cannot have their beaks cut (beak cutting is allowed in all the previous definitions and is very common). Eggs from these farms are most commonly found at specialty or health food stores and at farmers' markets.

The following terms are unregulated and therefore mean nothing:

- Natural
- Naturally Raised
- No Hormones
- No Antibiotics

## Dairy Products

All dairy foods are not created equal. Although they are generally rich in calcium and protein, some higher-fat varieties can also be high in artery-clogging saturated fat and cholesterol. So enjoy your dairy, but choose wisely, using the list below as a guide.

## Buttermilk

Commercially prepared buttermilk has a delicious and distinctive tang. It is made by culturing 1% milk with bacteria. When added to baked goods, it yields a tender, moist result and a slightly buttery flavor.

If you don't have buttermilk, it's easy to make a substitute. Mix 1 tbsp (15 mL) lemon juice or white vinegar into 1 cup (250 mL) milk. Let stand for at least 15 minutes before using, to allow the milk to curdle. Any extra can be stored in the refrigerator for the same amount of time as the milk from which it was made.

### Lower-Fat Dairy Products

Dairy products are used in a wide range of recipes in this book. All of the recipes were tested with lower-fat dairy products, but you may use regular dairy products if you prefer.

## Evaporated Milk

Produced by evaporating nearly half the water from fresh milk, evaporated milk is a shelf-stable canned milk. It is an excellent option for adding richness to recipes in place of cream.

## Yogurt

Yogurt, like buttermilk, is acidic and adds a distinctive tang to recipes. It tenderizes meats and baked goods, and makes an excellent substitution for sour cream in a wide range of recipes.

Greek yogurt is a thick, creamy yogurt similar in texture to sour cream. It is made by straining the whey from yogurt and is very high in protein, not to mention incredibly delicious.

## Ricotta Cheese

Ricotta is a rich, fresh cheese with a texture that is slightly grainy but still far smoother than cottage cheese. It is white and moist and has a slightly sweet flavor. A lower-fat variety is readily available and adds richness without fat to a wide range of dishes. It also has significantly fewer calories than the full-fat variety.

## Cottage Cheese

Cottage cheese is used in many recipes in this collection, from morning muffins to evening main dishes. In addition to its versatility, it has significant nutritional value (most notably in protein and calcium).

# Non-Dairy Milks

Non-dairy milks are essential for vegans, as well as those who are lactose intolerant or are allergic to dairy. But they are also a delicious option for all of us, whether to use in cooking or baking, or to drink straight up. The variety and availability of non-dairy milks is greater than ever, and you cannot beat their shelf-stable convenience. Although non-dairy milks are available in a variety of flavors, opt for plain when substituting for milk in any of the recipes in this collection.

### Soy Milk

Soy milk is made by combining ground soybeans with water and cooking the mixture. Finally, the liquid is pressed from the solids and then filtered.

### Almond Milk

Almond milk is made from almonds, water, sea salt and typically a small amount of sweetener. It works particularly well as a substitute for dairy milk in baked good recipes.

### Rice Milk

Rice milk is made from brown rice, water, sea salt and typically a small amount of oil. It is a very light, sweet beverage that can replace cow's milk in most recipes.

### Hemp Milk

Hemp milk is a thick, rich milk made from hemp seeds, water and a touch of brown rice syrup. It is rich in healthy omega-3 fatty acids, protein and essential vitamins and minerals. Because of its neutral taste, it can be used in a broad range of sweet and savory dishes.

### Light Coconut Milk

Typically available canned or in Tetra Paks, coconut milk adds instant exotic flair to curries, soups and sauces; it is also fantastic in desserts, such as ice cream, that usually rely on heavy dairy products. It is readily available and very affordable at supermarkets. All of the recipes in this collection were tested using light coconut milk, which has 50% to 75% less fat than regular coconut milk, but regular coconut milk may be used if you prefer.

# Fats and Oils

Fats and oils can be healthy or unhealthy; it all depends on the type you use and how much you consume. Some oils, such as those that contain essential fatty acids (omega-3 and omega-6, for example), are an absolutely necessary part of your diet. And when it comes to eating healthier over the long term, you'll feel happy and satisfied when you cook your food with a healthy amount of good fats.

## Unrefined Virgin Coconut Oil

Virgin coconut oil can be used in both cooking and baking. It is semi-solid at room temperature and must be melted slowly, over low heat, to avoid burning.

## Butter

Fresh butter has a delicate cream flavor and a pale yellow color, and adds tremendous flavor to a wide range of recipes.

Butter quickly picks up off-flavors during storage and when exposed to oxygen, so once the carton or wrap is opened, place it in a sealable plastic food bag or other airtight container. Store it away from foods with strong odors, especially items such as onions or garlic.

I recommend buying and using only unsalted butter for the recipes in this collection. The obvious reason is the added salt. Different manufacturers use different amounts of salt in their butter, so it's not possible to reliably determine how much salt is in any given stick or cube. The less obvious reason is that salt is a preservative: salted butter has a longer shelf life in the refrigerator (as much as 2 or 3 months). As such, the salted butter at the supermarket may be far less fresh than the unsalted option, and has sometimes been made from cream that is less fresh too. If you are concerned about keeping unsalted butter fresh once you've purchased it, you can store it in the freezer for up to 6 months.

## Substituting Margarine for Butter

Margarine may be substituted for butter, but I don't recommend doing so. Margarine is highly processed and lacks the rich flavor that butter offers. In addition, some brands contain high levels of unhealthy trans fats. If, however, you need to substitute margarine for butter because of specific dietary requirements (notably, to eliminate casein from the diet), avoid spreads in tub form; to make them spreadable, these products have a much higher percentage of water than sticks. Using a spread will alter the liquid and fat combination of the recipe, leading to either unsatisfactory or downright disastrous results. For best results, choose high-quality margarine sticks with at least an 80% fat content.

## Nonstick Cooking Spray

A number of recipes in this collection call for the use of nonstick cooking spray, which helps keep foods from sticking while simultaneously cutting back on fat and calories in a dish. While any variety of cooking spray may be used, I recommend using an organic cooking spray for two reasons: first, these sprays are typically made with higher-quality oils (in many cases expeller-pressed or cold-pressed oils) than most commercial brands; second, they are more likely to use compressed gas to expel the propellant, so no hydrocarbons are released into the environment. Read the label and choose wisely.

## Vegetable Oil

"Vegetable oil" is a generic term used to describe any neutral, plant-based oil that is liquid at room temperature. You can choose from a variety of vegetable oils (e.g., safflower, sunflower, canola), but opt for those that are:

1. Expeller-pressed or cold-pressed. Expeller-pressed oils are pressed simply by crushing the seeds, while cold-pressed oils are expeller-pressed oils that are produced in a heat-controlled environment.
2. High in healthful unsaturated fats (no more than 7% saturated fat).

## Olive Oil

Olive oil is a monounsaturated oil that is prized for its use in a wide range of dishes. Extra virgin olive oil is the cold-pressed result of the first pressing of the olives and is considered the finest and fruitiest of the olive oils. Its subtle nuances shine best when it is uncooked, whether in salad dressings or drizzled on top of soup. Consider using olive oil simply labeled "olive oil" — produced from additional pressings of the olives and far less expensive than extra virgin — for general cooking purposes.

## Toasted Sesame Oil

Toasted sesame oil has a dark brown color and a rich, nutty flavor. It is used sparingly, mostly in Asian recipes.

# Natural Sweeteners

Natural sweeteners are closer to their whole form than refined sweeteners, which have most or all of their natural vitamins and minerals removed during the refining process. From a flavor perspective, natural sweeteners contain a broader spectrum of flavors than refined sugar; hence, they add more than sweetness alone to sweet and savory dishes.

## Natural Cane Sugar

Natural cane sugar, also called whole cane sugar or evaporated cane juice, is made by extracting, clarifying, evaporating and crystallizing sugar cane juice. Many of the minerals from the plant are still present, which helps the human body digest the sugars.

Natural cane sugar comes in a wide variety of colors — from pale blond to dark brown — and in textures from coarse and dry to fine and somewhat moist. At present, there is no standardization for the processing and labeling of natural cane sugars, so choose the type that best suits your needs and tastes.

The recipes in this collection were tested using natural cane sugar that is fine-grained and somewhat moist, akin to light or dark brown sugar. Sucanat (an abbreviation of SUgar CAne NATural) is a trade name for this type of sugar, as is Rapadura. You can use other varieties of natural cane sugar, so long as it is fairly fine in texture (large crystals do not dissolve well in baking recipes). Alternatively, use packed light brown sugar, as is suggested throughout the recipes.

## Turbinado Sugar

Turbinado sugar is raw sugar that has been steam-cleaned. The coarse crystals are blond in color and have a delicate molasses flavor. They are typically used for decoration and texture atop baked goods.

## Brown Rice Syrup

Brown rice syrup is made from brown rice that has been soaked, sprouted and cooked with an enzyme that breaks the starches into maltose. Brown rice syrup has a light, mild flavor and a similar appearance to honey, though it is less sweet. Rice syrup can be substituted one for one for honey or maple syrup.

## Honey

Honey is plant nectar that has been gathered and concentrated by honey bees. Any variety of honey may be used in the recipes in this collection. Unopened containers of honey may be stored at room temperature. After opening, store honey in the refrigerator to protect against mold. Honey will keep indefinitely when stored properly.

## Maple Syrup

Maple syrup is a thick liquid sweetener made by boiling the sap from maple trees. It has a strong, pure maple flavor. Maple-flavored pancake syrup is just corn syrup with coloring and artificial maple flavoring added, and it is not recommended as a substitute for pure maple syrup. Unopened containers of maple syrup may be stored at room temperature. After opening, store maple syrup in the refrigerator to protect against mold. Maple syrup will keep indefinitely when stored properly.

## Molasses

Molasses is made from the juice of sugar cane or sugar beets, which is boiled until a syrupy mixture remains. The recipes in this collection were tested using dark (cooking) molasses, but you can substitute light (fancy) molasses if you prefer. Blackstrap molasses is thick and very dark, and it has a bitter flavor; it is not recommended for the recipes in this collection. Unopened containers of molasses may be stored at room temperature. After opening, store molasses in the refrigerator to protect against mold. Molasses will keep indefinitely when stored properly.

## Agave Nectar

Agave nectar (or agave syrup) is a plant-based sweetener derived from the agave cactus, native to Mexico. Used for centuries to make tequila, agave juice produces a light golden syrup.

## Stevia

Stevia is derived from the leaves of a South American shrub, *Stevia rebaudiana*. It is about 300 times sweeter than cane sugar, or sucrose. Stevia is not absorbed through the digestive tract, and therefore has no calories. Stevia comes in several forms: dried leaf, liquid extract and powdered extract. The few recipes in this collection that call for stevia use it in powdered form.

## Fresh Dates

Fresh dates — the fruit of the date palm tree — are among the sweetest fruits in the world, with a flavor similar to brown sugar. They can be used in desserts, snacks, sauces and even soups, stews and chilis to add sweetness. The most commonly available dates in the United States and Canada are Medjool dates, which are plump and tender, and Deglet Noor dates, which are semi-soft, slender and a bit chewy; both varieties have often been left on the tree for a while after they are ripe to dry a bit (and thus last longer after harvest). When choosing fresh dates, select those that are plump-looking; it is okay if they are slightly wrinkled, but they shouldn't feel hard.

# Fresh Herbs

Fresh herbs add an aromatic backbone to cooked food. When added during the cooking process, they willingly surrender their flavors and aromas in minutes. Alternatively, you can add them as a final flourish for a bright note of fresh flavor and color.

Flat-leaf (Italian) parsley, cilantro and chives are readily available and inexpensive, and they store well in the produce bin of the refrigerator, so keep them on hand year-round. Basil, mint and thyme are best in the spring and summer, when they are in season in your own garden or at the farmers' market.

# Chemical Leaveners

Chemical leaveners lighten dough, causing it to rise. In the baking recipes in this collection, baking powder and baking soda are used as the leaveners.

## Baking Powder

Baking powder is a chemical leavening agent made from a blend of alkali (sodium bicarbonate, known commonly as baking soda) and acid (most commonly calcium acid phosphate, sodium aluminum sulfate or cream of tartar), plus some form of starch to absorb any moisture so a reaction does not take place until a liquid is added. When baking powder is combined with a liquid, a chemical reaction produces carbon dioxide, which is trapped in tiny air pockets in the dough or batter. Heat releases additional carbon dioxide and expands the trapped gas and air to create steam. The pressure expands the air pockets, thus expanding the food.

The alkali and acid components of baking powder are naturally gluten-free, but in some cases, the starch that is added contains gluten. Most of the brands found in supermarkets are gluten-free, but if you are following a gluten-free diet, check with the manufacturer to be certain.

If you find yourself without baking powder as you prepare to bake, use this simple substitution: for every 1 tsp (5 mL) commercial baking powder, use a combination of $\frac{1}{4}$ tsp (1 mL) baking soda, $\frac{1}{2}$ tsp (2 mL) cream of tartar and $\frac{1}{4}$ tsp (1 mL) cornstarch.

## Baking Soda

Baking soda is a chemical leavener consisting of bicarbonate of soda. It is alkaline in nature and, when combined with an acidic ingredient such as buttermilk, yogurt, citrus juice, honey or molasses, it creates carbon dioxide bubbles, giving baked goods a dramatic rise. Baking soda is a naturally gluten-free.

# Flavorings

Elevating healthy, everyday dishes to exceptional levels of deliciousness can be as easy as creating a harmonious balance of simple flavorings — even if you're just adding salt and pepper. Here are my top recommendations for ingredients that will make the ordinary extraordinary.

## Fine Sea Salt

Unless otherwise specified, the recipes in this collection were tested using fine-grain sea salt. Conventional salt production uses chemicals, additives and heat processing to achieve the end product commonly called table salt. By contrast, unrefined sea salt contains an abundance of naturally occurring trace minerals.

## Black Pepper

Black pepper is made by grinding black peppercorns, which have been picked when the berry is not quite ripe, then dried until it shrivels and the skin turns dark brown to black. Black pepper has a strong, slightly hot flavor, with a hint of sweetness.

## Spices and Dried Herbs

Spices and dried herbs can turn the simplest of meals into masterpieces. They should be stored in light- and airproof containers, away from direct sunlight and heat, to preserve their flavors. Co-ops, health food stores and mail order sources that sell herbs and spices in bulk are all excellent options for purchasing very fresh, organic spices and dried herbs, often at a low cost.

With ground spices and dried herbs, freshness is everything. To determine whether a ground spice or dried herb is fresh, open the container and sniff. A strong fragrance means it is still acceptable for use.

Note that ground spices, not whole, are used throughout this collection. Here are my favorite ground spices and dried herbs:

### Ground Spices
- Black pepper (cracked and ground)
- Cardamom
- Cayenne pepper (also labeled "ground red pepper")
- Chili powder
- Chinese five-spice powder
- Chipotle chile powder
- Cinnamon
- Coriander
- Cumin
- Garam masala
- Ginger

### Ground Spices
- Hot pepper flakes
- Mild curry powder
- Nutmeg
- Paprika
- Smoked paprika (both hot and sweet)
- Turmeric

### Dried Herbs
- Bay leaves
- Oregano
- Rosemary
- Rubbed sage
- Thyme

## Citrus Zest

Zest is the name for the colored outer layer of citrus peel. The oils in zest are intense in flavor. Use a zester, a Microplane-style grater or the small holes of a box grater to grate zest. Avoid grating the white layer (pith) just below the zest; it is very bitter.

## Cocoa Powder

Select natural cocoa powder rather than Dutch process for the recipes in this collection. Natural cocoa powder has a deep, true chocolate flavor. The packaging should state whether it is Dutch process or not, but you can also tell the difference by sight: if it is dark to almost black, it is Dutch process; natural cocoa powder is much lighter and is typically brownish red in color.

## Chocolate

At its most basic, chocolate is made up of cocoa butter and cocoa powder — which together are called cacao liquor and determine cacao content — along with sugar. As cacao content goes up, sugar content goes down. Semisweet chocolate is the most common chocolate used in baking recipes and has a typical cacao content of 35% to 40%. It is the variety of chocolate called for throughout this collection.

### Gluten-Free Chocolate

It is becoming easier to find gluten-free chocolate, in both bar and chip form. Nevertheless, if you are following a gluten-free diet, the best way to make sure your chocolate is gluten-free is to double-check the label and contact the manufacturer if necessary. Bars of gluten-free chocolate are sometimes easier to find than gluten-free chocolate chips. If necessary, use 3 oz (90 g) chocolate, chopped, for every $\frac{1}{2}$ cup (125 mL) chocolate chips.

Chocolate chips are small chunks of chocolate that are typically sold in a round, flat-bottomed teardrop shape. They are available in numerous sizes, from large to miniature, but are usually around $\frac{1}{2}$ inch (1 cm) in diameter.

## Vanilla Extract

Vanilla extract adds a sweet, fragrant flavor to dishes, especially baked goods. It is produced by combining an extraction from dried vanilla beans with an alcohol and water mixture. It is then aged for several months. The three most common types of vanilla beans used to make vanilla extract are Bourbon-Madagascar, Mexican and Tahitian. Select a brand that is clearly labeled as gluten-free if you're following a gluten-free diet.

## Almond Extract

Almond extract is a flavoring manufactured by combining bitter almond oil with ethyl alcohol. It is used in much the same way as vanilla extract. Almond extract has a highly concentrated, intense flavor, so measure with care. Select a brand that is clearly labeled as gluten-free if you're following a gluten-free diet.

## Tamari and Soy Sauce

Both tamari and soy sauce are natural products made from soybeans, water and sea salt; the two are very similar, but tamari has a deeper color and flavor. Wheat is sometimes added to the mix of ingredients in the fermenting process, so select a brand that is clearly labeled as gluten-free if you're following a gluten-free diet.

## Miso

Miso is a sweet, fermented soybean paste. It comes unpasteurized and in several varieties, from golden yellow to deep red to sweet white. It can be made into a soup or a sauce or used as a salt substitute. Select a variety that is clearly labeled as gluten-free if you are following a gluten-free diet.

## Wasabi

Wasabi is a Japanese horseradish. It is dried into a pale green powder that, when mixed with water, makes a potent, fiery paste. Store it in a tightly covered glass jar, away from heat or light, to preserve its flavor.

## Thai Curry Paste

Available in small jars, Thai curry paste is a blend of Thai chiles, garlic, lemongrass, galangal, ginger and wild lime leaves. It is a fast and delicious way to add Southeast Asian flavor to a broad spectrum of recipes in a single step. Panang and yellow curry pastes tend to be the mildest. Red curry paste is medium hot, and green curry paste is typically the hottest.

### Gluten-Free Reminders

If you're following a gluten-free diet, you'll appreciate the handy note "GF, if needed" I've included in the ingredient lists to remind you that you'll need to pay special attention to buying gluten-free versions of those ingredients when shopping.

# Dijon Mustard

Dijon mustard adds depth of flavor to a wide range of dishes. It is most commonly used in this collection for salad dressing because it facilitates the emulsification of oil and vinegar.

# Vinegars

Vinegars are multipurpose flavor powerhouses. Delicious in vinaigrettes and dressings, they are also stealth ingredients for use at the end of cooking time to enhance and balance the natural flavors of dishes. Store vinegars in a dark place, away from heat or light.

## Cider Vinegar

Cider vinegar is made from the juice of crushed apples. After the juice is collected, it is allowed to age in wooden barrels.

## Unseasoned Rice Vinegar

Rice vinegar is made from an alcohol fermentation of mashed rice. It then undergoes another fermentation to produce vinegar. In general, rice vinegar tends to be more acidic than other vinegars. Be sure to check the label to make sure it is unseasoned; seasoned rice vinegar has added salt and sugar.

## Red Wine Vinegar

Red wine vinegar is produced by fermenting red wine in wooden barrels. This produces acetic acid, which gives red wine vinegar its distinctive taste. Red wine vinegar has a characteristic dark red color and red wine flavor.

## White Wine Vinegar

White wine vinegar is a moderately tangy vinegar made from a blend of white wines. The wine is fermented, aged and filtered to produce a vinegar with a slightly lower acidity level than red wine vinegar.

## Sherry Vinegar

Sherry vinegar has a deep, complex flavor and a dark reddish color. It is made from three different white grape varieties grown in the Jerez region of Spain. Most of the sherry vinegar produced comes from this region, making it a popular ingredient in Spanish cooking.

## Balsamic Vinegar

Balsamic vinegar is a thick, aromatic vinegar made from concentrated grape must. Grape must is the freshly pressed juice of the grape, and also contains pulp, skins, stems and seeds. The must is boiled down to a sap and aged in wooden barrels for 6 months to 12 years. Some very expensive balsamic vinegars are aged for up to 25 years.

## Ready-to-Use Broths

Ready-made chicken, beef and vegetable broths are essential for many of the recipes in this collection. Opt for certified organic broths that are all-natural, reduced-sodium and MSG-free. For chicken and beef broths, look for brands that are made from chicken or cattle raised without hormones or antibiotics. If you're following a gluten-free diet, select a brand that is clearly labeled as gluten-free.

For convenience, look for broths in Tetra Paks, which typically come in 32-oz (1 L), 48-oz (1.5 L) and occasionally 16-oz (500 mL) sizes. Once opened, these can be stored in the refrigerator for up to 1 week.

# Measuring Ingredients

Accurate measurements are important for cooking — and essential for baking — to achieve consistent results time and again. So take both time and care as you measure.

## Measuring Dry Ingredients

When measuring a dry ingredient, such as flour, cocoa powder, sugar, spices or salt, spoon it into the appropriate-size dry measuring cup or measuring spoon, heaping it up over the top. Slide a straight-edged utensil, such as a knife, across the top to level off the extra. Be careful not to shake or tap the cup or spoon to settle the ingredient, or you will have more than you need.

## Measuring Moist Ingredients

Moist ingredients, such as brown sugar, coconut and dried fruit, must be firmly packed in a measuring cup or spoon to be measured accurately. Use a dry measuring cup for these ingredients. Fill the measuring cup to slightly overflowing, then pack down the ingredient firmly with the back of a spoon. Add more of the ingredient and pack down again until the cup is full and even with the top of the measure.

## Measuring Liquid Ingredients

Use a clear plastic or glass measuring cup or container with lines up the sides to measure liquid ingredients. Set the container on the counter and pour the liquid to the appropriate mark. Lower your head to read the measurement at eye level.

# Breakfasts

# Quinoa Flake Granola

*Prepare yourself for the crispiest, crunchiest, most delectable granola you've ever had. It's all about the quinoa flakes, which are lighter in texture than oats and readily form the kinds of clusters you're looking for when making granola. The possibilities for variation are endless, so have fun with spices, sweeteners, nuts, seeds, flaked coconut and dried fruit.*

- **Preheat oven to 325°F (160°C)**
- **Large rimmed baking sheet, lined with parchment paper**

| | | |
|---|---|---|
| 2 cups | quinoa flakes | 500 mL |
| ½ cup | chopped pecans | 125 mL |
| ¼ cup | ground flax seeds (flaxseed meal) | 60 mL |
| 2 tsp | ground cinnamon | 10 mL |
| ½ cup | pure maple syrup, liquid honey or brown rice syrup | 125 mL |
| 2 tbsp | vegetable oil or unsalted butter, melted | 30 mL |
| 2 tsp | vanilla extract (GF, if needed) | 10 mL |
| ½ cup | dried blueberries, cranberries or chopped cherries | 125 mL |

1. In a large bowl, combine quinoa flakes, pecans, flax seeds and cinnamon.
2. In a medium bowl, whisk together maple syrup, oil and vanilla until well blended.
3. Add the maple mixture to the quinoa mixture and stir until well coated. Spread mixture in a single layer on prepared baking sheet.
4. Bake in preheated oven for 22 to 27 minutes or until quinoa flakes are golden brown. Let cool completely on pan.
5. Transfer granola to an airtight container and stir in blueberries. Store at room temperature for up to 2 weeks.

# Peanut Butter and Quinoa Granola

**Makes about 4 cups (1 L)**

*I have fond memories of my mother's homemade granola, rich with nuts, honey and toasted oats. My version ups the flavor and nutrition ante with quinoa, peanut butter and dried cranberries. Spoon it up with milk, sprinkle it on yogurt or pack a handful in a small plastic bag for a mid-morning boost.*

## Tip

Any unsweetened natural nut or seed butter (such as cashew, almond, sunflower seed or tahini) may be used in place of the peanut butter.

- **Preheat oven to 325°F (160°C)**
- **Large rimmed baking sheet, lined with parchment paper**

| | | |
|---|---|---|
| 2 cups | large-flake (old-fashioned) rolled oats (certified GF, if needed) | 500 mL |
| ¾ cup | quinoa, rinsed | 175 mL |
| ¾ cup | lightly salted roasted peanuts, coarsely chopped | 175 mL |
| ½ tsp | fine sea salt | 2 mL |
| ½ tsp | ground cinnamon | 2 mL |
| ¼ cup | natural cane sugar or packed light brown sugar | 60 mL |
| ¼ cup | liquid honey or brown rice syrup | 60 mL |
| ½ cup | unsweetened natural peanut butter | 125 mL |
| ⅓ cup | vegetable oil | 75 mL |
| 1 tsp | vanilla extract (GF, if needed) | 5 mL |
| ⅔ cup | dried cranberries | 150 mL |

1. In a large bowl, combine oats, quinoa, peanuts, salt and cinnamon.
2. In a small saucepan, combine sugar and honey. Bring to a simmer over medium heat, stirring constantly. Turn off heat and stir in peanut butter, oil and vanilla until blended.
3. Pour peanut butter mixture over oat mixture and stir until coated. Spread mixture in a single layer on prepared baking sheet.
4. Bake in preheated oven for 40 minutes, stirring twice, until golden brown. Let cool completely on pan.
5. Transfer granola to an airtight container and stir in cranberries. Store at room temperature for up to 2 weeks.

## Variation

*Chocolate and Peanut Butter Granola:* Add ½ cup (125 mL) miniature semisweet chocolate chips (GF, if needed) after the granola has cooled completely.

# Coconut Quinoa Oat Granola

*Outcast in the 1990s
as an artery-clogging
villain, virgin coconut oil
has been newly embraced
by health-conscious
eaters everywhere. It's
praised for its high
levels of lauric acid,
which is believed to
help increase levels of
"good" cholesterol, but
it's the oil's delicate sweet,
tropical, almost vanilla-
like flavor that has really
won people over. Here,
it enhances oats and
quinoa, coaxing out their
natural nuttiness in a
most delicious way.*

- **Preheat oven to 300°F (150°C)**
- **Large rimmed baking sheet, lined with parchment paper**

| | | |
|---|---|---|
| 2 cups | large-flake (old-fashioned) rolled oats (certified GF, if needed) | 500 mL |
| 1 cup | quinoa, rinsed | 250 mL |
| 1 cup | unsweetened flaked coconut | 250 mL |
| ¾ cup | almonds, coarsely chopped | 175 mL |
| 1½ tsp | ground cardamom or ginger | 7 mL |
| ½ cup | coconut oil, warmed | 125 mL |
| ½ cup | liquid honey or brown rice syrup | 125 mL |
| ⅔ cup | chopped dried apricots or golden raisins | 150 mL |

1. In a large bowl, combine oats, quinoa, coconut, almonds and cardamom.
2. In a medium bowl, whisk together oil and honey until well blended.
3. Add the honey mixture to the oats mixture and stir until well coated. Spread mixture in a single layer on prepared baking sheet.
4. Bake in preheated oven for 20 to 25 minutes or until oats are golden brown. Let cool completely on pan.
5. Transfer granola to an airtight container and stir in apricots. Store at room temperature for up to 2 weeks.

# Spiced Fruit and Grain Cereal

*Superstar powers, activate! A serving of this über-healthy cereal will make you feel like you can leap tall buildings in a single bound, or at least sail through to lunchtime without feeling hungry. But it's the pleasing mix of flavors and textures that will make this your new favorite breakfast.*

| | | |
|---|---|---|
| ½ cup | quinoa, rinsed | 125 mL |
| ⅛ tsp | fine sea salt | 0.5 mL |
| 1 cup | water | 250 mL |
| ¾ cup | milk or plain non-dairy milk (such as soy, almond, rice or hemp) | 175 mL |
| ½ cup | large-flake (old-fashioned) rolled oats (certified GF, if needed) | 125 mL |
| 3 tbsp | chopped dried figs or dried apricots | 45 mL |
| 2 tbsp | ground flax seeds (flaxseed meal) | 30 mL |
| ¼ tsp | ground ginger | 1 mL |
| ¼ tsp | ground cloves | 1 mL |
| 2 tbsp | chopped toasted walnuts | 30 mL |
| 2 tbsp | liquid honey | 30 mL |

1. In a medium saucepan, combine quinoa, salt, water and milk. Bring to a boil over medium-high heat. Reduce heat to low, cover and simmer for 10 minutes.

2. Stir in oats, figs, flax seeds, ginger and cloves. Cover and simmer for 5 to 8 minutes or until most of the liquid is absorbed and quinoa and oats are cooked through. Stir in walnuts and drizzle with honey.

# Fruit and Quinoa Muesli

*Muesli was developed by Swiss nutritionist Dr. Bircher-Benner more than a century ago. It can include cereals, fruits, nuts, bran and wheat germ.*

## Tip

For the fresh fruit, try mangos, pear, kiwi, strawberries and/or blueberries.

| | | |
|---|---|---|
| 1¼ cups | quinoa flakes | 300 mL |
| ⅔ cup | milk | 150 mL |
| ⅔ cup | plain yogurt | 150 mL |
| 1 tsp | vanilla extract (GF, if needed) | 5 mL |
| ⅔ cup | freshly squeezed orange juice | 150 mL |
| ¼ cup | liquid honey or agave nectar | 60 mL |
| 3 cups | chopped fresh fruit or berries | 750 mL |
| 1½ cups | shredded peeled tart-sweet apples (such as Braeburn or Gala) | 375 mL |
| 1 cup | chopped toasted walnuts or pecans | 250 mL |

1. In a large bowl, combine quinoa flakes, milk, yogurt and vanilla. Let stand for 5 minutes to soften flakes.

2. In a medium bowl, whisk together orange juice and honey. Stir in chopped fruit, apples and walnuts.

3. Stir fruit mixture into oat mixture. Serve immediately or cover and refrigerate for up to 8 hours.

# Baked Pumpkin Quinoa

*A bite of this baked
breakfast cereal, fragrant
with traditional pumpkin
pie spices and packed
with two superstar
superfoods — quinoa
and pumpkin — is very
comforting despite the
dish's modern look. Serve
it straight up or with
any of the suggested
accompaniments for
a super-energizing
breakfast.*

## Storage Tip

Let cool completely,
cover and refrigerate for
up to 2 days. Warm in
the microwave.

- **Preheat oven to 375°F (190°C)**
- **8- or 9-inch (20 or 23 cm) square glass baking dish,
  sprayed with nonstick cooking spray**

| | | |
|---|---|---|
| 1 tbsp | unsalted butter or coconut oil | 15 mL |
| 1 cup | quinoa, rinsed | 250 mL |
| ¼ cup | natural cane sugar or packed dark brown sugar | 60 mL |
| 1 tsp | ground cinnamon | 5 mL |
| ¾ tsp | ground ginger | 3 mL |
| ½ tsp | salt | 2 mL |
| ¼ tsp | ground cloves | 1 mL |
| 2 cups | milk or plain non-dairy milk (such as soy, almond, rice or hemp) | 500 mL |
| ¾ cup | pumpkin purée (not pie filling) | 175 mL |
| ½ cup | water | 125 mL |
| 1 tsp | vanilla extract (GF, if needed) | 5 mL |

### Suggested Accompaniments

Pure maple syrup

Milk or plain non-dairy milk

Blueberries

Dried cranberries or dried cherries

1. In a medium saucepan, melt butter over medium heat. Add quinoa and cook, stirring, for 2 to 3 minutes or until fragrant and golden. Whisk in sugar, cinnamon, ginger, salt, cloves, milk, pumpkin, water and vanilla. Pour into prepared baking dish and cover tightly with foil.

2. Bake in preheated oven for 35 minutes. Transfer to a wire rack and carefully remove foil (steam will be released). Stir and let stand for 5 minutes.

3. Spoon into bowls and serve with any of the suggested accompaniments, as desired.

# Toasted Quinoa Porridge

*This power breakfast
is an easy bowlful of
deliciousness. Not as
heavy as other grain
porridges, it's one of those
magical breakfast dishes
that works for any season
of the year.*

| | | |
|---|---|---|
| ½ cup | quinoa, rinsed | 125 mL |
| ½ tsp | ground cinnamon | 2 mL |
| ⅛ tsp | fine sea salt | 0.5 mL |
| 1¼ cups | milk or plain non-dairy milk (such as soy, almond, rice or hemp), divided | 300 mL |
| 1 cup | water | 250 mL |

**Suggested Accompaniments**

Agave nectar, liquid honey, brown rice syrup or pure maple syrup

Fresh or dried fruit

1. In a small saucepan, over medium heat, toast quinoa, stirring, for 2 to 3 minutes or until golden and fragrant. Add cinnamon, salt, 1 cup (250 mL) of the milk and water; bring to a boil. Reduce heat to low, cover and simmer, stirring occasionally, for about 25 minutes or until liquid is absorbed.

2. Serve drizzled with the remaining milk and any of the suggested accompaniments, as desired.

# Indian Carrot and Quinoa Porridge

*This delectable
porridge is based on a
popular Indian dessert,
gajar halva.*

## Storage Tip

Store the cooled porridge in an airtight container in the refrigerator for up to 3 days. Reheat individual portions in the microwave on High for 45 to 60 seconds or until warm, then sprinkle with pistachios.

| | | |
|---|---|---|
| 12 oz | carrots, finely shredded (about 2½ cups/625 mL) | 375 g |
| ½ cup | quinoa, rinsed | 125 mL |
| ¾ tsp | ground cardamom | 3 mL |
| ¼ tsp | fine sea salt | 1 mL |
| 2½ cups | milk or plain non-dairy milk (such as soy, almond, rice, coconut or hemp) | 625 mL |
| 1 cup | water | 250 mL |
| ¼ cup | liquid honey, brown rice syrup or agave nectar | 60 mL |
| 1 tbsp | unsalted butter or coconut oil | 15 mL |
| ¼ cup | lightly salted roasted pistachios or cashews | 60 mL |

1. In a medium saucepan, combine carrots, quinoa, cardamom, salt, milk, water and honey. Bring to a gentle boil, stirring, over medium-high heat. Reduce heat and simmer, stirring occasionally, for 35 to 40 minutes or until carrots are very tender and mixture is thickened. Remove from heat and stir in butter until blended. Let cool completely. Sprinkle with pistachios just before serving.

# Chicken and Apple Breakfast Sausages

*Ground chicken, tart-sweet apple and two types of quinoa add up to a sensational breakfast patty that is especially pleasing during the transitional months of autumn.*

## Tip

For the apple, try Braeburn or Gala.

| | | |
|---|---|---|
| 4 tsp | olive oil, divided | 20 mL |
| 1 cup | chopped peeled tart-sweet apple | 250 mL |
| 1 cup | chopped green onions | 250 mL |
| ½ cup | quinoa flakes | 125 mL |
| 8 oz | lean ground chicken or turkey | 250 g |
| 1¼ cups | cooked quinoa (see page 10), cooled | 300 mL |
| 2 tsp | dried sage | 10 mL |
| 1½ tsp | dried thyme | 7 mL |
| 1 tsp | fine sea salt | 5 mL |
| ¼ tsp | freshly cracked black pepper | 1 mL |
| 1 | large egg, lightly beaten | 1 |
| 1 tbsp | pure maple syrup or liquid honey | 15 mL |
| | Nonstick cooking spray | |

1. In a large nonstick skillet, heat half the oil over medium-high heat. Add apple and green onions; cook, stirring, for 4 to 5 minutes or until apple is just softened. Transfer to a large bowl and let cool 5 minutes. Wipe out skillet.

2. Add quinoa flakes to skillet and cook, stirring, over medium heat for 3 to 4 minutes or until golden and fragrant. Add to apple mixture.

3. To the apple mixture, add chicken, cooked quinoa, sage, thyme, salt, pepper, egg and maple syrup, gently stirring to combine.

4. Add the remaining oil to the skillet and heat over medium heat. Using a ⅓-cup (75 mL) measure, scoop five portions of sausage mixture into the pan, using a spatula to flatten each into a 3-inch (7.5 cm) patty. Cook for about 3 minutes per side or until browned and no longer pink inside. Spray the skillet with cooking spray and repeat with remaining sausage mixture.

# Andean Hash

*Peppers and potatoes
share quinoa's Andean
pedigree. Here, the trio
shines in a quick hash
that can be dressed up
(with eggs, herbs, yogurt
or salsa, for example) or
served unadorned.*

| 1 tbsp | olive oil | 15 mL |
|---|---|---|
| 1½ cups | chopped onions | 375 mL |
| 1 | small green bell pepper, chopped | 1 |
| 1 | small red bell pepper, chopped | 1 |
| 2 | cloves garlic, minced | 2 |
| 1 cup | quinoa, rinsed | 250 mL |
| 2 cups | diced peeled yellow-fleshed potatoes (such as Yukon gold) | 500 mL |
| 2¼ cups | reduced-sodium ready-to-use vegetable or chicken broth | 550 mL |
| | Fine sea salt and cracked black pepper | |

**Suggested Accompaniments**

Chopped fresh cilantro or flat-leaf (Italian) parsley

Chopped fresh chives or green onions

Crumbled queso fresco

Poached eggs

Plain Greek yogurt

Salsa

1. In a large saucepan, heat oil over medium-high heat. Add onions, green pepper and red pepper; cook, stirring, for 6 to 8 minutes or until softened. Add garlic and quinoa; cook, stirring, for 1 minute.

2. Stir in potatoes and broth; bring to a boil. Reduce heat, cover and simmer, without stirring, for 12 minutes. Uncover and fluff hash with a spatula. Cook, stirring, for 2 to 3 minutes or until liquid is absorbed and quinoa and potatoes are tender and slightly browned. Cover and let stand for 5 minutes. Season to taste with salt and pepper. Serve warm with any of the suggested accompaniments, as desired.

# Red Flannel Quinoa Hash

**Tip**

To poach the eggs, pour enough water into a medium skillet to reach a depth of 1½ inches (4 cm). Add ½ tsp (2 mL) salt and bring to simmer over medium heat. Crack each egg into a separate custard cup. Gently slide one egg at a time into the simmering water and simmer for about 1 minute or until egg whites are set (the yolks will be only partially cooked); cook longer for more firmly set yolks.

| | | |
|---|---|---|
| ½ cup | quinoa, rinsed | 125 mL |
| 2 | slices bacon, chopped | 2 |
| 1 cup | chopped onion | 250 mL |
| 1 | can (15 oz/425 mL) whole beets, drained and diced | 1 |
| ½ cup | milk | 125 mL |
| 2 | large eggs, poached (see tip, at left) | 2 |
| 2 tbsp | chopped fresh flat-leaf (Italian) parsley | 30 mL |

1. In a large pot of boiling salted water, cook quinoa for 10 minutes. Drain.
2. Meanwhile, in a large skillet over medium heat, cook bacon until crisp. Using a slotted spoon, transfer bacon to a plate lined with paper towels. Drain off all but 1 tsp (5 mL) fat from skillet.
3. Add onion to the skillet and cook, stirring, for 5 to 6 minutes or until softened. Add quinoa, beets and milk. Cook, stirring up bottom crust two to three times, for 10 to 12 minutes or until warmed through and browned.
4. Divide hash between two plates. Top each with a poached egg and sprinkle with bacon and parsley.

# Parmesan Quinoa Omelet for One

*In this easily assembled omelet, the delicate onion flavor of chives fuses with the eggs, quinoa and Parmesan in perfect harmony.*

| | | |
|---|---|---|
| 3 | large egg whites | 3 |
| 1 | large egg | 1 |
| Pinch | fine sea salt | Pinch |
| ⅓ cup | cooked quinoa (see page 10), cooled | 75 mL |
| 1 tbsp | minced fresh chives or green onions | 15 mL |
| 2 tsp | olive oil | 10 mL |
| 2 tbsp | freshly grated Parmesan cheese | 30 mL |
| | Nonstick cooking spray | |

1. In a small bowl, beat egg whites, egg and salt until blended. Stir in quinoa and chives.
2. In a small skillet, heat oil over medium heat. Pour in egg mixture and sprinkle with cheese. Cook, without stirring, for 2 to 4 minutes or until eggs are set. Remove from heat and invert onto a plate. Spray skillet with cooking spray and return omelet, browned side up, to skillet. Cook for 1 minute. Invert onto plate and serve.

# Broccoli, Quinoa and Feta Omelet

*Breakfast, lunch, dinner — this recipe is the all-in-one answer for leftover quinoa. A bevy of broccoli florets and a sprinkle of tangy feta cheese makes it irresistible any time of day.*

| | | |
|---|---|---|
| 5 | large eggs | 5 |
| 1/4 tsp | fine sea salt | 1 mL |
| 1/4 tsp | freshly cracked black pepper | 1 mL |
| 2 tsp | extra virgin olive oil | 10 mL |
| 2 cups | coarsely chopped broccoli florets | 500 mL |
| 2 | cloves garlic, minced | 2 |
| 1 1/4 cups | cooked quinoa (see page 10), cooled | 300 mL |
| 1/2 cup | crumbled feta cheese | 125 mL |
| 1/4 cup | packed fresh flat-leaf (Italian) parsley leaves | 60 mL |

1. In a large bowl, beat eggs, salt and pepper until blended. Set aside.

2. In a large skillet, heat oil over medium-high heat. Add broccoli and cook, stirring, for 4 to 5 minutes or until tender. Reduce heat to medium and add garlic and quinoa; cook, stirring, for 30 seconds.

3. Pour egg mixture over broccoli mixture. Cook, lifting edges to allow uncooked eggs to run underneath and shaking skillet occasionally to loosen omelet, for 4 to 5 minutes or until almost set. Slide out onto a large plate.

4. Invert skillet over omelet and, using pot holders, firmly hold plate and skillet together. Invert omelet back into skillet and cook for 1 to 2 minutes to set eggs. Slide out onto plate and sprinkle with cheese and parsley.

# Mushroom Quinoa Frittata

*A frittata is an Italian omelet in which the filling ingredients are mixed with the beaten eggs and the mixture is baked or broiled until set. Don't relegate it to the land of brunches: make it ahead, let it cool, then store it in the refrigerator for weekday frittata squares on the go.*

## Tip

When selecting mushrooms, choose those with a fresh, smooth appearance, free from major blemishes and with a dry surface. Once home, keep mushrooms refrigerated; they're best when used within a few days after purchase. When ready to use, gently wipe mushrooms with a damp cloth or soft brush to remove dirt particles. Alternatively, rinse mushrooms quickly with cold water, then immediately pat dry with paper towels.

- **Preheat oven to 350°F (180°C)**
- **8-inch (20 cm) square glass baking dish, sprayed with nonstick cooking spray (preferably olive oil)**

| | | |
|---|---|---|
| 6 | large eggs | 6 |
| ½ tsp | fine sea salt | 2 mL |
| ¼ tsp | freshly ground black pepper | 1 mL |
| 2 tsp | extra virgin olive oil | 10 mL |
| 8 oz | cremini or button mushrooms, sliced | 250 g |
| 1½ cups | chopped green onions | 375 mL |
| 1½ cups | cooked quinoa (see page 10), cooled | 375 mL |
| ¼ cup | freshly grated Parmesan cheese | 60 mL |

1. In a large bowl, beat eggs, salt and pepper until blended. Set aside.

2. In a large skillet, heat oil over medium-high heat. Add mushrooms and green onions; cook, stirring, for 5 to 7 minutes or until softened. Stir in quinoa and cook, stirring, for 1 minute.

3. Spread quinoa mixture in prepared baking dish and pour egg mixture over top. Sprinkle with cheese.

4. Bake in preheated oven for 23 to 28 minutes or until golden and set. Let cool on a wire rack for at least 10 minutes before cutting. Serve warm or let cool completely.

# Chorizo and Kale Breakfast Casserole

*Here's a zippy, modern twist on the savory breakfast casserole. For a less spicy but equally delicious dish, use sweet Italian sausage (turkey or pork) in place of the chorizo.*

## Tip

Unlike other greens, kale stems are so tough they are virtually inedible. Hence, they, along with the tougher part of the center rib, must be removed before cooking. To do so, lay a leaf upside down on a cutting board and use a paring knife to cut a V shape along both sides of the rib, cutting it and the stem free from the leaf.

- Preheat oven to 350°F (180°C)
- 8- or 9-inch (20 or 23 cm) square glass baking dish, sprayed with nonstick cooking spray (preferably olive oil)

| | | |
|---|---|---|
| 8 oz | fresh chorizo sausage (bulk or casings removed) | 250 g |
| 8 | large eggs | 8 |
| 1¼ cups | milk | 300 mL |
| 1 tsp | dried oregano | 5 mL |
| ½ tsp | fine sea salt | 2 mL |
| 2½ cups | coarsely chopped kale (tough stems and center ribs removed) | 625 mL |
| ½ cup | quinoa, rinsed | 125 mL |
| ½ cup | freshly grated manchego or Parmesan cheese | 125 mL |

1. In a large skillet, cook chorizo over medium-high heat, breaking it up with a spoon, for 4 to 6 minutes or until no longer pink. Drain off any excess fat.
2. In a large bowl, whisk together eggs, milk, oregano and salt. Stir in chorizo, kale and quinoa. Pour into prepared baking dish and cover tightly with foil.
3. Bake in preheated oven for 40 to 45 minutes or until just set. Remove foil and sprinkle with cheese. Bake, uncovered, for 10 to 15 minutes or until golden brown. Let cool on a wire rack for at least 10 minutes before serving.

## Variation

For a meatless dish, use soy chorizo (soyrizo) in place of the fresh chorizo. Brown as directed on the package, then continue with step 2.

# Baked Apple Quinoa

*Apples times two — diced
and applesauce — add
moistness and natural
sweetness to this
delicious, healthful baked
quinoa breakfast. A light
sprinkling of turbinado
sugar adds a beautiful
and tasty touch.*

## Tip

For the apples, try Gala,
Braeburn or Cortland.

- **Preheat oven to 400°F (200°C)**
- **8-inch (20 cm) square glass baking dish, sprayed with nonstick cooking spray**

| | | |
|---|---|---|
| 1 cup | quinoa, rinsed | 250 mL |
| 1½ tsp | ground cinnamon | 7 mL |
| ½ tsp | fine sea salt | 2 mL |
| 2 cups | milk or plain non-dairy milk (such as soy, almond, rice or hemp) | 500 mL |
| 2 | large eggs | 2 |
| ½ cup | unsweetened applesauce | 125 mL |
| ¼ cup | pure maple syrup or liquid honey | 60 mL |
| 1 tsp | vanilla extract (GF, if needed) | 5 mL |
| 2 cups | diced peeled tart-sweet apples | 500 mL |
| ½ cup | dried cranberries, cherries or raisins (optional) | 125 mL |
| 1 tbsp | turbinado sugar | 15 mL |

### Suggested Accompaniments

Warm or cold milk or plain non-dairy milk (such as soy, almond, rice or hemp)

Liquid honey or pure maple syrup

1. In a medium saucepan, combine quinoa, cinnamon, salt and milk. Bring to a boil over medium-high heat. Reduce heat to low, cover and simmer for 15 minutes.

2. Meanwhile, in a small bowl, whisk together eggs, applesauce, maple syrup and vanilla until blended.

3. Add the egg mixture to the quinoa mixture and stir until just blended. Gently fold in apples and cranberries (if using). Spread evenly in prepared baking dish and sprinkle with sugar.

4. Bake in preheated oven for 20 to 25 minutes or until set at the center and golden. Let cool in pan on a wire rack for 5 minutes. Serve warm with any of the suggested accompaniments, as desired.

# Spinach Quinoa Breakfast Bake

**Makes
8 servings**

*Easy, healthy and delicious, this hearty breakfast bake can be taken on the go: make it ahead of time, let it cool completely, then cut it into squares. Wrap the squares tightly in plastic wrap and store in the refrigerator. The squares are delicious cold, but you can also zap them in the microwave to warm them up.*

- **Preheat oven to 350°F (180°C)**
- **Blender**
- **8- or 9-inch (20 or 23 cm) square glass baking dish, sprayed with nonstick cooking spray (preferably olive oil)**

| | | |
|---|---|---:|
| 6 | large eggs | 6 |
| 2 cups | cottage cheese | 500 mL |
| 1 | package (10 oz/300 g) frozen chopped spinach, thawed and squeezed dry | 1 |
| 1¼ cups | cooked quinoa (see page 10), cooled | 300 mL |
| 1 cup | chopped green onions | 250 mL |
| 1 cup | crumbled feta cheese | 250 mL |
| ⅛ tsp | freshly ground black pepper | 0.5 mL |

1. In blender, combine eggs and cottage cheese; purée until smooth.
2. Transfer purée to medium bowl and stir in spinach, quinoa, green onions, feta and pepper. Spread evenly in prepared baking dish.
3. Bake in preheated oven for 35 to 40 minutes or until golden brown and set.

# Tofu Quinoa Scramble

**Makes
4 servings**

*Health food gets fancy, turning tofu, quinoa and vegetables into a truly delectable morning meal.*

| | | |
|---|---|---:|
| 1 tbsp | extra virgin olive oil | 15 mL |
| 1 | large red bell pepper, chopped | 1 |
| 1 cup | chopped mushrooms | 250 mL |
| 16 oz | extra-firm or firm tofu, drained and coarsely mashed with a fork | 500 g |
| 1 cup | cooked quinoa (see page 10), cooled | 250 mL |
| ¼ cup | chopped green onions | 60 mL |
| 1 tbsp | reduced-sodium tamari or soy sauce | 15 mL |
| Pinch | freshly ground black pepper | Pinch |

1. In a small skillet, heat oil over medium-high heat. Add red pepper and mushrooms; cook, stirring, for 4 to 5 minutes or until softened. Add tofu, quinoa, green onions and tamari; cook, stirring, for 5 to 6 minutes or until tofu is golden brown. Season with pepper.

# Sweet Potato and Quinoa Breakfast Tortilla

**Makes 6 servings**

*I've swapped in sweet potatoes and quinoa for the traditional white potatoes in this Spanish skillet dish. It's one of Spain's favorite vegetarian meals, and with these newfangled twists, it will become one of yours, too. Serve with roasted pepper sauce.*

- **Preheat broiler, with rack set 4 to 6 inches (10 to 15 cm) from heat source**
- **Large ovenproof skillet**

| | | |
|---|---|---|
| 6 | large eggs | 6 |
| 1 tsp | fine sea salt | 5 mL |
| 1 tbsp | extra virgin olive oil | 15 mL |
| 2 cups | coarsely shredded peeled sweet potato (about 1 medium) | 500 mL |
| 1 cup | chopped green onions | 250 mL |
| 1¼ cups | cooked quinoa (see page 10), cooled | 300 mL |

1. In a medium bowl, whisk together eggs and salt.

2. In ovenproof skillet, heat oil over medium-high heat. Add sweet potato and cook, stirring, for 8 to 10 minutes or until softened. Add egg mixture, green onions and quinoa, gently shaking pan to distribute eggs. Reduce heat to medium and cook for about 8 minutes, gently shaking pan every minute, until eggs are almost set.

3. Place skillet under preheated broiler and broil for 1 to 2 minutes or until lightly browned. Slide out of the pan onto a cutting board and cut into wedges.

# Tex-Mex Power Pitas

*Using chipotle salsa to top these Southwestern pitas adds smoky flavor without the hassle of mincing canned chipotle chiles.*

**Tip**

GF or whole wheat tortillas may be used in place of the pitas.

| | | |
|---|---|---|
| 3 | large egg whites | 3 |
| 1 | large egg | 1 |
| ½ tsp | ground cumin | 2 mL |
| ⅔ cup | cooked quinoa (see page 10), cooled | 150 mL |
| | Fine sea salt and ground black pepper | |
| 1 tsp | extra virgin olive oil | 5 mL |
| 2 | 6-inch (15 cm) GF or whole wheat pitas, warmed and split at top | 2 |
| ½ | small ripe Hass avocado, sliced | ½ |
| ¼ cup | reduced-sodium chipotle salsa | 60 mL |

1. In a small bowl, beat egg whites, egg and cumin until blended. Stir in quinoa. Season with salt and pepper.
2. In a small skillet, heat oil over medium-high heat. Add egg mixture and cook, stirring gently with a spatula, for 2 to 4 minutes or until eggs are set.
3. Spoon egg mixture into warm pitas and top with avocado and salsa. Serve immediately or wrap in foil to eat on the go.

# Quinoa and Raspberry Flan

**Tip**

The flan will continue to firm up as it cools. For a loose, pudding-like dessert, serve it while still warm from the oven. For a firmer custard, let it cool to room temperature or chill it.

- **Preheat oven to 350°F (180°C)**
- **8-inch (20 cm) square glass baking dish, sprayed with nonstick cooking spray**

| | | |
|---|---|---|
| ⅓ cup | natural cane sugar or granulated sugar | 75 mL |
| ¼ tsp | fine sea salt | 1 mL |
| 3 | large eggs | 3 |
| 1¼ cups | milk or plain non-dairy milk | 300 mL |
| 2 tsp | finely grated lemon zest | 10 mL |
| ½ cup | quinoa flakes | 125 mL |
| 1½ cups | raspberries, blackberries or blueberries | 375 mL |

1. In a large bowl, whisk together sugar, salt, eggs, milk and lemon zest until blended. Stir in quinoa flakes. Pour mixture into prepared baking dish and sprinkle evenly with raspberries.
2. Bake in preheated oven for 35 to 40 minutes or until set at the center and golden. Let cool on a wire rack for 20 minutes. Cut into servings and serve warm.

# Morning Clafouti with Fruit and Nuts

*This amazingly delicious and healthy baked breakfast is filling and satisfying without being heavy. The possibilities for variation are endless, so pick and choose the fruits, nuts and flavorings of your choice. Cinnamon and natural cane sugar boost the flavor of the fruit, making this breakfast an absolute knockout.*

## Tip

Other fruits, such as diced bananas, pears, peaches or berries, may be used in place of the apples.

## Storage Tip

Let clafouti cool completely, then wrap individual portions in plastic wrap and store in an airtight container in the refrigerator for up to 3 days or in the freezer for up to 1 month.

- **Preheat oven to 350°F (180°C)**
- **13- by 9-inch (33 by 23 cm) glass baking dish, sprayed with nonstick cooking spray**

| | | |
|---|---|---|
| 2½ cups | quinoa flakes | 625 mL |
| ⅔ cup | natural cane sugar or packed light brown sugar | 150 mL |
| ¾ cup | dried fruit (such as raisins, cranberries or blueberries) | 175 mL |
| ⅓ cup | chopped toasted nuts (such as walnuts, pecans or hazelnuts) | 75 mL |
| 1 tsp | ground cinnamon | 5 mL |
| ½ tsp | fine sea salt | 2 mL |
| 3 | large eggs, lightly beaten | 3 |
| 3¼ cups | milk or plain non-dairy milk (such as soy, almond, rice or hemp) | 800 mL |
| 2 tsp | vanilla extract (GF, if needed) | 10 mL |
| 1½ cups | chopped peeled apples | 375 mL |

1. In a large bowl, combine quinoa flakes, sugar, dried fruit and nuts.
2. In a small bowl, whisk together cinnamon, salt, eggs, milk and vanilla.
3. Pour egg mixture over quinoa mixture and stir until combined. Stir in apples. Pour mixture into prepared baking dish, spreading evenly.
4. Bake in preheated oven for 55 to 60 minutes or until set at the center and golden. Let cool on a wire rack for 20 minutes. Cut into servings and serve warm.

# Quinoa Coconut Fruit Sushi

This playful breakfast
is perfect for breakfast
on the run — and for
satisfying a morning
sweet tooth. Use any
fresh or canned fruit
you like, or use colorful
dried fruits, such as diced
dried apricots, dates
or cherries.

## Tip

For the fruit, try
raspberries, blueberries,
kiwifruit and/or mandarin
oranges.

- **Large baking sheet, lined with waxed paper or foil**

| | | |
|---|---|---|
| ⅔ cup | sushi rice or other short-grain white rice | 150 mL |
| ⅓ cup | black or white quinoa, rinsed | 75 mL |
| 1 tbsp | cornstarch or arrowroot starch | 15 mL |
| ⅛ tsp | fine sea salt | 0.5 mL |
| 1 cup | water | 250 mL |
| ¾ cup | light coconut milk, divided | 175 mL |
| ¼ cup | agave nectar or liquid honey | 60 mL |
| | Nonstick cooking spray | |
| | Assorted small-diced fruit or berries | |
| ⅔ cup | vanilla-flavored yogurt or cultured non-dairy yogurt (such as soy or rice) | 150 mL |

1. In a medium saucepan, combine rice, quinoa, cornstarch, salt, water, $\frac{1}{2}$ cup (125 mL) of the coconut milk, and agave nectar. Bring to a boil over medium-high heat. Reduce heat to low, cover and simmer for 15 minutes. Remove from heat and gently stir in the remaining coconut milk. Cover and let stand for 30 minutes.

2. Lightly coat your hands with cooking spray. Using your hands, press $1\frac{1}{2}$-tbsp (22 mL) portions of rice mixture into an oval shape. Place on prepared baking sheet. Cover and refrigerate for at least 1 hour, until chilled, or for up to 24 hours.

3. Just before serving, top each oval with a few pieces of fruit or berries, gently pressing them into the rice mixture so they adhere. Serve with yogurt for dipping.

# Multigrain Pancake and Waffle Mix

**Makes about
4½ cups
(1.125 L)**

*Hearty, healthy and highly addictive, pancakes and waffles made from this make-ahead mix are an ideal start to an action-packed day.*

| | | |
|---|---|---|
| 1½ cups | quinoa flour | 375 mL |
| 1½ cups | finely ground cornmeal (GF, if needed) | 375 mL |
| ½ cup | quick-cooking rolled oats (certified GF, if needed) | 125 mL |
| ½ cup | ground flax seeds (flaxseed meal) | 125 mL |
| ½ cup | instant skim milk powder or soy milk powder | 125 mL |
| 2 tbsp | natural cane sugar | 30 mL |
| 2 tbsp | baking powder (GF, if needed) | 30 mL |
| 1 tsp | fine sea salt | 5 mL |
| ¾ tsp | baking soda | 3 mL |

1. In a large bowl, whisk together quinoa flour, cornmeal, oats, flax seeds, milk powder, sugar, baking powder, salt and baking soda.
2. Transfer to a large airtight container and store in the refrigerator for up to 1 month.

## To Prepare Multigrain Pancakes

**Makes
6 pancakes**

| | | |
|---|---|---|
| 1 cup | Multigrain Pancake and Waffle Mix | 250 mL |
| 1 | large egg | 1 |
| ⅔ cup | milk | 150 mL |
| 2 tsp | vegetable oil or unsalted butter, melted | 10 mL |
| | Nonstick cooking spray | |

1. In a medium bowl, combine pancake mix, egg, milk and oil until blended. Let stand for 1 minute.
2. Heat a griddle or skillet over medium heat. Spray with cooking spray. For each pancake, pour about ¼ cup (60 mL) batter onto griddle. Cook until bubbles appear on top. Turn pancake over and cook for about 1 minute or until golden brown. Repeat with the remaining batter, spraying griddle and adjusting heat as necessary between batches.

## Storage Tip

Let pancakes or waffles cool completely on a wire rack, then wrap individually in plastic wrap and store in an airtight container in the refrigerator for up to 3 days or the freezer for up to 1 month. Reheat in the microwave on High for 45 seconds, until warmed through (no need to thaw), or toast in the toaster oven for 1 to 2 minutes or until toasted and warmed though.

# To Prepare Waffles

- **Preheat waffle maker to medium-high**

| | | |
|---|---|---|
| 1 cup | Multigrain Pancake and Waffle Mix | 250 mL |
| 1 | large egg | 1 |
| $\frac{2}{3}$ cup | milk | 150 mL |
| 2 tsp | vegetable oil or unsalted butter, melted | 10 mL |
| | Nonstick cooking spray | |

1. In a medium bowl, combine pancake mix, egg, milk and oil until blended.
2. Spray preheated waffle maker with cooking spray. For each waffle, pour about $\frac{1}{3}$ cup (75 mL) batter into waffle maker. Cook according to manufacturer's instructions until golden brown.

# Oatmeal Quinoa Pancakes

*Ladies and gentlemen, prepare your griddles. These scrumptious pancakes capture the comfort of a warming bowl of oatmeal in golden pancake form. Drizzle with warm maple syrup or honey, or top with vanilla yogurt and fresh fruit.*

## Tip

An equal amount of brown rice syrup, pure maple syrup or agave nectar may be used in place of the honey.

## Storage Tip

See tip, page 52.

| | | |
|---|---|---|
| 1 cup | quick-cooking rolled oats (certified GF, if needed) | 250 mL |
| 2 cups | buttermilk, divided | 500 mL |
| $\frac{3}{4}$ cup | quinoa flour | 175 mL |
| $1\frac{1}{2}$ tsp | baking powder (GF, if needed) | 7 mL |
| 1 tsp | ground cinnamon | 5 mL |
| $\frac{3}{4}$ tsp | baking soda | 3 mL |
| $\frac{1}{2}$ tsp | fine sea salt | 2 mL |
| 1 | large egg | 1 |
| 2 tbsp | vegetable oil | 30 mL |
| 1 tbsp | liquid honey | 15 mL |
| | Nonstick cooking spray | |

1. In a small bowl, combine oats and half the buttermilk. Let stand for 10 minutes.
2. In a large bowl, whisk together quinoa flour, baking powder, cinnamon, baking soda and salt. Add oat mixture, the remaining buttermilk, egg, oil and honey, stirring until blended.
3. Heat a griddle or skillet over medium heat. Spray with cooking spray. For each pancake, pour about $\frac{1}{4}$ cup (60 mL) batter onto griddle. Cook until bubbles appear on top. Turn pancake over and cook for about 1 minute or until golden brown. Repeat with the remaining batter, spraying griddle and adjusting heat as necessary between batches.

# Blueberry Buttermilk Pancakes

*If you think blueberry
pancakes are fussy fare
for brunch, you need
to whip up a batch of
these hearty flapjacks.
Chock full of good-for-
you and good-tasting
things, they'll sustain you
through the most rigorous
of activities.*

## Storage Tip

Let pancakes cool
completely on a wire rack,
then wrap individually in
plastic wrap and store in
an airtight container in
the refrigerator for up to
2 days or the freezer for
up to 1 month. Reheat
in the microwave on
High for 45 seconds, until
warmed through (no
need to thaw), or toast in
the toaster oven for 1 to
2 minutes or until toasted
and warmed though.

| | | |
|---|---|---|
| 1½ cups | quinoa flour | 375 mL |
| 2 tsp | baking powder (GF, if needed) | 10 mL |
| 1 tsp | baking soda | 5 mL |
| ⅛ tsp | fine sea salt | 0.5 mL |
| 2 | large eggs | 2 |
| 1⅔ cups | buttermilk | 400 mL |
| 2 tbsp | vegetable oil | 30 mL |
| 1 tbsp | liquid honey or pure maple syrup | 15 mL |
| | Nonstick cooking spray | |
| 2 cups | blueberries | 500 mL |

1. In a large bowl, whisk together quinoa flour, baking powder, baking soda and salt.
2. In a medium bowl, whisk together eggs, buttermilk, oil and honey.
3. Add the egg mixture to the flour mixture and stir until just blended.
4. Heat a griddle or skillet over medium heat. Spray with cooking spray. For each pancake, pour about ¼ cup (60 mL) batter onto griddle and top with 8 to 10 blueberries. Cook until bubbles appear on top. Turn pancake over and cook for about 1 minute or until golden brown. Repeat with the remaining batter, spraying griddle and adjusting heat as necessary between batches.

## Variations

*Quinoa Buttermilk Pancakes:* Omit the blueberries.

*Chocolate Chip Quinoa Pancakes:* Use ¾ cup (175 mL) semisweet chocolate chips (GF, if needed) in place of the blueberries. Sprinkle 8 to 10 chocolate chips on each pancake in step 4.

# Blintz Pancakes with Yogurt and Jam

*These pretty puffed pancakes — beautifully textured and absolutely delicious — have much of the flavor of cheese-stuffed blintzes, sans fuss. The key is cottage cheese in the batter, which, together with the quinoa flour, power-packs each pancake. Tart yogurt and fruit preserves top things off with delectable ease.*

## Storage Tip

Let pancakes cool completely on a wire rack, then wrap individually in plastic wrap and store in an airtight container in the refrigerator for up to 2 days or the freezer for up to 1 month. Reheat in the microwave on High for 45 seconds, until warmed through (no need to thaw), or toast in the toaster oven for 1 to 2 minutes or until toasted and warmed though.

| | | |
|---|---|---:|
| 1 cup | quinoa flour | 250 mL |
| ½ tsp | baking soda | 2 mL |
| ¼ tsp | fine sea salt | 1 mL |
| 4 | large eggs | 4 |
| 1 cup | cottage cheese | 250 mL |
| ½ cup | milk | 125 mL |
| 2 tbsp | vegetable oil | 30 mL |
| 2 tbsp | pure maple syrup or liquid honey | 30 mL |
| | Nonstick cooking spray | |
| 1 cup | plain yogurt | 250 mL |
| ¼ cup | fruit-sweetened blackberry or raspberry jam | 60 mL |

1. In a large bowl, whisk together quinoa flour, baking soda and salt.
2. In a medium bowl, whisk together eggs, cottage cheese, milk, oil and maple syrup until blended.
3. Add the egg mixture to the flour mixture and stir until just blended.
4. Heat a griddle or skillet over medium heat. Spray with cooking spray. For each pancake, pour about ¼ cup (60 mL) batter onto griddle. Cook until bubbles appear on top. Turn pancake over and cook for about 1 minute or until golden brown. Repeat with the remaining batter, spraying griddle and adjusting heat as necessary between batches.
5. Serve pancakes topped with yogurt and jam.

# Quinoa Dutch Baby

*A cross between a pancake and a popover, Dutch babies thrill adults and children alike. Quinoa flour renders the pancake especially light while also adding a subtle sesame flavor that works harmoniously with the cinnamon and nutmeg in the batter.*

**• Large ovenproof skillet**

| | | |
|---|---|---|
| 3 | large eggs, at room temperature | 3 |
| ⅔ cup | quinoa flour | 150 mL |
| ⅛ tsp | ground cinnamon | 0.5 mL |
| ⅛ tsp | ground nutmeg | 0.5 mL |
| ⅛ tsp | fine sea salt | 0.5 mL |
| ¾ cup | milk, at room temperature | 175 mL |
| ¼ tsp | vanilla extract (GF, if needed) | 1 mL |
| 2 tbsp | unsalted butter | 30 mL |

**Suggested Accompaniments**

Pure maple syrup or liquid honey

Confectioners' (icing) sugar and freshly squeezed lemon juice

Fresh fruits and berries

**1.** Place skillet in oven. Preheat oven to 450°F (230°C).

**2.** In a large bowl, using an electric mixer, beat eggs on high speed for 1 to 2 minutes or until frothy. Add quinoa flour, cinnamon, nutmeg, salt, milk and vanilla; beat on medium-high speed for about 1 minute, stopping once to scrape down bottom and sides of bowl with a spatula, until smooth (batter will be thin).

**3.** Remove skillet from oven. Add butter and melt, swirling to coat. Add batter and immediately return skillet to oven. Bake for 19 to 24 minutes or until puffed and golden brown. Serve with any of the suggested accompaniments, as desired.

# Quinoa Crêpes

**Makes
12 crêpes**

*Quinoa flour produces
a light crêpe with lots
of nutty flavor. You can
forget what you've heard
about crêpes being fussy
or challenging — they're
very easy to make.
Moreover, a regular
nonstick skillet works
just as well as any
crêpe pan or specialty
crêpe griddle.*

## Tip

Refrigerating the batter
before use allows the
bubbles that form during
blending to subside,
making the crêpes less
likely to tear during
cooking. The batter will
keep for up to 48 hours.

## Storage Tip

Refrigerate crêpes
between sheets of waxed
paper, tightly covered
in plastic wrap, for up to
2 days or freeze, enclosed
in a sealable plastic bag,
for up to 1 month.

- **Blender**

| | | |
|---|---|---|
| 2 | large eggs | 2 |
| ¾ cup | milk | 175 mL |
| ½ cup | water | 125 mL |
| 3 tbsp | unsalted butter, melted and cooled | 45 mL |
| ¼ tsp | fine sea salt | 1 mL |
| 1 cup | quinoa flour | 250 mL |
| | Nonstick cooking spray | |

1. In blender, combine eggs, milk, water, butter and salt.
   Add quinoa flour and blend until smooth. Transfer to a
   bowl, cover and refrigerate for 1 hour.

2. Heat a large nonstick skillet over medium-high heat.
   Remove from heat and lightly coat pan with cooking
   spray. Whisk the batter slightly. For each crêpe, pour
   about ¼ cup (60 mL) batter into pan, quickly tilting in
   all directions to cover bottom of pan. Cook for about
   45 seconds or until just golden at the edges. With a
   spatula, carefully lift edge of crêpe to test for doneness.
   The crêpe is ready to turn when it is golden brown on
   the bottom and can be shaken loose from the pan. Turn
   crêpe over and cook for about 15 to 30 seconds or until
   golden brown.

3. Transfer crêpe to an unfolded kitchen towel to cool
   completely. Repeat with the remaining batter, spraying
   skillet and adjusting heat as necessary between crêpes,
   stacking cooled crêpes between sheets of waxed paper
   to prevent sticking.

### Crêpe Filling Ideas

Lemon juice and a drizzle of honey; a thin spread of nut or
seed butter and all-fruit jam; Greek yogurt and fresh fruit
or jam; ricotta or cottage cheese and a drizzle of honey or
agave nectar; grated bittersweet chocolate (GF, if needed)
and toasted nuts; thinly sliced ham and shredded Gruyère
or Swiss cheese; sautéed spinach and freshly grated
Parmesan cheese; shredded sharp (old) Cheddar cheese
and thinly sliced or grated tart-sweet apples; thinly sliced
pears and a drizzle of pure maple syrup; scrambled eggs
or egg whites, or scrambled tofu.

# Banana Cinnamon Quinoa Waffles

**Makes
10 waffles**

*These banana and cinnamon waffles make ordinary varieties taste ho-hum. They are extra-wonderful with a drizzle of maple syrup on top.*

## Storage Tip

Let waffles cool completely on a wire rack, then wrap individually in plastic wrap and store in an airtight container in the refrigerator for up to 2 days or the freezer for up to 1 month. Reheat in the microwave on High for 45 seconds, until warmed through (no need to thaw), or toast in the toaster oven for 1 to 2 minutes or until toasted and warmed though.

- **Preheat waffle maker to medium-high**

| | | |
|---|---|---|
| 1¾ cups | quinoa flour | 425 mL |
| ¼ cup | ground flax seeds (flaxseed meal) | 60 mL |
| 1½ tsp | baking powder (GF, if needed) | 7 mL |
| 1 tsp | ground cinnamon | 5 mL |
| ¼ tsp | fine sea salt | 1 mL |
| 2 | large eggs | 2 |
| 1 cup | milk | 250 mL |
| 3 tbsp | unsalted butter, melted | 45 mL |
| 2 tbsp | pure maple syrup or liquid honey | 30 mL |
| 2 tsp | vanilla extract (GF, if needed) | 10 mL |
| ¾ cup | mashed ripe bananas | 175 mL |
| | Nonstick cooking spray | |

1. In a large bowl, whisk together quinoa flour, flax seeds, baking powder, cinnamon and salt.
2. In a medium bowl, whisk together eggs, milk, butter, maple syrup and vanilla. Stir in banana.
3. Add the egg mixture to the flour mixture and stir until just blended.
4. Spray preheated waffle maker with cooking spray. For each waffle, pour about $1/3$ cup (75 mL) batter into waffle maker. Cook according to manufacturer's instructions until golden brown.

# Pumpkin Maple Waffles

**Makes
10 waffles**

*Just right for super-
charging your breakfast
any day of the week,
these waffles are subtly
spiced, tender and gently
sweetened with a touch of
maple syrup.*

## Storage Tip

Let waffles cool
completely on a wire rack,
then wrap individually in
plastic wrap and store in
an airtight container in
the refrigerator for up to
2 days or the freezer for
up to 1 month. Reheat
in the microwave on
High for 45 seconds, until
warmed through (no
need to thaw), or toast in
the toaster oven for 1 to
2 minutes or until toasted
and warmed though.

- **Preheat waffle maker to medium-high**

| | | |
|---|---|---:|
| 1¼ cups | quinoa flour | 300 mL |
| 2 tbsp | ground flax seeds (flaxseed meal) | 30 mL |
| 2 tsp | pumpkin pie spice | 10 mL |
| 1½ tsp | baking powder (GF, if needed) | 7 mL |
| ¼ tsp | baking soda | 1 mL |
| ¼ tsp | fine sea salt | 1 mL |
| 1 | large egg | 1 |
| 1 cup | buttermilk | 250 mL |
| 1 cup | pumpkin purée (not pie filling) | 250 mL |
| 2 tbsp | unsalted butter, melted, or vegetable oil | 30 mL |
| 2 tbsp | pure maple syrup or liquid honey | 30 mL |
| | Nonstick cooking spray | |

1. In a large bowl, whisk together quinoa flour, flax
   seeds, pumpkin pie spice, baking powder, baking soda
   and salt.
2. In a medium bowl, whisk together egg, buttermilk,
   pumpkin, butter and maple syrup.
3. Add the egg mixture to the flour mixture and stir until
   just blended.
4. Spray preheated waffle maker with cooking spray.
   For each waffle, pour about ⅓ cup (75 mL) batter
   into waffle maker. Cook according to manufacturer's
   instructions until golden brown.

# Maple Blueberry Coffee Cake

*Buttermilk, quinoa
flour and plump, fresh
berries are a sublime
combination in this pretty
coffee cake. The mellow
sweetness of maple syrup
makes the cake special
enough for brunch
with guests.*

## Tip

An equal amount of liquid
honey or brown rice syrup
may be used in place of
the maple syrup.

## Storage Tip

Store cooled coffee cake
tightly covered or in an
airtight container in the
refrigerator for up to
3 days.

- **Preheat oven to 350°F (180°C)**
- **Food processor**
- **9-inch (23 cm) square metal baking pan, sprayed with
  nonstick cooking spray**

| | | |
|---|---|---|
| 1½ cups | large-flake (old-fashioned) rolled oats (certified GF, if needed) | 375 mL |
| 1 cup | quinoa flour | 250 mL |
| 2 tsp | ground cinnamon | 10 mL |
| 1 tsp | baking powder (GF, if needed) | 5 mL |
| 1 tsp | baking soda | 5 mL |
| ¾ tsp | fine sea salt | 3 mL |
| 2 | large eggs | 2 |
| ⅔ cup | pure maple syrup | 150 mL |
| ¼ cup | unsalted butter, melted | 60 mL |
| 2 tsp | vanilla extract (GF, if needed) | 10 mL |
| 1½ cups | buttermilk | 375 mL |
| 1½ cups | blueberries | 375 mL |
| ½ cup | finely chopped pecans | 125 mL |
| 1 tbsp | turbinado sugar | 15 mL |

1. In food processor, pulse oats five or six times, until oats resemble coarse meal.
2. Transfer oats to a large bowl and whisk in quinoa flour, cinnamon, baking powder, baking soda and salt.
3. In a medium bowl, whisk together eggs, maple syrup, butter and vanilla until well blended. Whisk in buttermilk until blended.
4. Add the egg mixture to the flour mixture and stir until just blended. Gently fold in blueberries.
5. Spread batter evenly in prepared pan and sprinkle with pecans and sugar.
6. Bake in preheated oven for 28 to 33 minutes or until a toothpick inserted in the center comes out clean. Let cool completely in pan on a wire rack.

# Cocoa Banana Mini Muffins

*Everyone needs a great breakfast recipe that can be thrown together in minutes the night before. These mini muffins are just such a recipe. Not too sweet, they are made with ingredients you likely always have on hand, and everybody will love them. Freeze the extras in a large zip-top bag — they thaw in about 5 minutes.*

## Tip

Natural cane confectioners' (icing) sugar is made using the same process as regular confectioners' sugar (granulated sugar is crushed to a fine white powder), but is made with less processed natural cane sugar. Regular confectioners' sugar may be used in its place.

## Storage Tip

Store cooled muffins in an airtight container in the refrigerator for up to 5 days.

- **Preheat oven to 400°F (200°C)**
- **Three 12-cup mini muffin pans, sprayed with nonstick cooking spray**

| | | |
|---|---|---|
| 1¼ cups | quinoa flour | 300 mL |
| 1 cup | quick-cooking rolled oats (certified GF, if needed) | 250 mL |
| ½ cup | natural cane sugar or packed light brown sugar | 125 mL |
| ⅓ cup | unsweetened cocoa powder (not Dutch process) | 75 mL |
| 1¼ tsp | baking powder (GF, if needed) | 6 mL |
| ½ tsp | baking soda | 2 mL |
| ¼ tsp | fine sea salt | 1 mL |
| 2 | large eggs | 2 |
| ⅔ cup | mashed ripe bananas | 150 mL |
| ½ cup | milk or plain non-dairy milk (such as soy, almond, rice or hemp) | 125 mL |
| ¼ cup | coconut oil, warmed, or unsalted butter, melted | 60 mL |
| 1 tsp | vanilla extract (GF, if needed) | 5 mL |
| 2 tbsp | natural cane confectioners' (icing) sugar (optional) | 30 mL |

1. In a large bowl, whisk together quinoa flour, oats, cane sugar, cocoa powder, baking powder, baking soda and salt.
2. In a medium bowl, whisk together eggs, bananas, milk, oil and vanilla until well blended.
3. Add the egg mixture to the flour mixture and stir until just blended.
4. Divide batter equally among prepared muffin cups.
5. Bake in preheated oven 10 to 12 minutes or until a toothpick inserted in the center comes out clean. Let cool in pans on a wire rack for 5 minutes, then transfer to the rack to cool. Sprinkle with confectioners' sugar, if desired.

# Cheese and Mushroom Frittata Muffins

*Part muffin, part frittata, these not-so-humble muffins pack a range of flavors: tangy, earthy and cheesy. They add up to irresistible.*

## Storage Tip

Store cooled muffins in an airtight container in the refrigerator for up to 3 days.

- **12-cup muffin pan, 9 cups greased**

| | | |
|---|---|---|
| 1 tsp | olive oil | 5 mL |
| 8 oz | cremini or button mushrooms, coarsely chopped | 250 g |
| 1 cup | quinoa flour | 250 mL |
| 1 tsp | baking powder (GF, if needed) | 5 mL |
| ¼ tsp | fine sea salt | 1 mL |
| ¼ tsp | freshly ground black pepper | 1 mL |
| 4 | large eggs | 4 |
| ⅔ cup | small-curd cottage cheese | 150 mL |
| 2 tbsp | freshly grated Parmesan cheese | 30 mL |
| ½ cup | crumbled feta cheese | 125 mL |
| ¼ cup | chopped green onions | 60 mL |

1. In a large skillet, heat oil over medium-high heat. Add mushrooms and cook, stirring, for 4 to 5 minutes or until starting to brown and liquid has evaporated. Remove from heat and let cool.
2. Preheat oven to 400°F (200°C).
3. In a large bowl, whisk together quinoa flour, baking powder, salt and pepper. Stir in eggs, cottage cheese and Parmesan until just blended. Fold in sautéed mushrooms, feta and green onions.
4. Divide batter equally among prepared muffin cups.
5. Bake for 23 to 25 minutes or until tops are golden and a toothpick inserted in the center comes out clean. Let cool in pan on a wire rack for 5 minutes, then transfer to the rack to cool slightly. Serve warm or let cool to room temperature.

# Maple Breakfast Biscotti

*Few people need an excuse to eat cookies for breakfast, but you certainly won't need one for these crisp biscotti: they have a plethora of good-for-you ingredients and are great on the go or slowly savored (and dunked) with a morning cup of joe.*

## Tips

For the nuts, you can also try walnuts, hazelnuts, pistachios or almonds. For the dried fruit, try raisins, cherries or chopped apricots.

The biscotti will continue to harden as they cool after the second bake.

## Storage Tip

Store the cooled biscotti in an airtight container at room temperature for up to 5 days.

- **Preheat oven to 300°F (150°C)**
- **Food processor**
- **Large rimmed baking sheet, lined with parchment paper**

| | | |
|---|---|---|
| 1½ cups | large-flake (old-fashioned) rolled oats (certified GF, if needed), divided | 375 mL |
| 1 cup | quinoa flour | 250 mL |
| 1 tsp | baking powder (GF, if needed) | 5 mL |
| ½ tsp | baking soda | 2 mL |
| ¼ tsp | fine sea salt | 1 mL |
| ⅔ cup | chopped toasted pecans | 150 mL |
| ⅔ cup | chopped pitted dates | 150 mL |
| ⅓ cup | natural cane sugar or packed light brown sugar | 75 mL |
| 2 | large eggs | 2 |
| ⅓ cup | pure maple syrup | 75 mL |
| 1 tsp | vanilla extract (GF, if needed) | 5 mL |

1. In food processor, pulse ¾ cup (175 mL) of the oats until they resemble fine flour.
2. Transfer ground oats to a medium bowl and whisk in the remaining oats, quinoa flour, baking powder, baking soda and salt. Stir in pecans and dates.
3. In a large bowl, whisk together sugar, eggs, maple syrup and vanilla until blended. Gradually add the flour mixture, stirring until just blended. Divide dough in half.
4. Place dough on prepared baking sheet and, using moistened hands, shape into two parallel 12- by 2-inch (30 by 5 cm) rectangles, spaced about 3 inches (7.5 cm) apart.
5. Bake in preheated oven for 30 to 35 minutes or until set at the center and golden. Let cool on pan on a wire rack for 15 minutes.
6. Cut rectangles crosswise into ½-inch (1 cm) slices. Place slices, cut side down, on baking sheet. Bake for 8 to 10 minutes or until edges are golden. Let cool on pan for 1 minute, then transfer to wire racks to cool completely.

# Superpower Breakfast Cookies

*Loaded with all of the essential amino acids, as well as vitamins and minerals, quinoa is a perfect way to start the day. It makes a delicious addition to these tender breakfast cookies. And dried blueberries are a smart way to enjoy this superfruit, in baked goods or out of hand, year-round.*

## Storage Tip

Store cooled cookies in an airtight container in the refrigerator for up to 5 days.

- **Preheat oven to 350°F (180°C)**
- **Baking sheets, lined with parchment paper**

| | | |
|---|---|---|
| ½ cup | quinoa, rinsed | 125 mL |
| 1¼ cups | quinoa flour | 300 mL |
| ¾ cup | quick-cooking rolled oats (certified GF, if needed) | 175 mL |
| 1½ tsp | baking powder (GF, if needed) | 7 mL |
| 1 tsp | fine sea salt | 5 mL |
| ½ tsp | baking soda | 2 mL |
| 1 | large egg, lightly beaten | 1 |
| ½ cup | liquid honey, pure maple syrup or brown rice syrup | 125 mL |
| ⅓ cup | plain yogurt | 75 mL |
| ¼ cup | coconut oil, warmed, or vegetable oil | 60 mL |
| 1 tsp | vanilla extract (GF, if needed) | 5 mL |
| ⅔ cup | dried cherries, cranberries or blueberries | 150 mL |

1. In a pot of boiling salted water, cook quinoa for 9 minutes. Drain and rinse under cold water until cool (quinoa will still be slightly chewy).

2. In a large bowl, whisk together quinoa flour, oats, baking powder, salt and baking soda. Stir in egg, honey, yogurt, oil and vanilla until just blended. Gently fold in quinoa and cherries.

3. Drop batter by 2 tbsp (30 mL) onto prepared baking sheets, spacing cookies 2 inches (5 cm) apart.

4. Bake one sheet at a time in preheated oven for 12 to 15 minutes or until just set at the center. Let cool in pan on a wire rack for 5 minutes, then transfer to the rack to cool.

# PB&Q Breakfast Cookies

*Peanut butter and quinoa: two great things that go great together. Here they come in an adorable little package loaded with additional superfood ingredients, including oats, banana and dried blueberries. A healthy breakfast on the go never tasted so good!*

## Tip

Any unsweetened natural nut or seed butter (such as cashew, almond, sunflower seed or tahini) may be used in place of the peanut butter.

## Storage Tip

Store cooled cookies in an airtight container in the refrigerator for up to 5 days.

- **Preheat oven to 350°F (180°C)**
- **Baking sheets, lined with parchment paper**

| | | |
|---|---|---|
| 1 cup | quick-cooking rolled oats (certified GF, if needed) or quinoa flakes | 250 mL |
| ½ cup | quinoa flour | 125 mL |
| ¼ cup | instant skim milk powder or soy milk powder | 60 mL |
| 2 tsp | ground cinnamon | 10 mL |
| ¼ tsp | baking soda | 1 mL |
| ¼ tsp | fine sea salt | 1 mL |
| 1 | large egg, lightly beaten | 1 |
| ½ cup | mashed ripe banana | 125 mL |
| ½ cup | unsweetened natural peanut butter | 125 mL |
| ½ cup | liquid honey, pure maple syrup or brown rice syrup | 125 mL |
| 1 tsp | vanilla extract (GF, if needed) | 5 mL |
| ¾ cup | dried blueberries or cranberries | 175 mL |

1. In a large bowl, whisk together oats, quinoa flour, milk powder, cinnamon, baking soda and salt. Stir in egg, banana, peanut butter, honey and vanilla until just blended. Gently fold in blueberries.

2. Drop batter by 2 tbsp (30 mL) onto prepared baking sheets, spacing cookies 2 inches (5 cm) apart. With a metal spatula, flatten each mound to ½-inch (1 cm) thickness.

3. Bake one sheet at a time in preheated oven for 12 to 15 minutes or until just set at the center. Let cool in pan on a wire rack for 5 minutes, then transfer to the rack to cool.

# Carrot Cake Breakfast Cookies

*I am hard-pressed to find someone who doesn't like carrot cake, so what better option for breakfast than a carrot cake cookie? These tender gems taste utterly decadent, but are in fact utterly nutritious, so help yourself to two.*

## Storage Tip

Store cooled cookies in an airtight container in the refrigerator for up to 5 days.

- **Preheat oven to 375°F (190°C)**
- **Baking sheets, lined with parchment paper**

| | | |
|---|---|---|
| 1½ cups | large-flake (old-fashioned) rolled oats (certified GF, if needed) | 375 mL |
| 1 cup | quinoa flour | 250 mL |
| ¼ cup | ground flax seeds (flaxseed meal) | 60 mL |
| 2 tsp | ground cinnamon | 10 mL |
| 1 tsp | baking soda | 5 mL |
| ¼ tsp | fine sea salt | 1 mL |
| 2 | large eggs, lightly beaten | 2 |
| ½ cup | unsweetened applesauce | 125 mL |
| ½ cup | liquid honey | 125 mL |
| ¼ cup | vegetable oil | 60 mL |
| 2 cups | shredded carrots | 500 mL |
| ⅔ cup | raisins | 150 mL |
| ½ cup | chopped toasted walnuts | 125 mL |

1. In a large bowl, whisk together oats, quinoa flour, flax seeds, cinnamon, baking soda and salt. Stir in eggs, applesauce, honey and oil until just blended. Gently fold in carrots, raisins and walnuts.

2. Drop batter by 2 tbsp (30 mL) onto prepared baking sheets, spacing cookies 2 inches (5 cm) apart.

3. Bake one sheet at a time in preheated oven for 12 to 15 minutes or until just set at the center. Let cool in pan on a wire rack for 5 minutes, then transfer to the rack to cool.

# Toasted Sesame Quinoa Bars

**Makes 16 bars**

*Weary of store-bought power bars and breakfast bars? Then give this no-bake bar a try. The tahini and honey base is amped up with toasted quinoa, sesame seeds and dried fruit, all to delicious, nutritious effect.*

## Tip

Lining a pan with foil is easy. Begin by turning the pan upside down. Tear off a piece of foil longer than the pan, then mold the foil over the pan. Remove the foil and set it aside. Flip the pan over and gently fit the shaped foil into the pan, allowing the foil to hang over the sides (the overhang ends will work as "handles" when the contents of the pan are removed).

## Storage Tip

Wrap bars individually and refrigerate for up to 2 weeks.

• **9-inch (23 cm) square metal baking pan, lined with foil (see tip, at left)**

| | | |
|---|---|---|
| ¾ cup | quinoa, rinsed | 175 mL |
| ¼ cup | sesame seeds | 60 mL |
| 4 cups | large-flake (old-fashioned) rolled oats (certified GF, if needed) | 1 L |
| ¾ cup | pitted dates, chopped | 175 mL |
| ¾ cup | chopped dried apricots | 175 mL |
| ¼ tsp | fine sea salt | 1 mL |
| 1 cup | tahini | 250 mL |
| ½ cup | liquid honey or brown rice syrup | 125 mL |
| 2 tsp | vanilla extract (GF, if needed) | 10 mL |

**1.** In a large skillet, over medium heat, toast quinoa and sesame seeds, stirring, for 4 to 5 minutes or until seeds are golden and beginning to pop. Transfer to a large bowl and let cool completely.

**2.** To the quinoa mixture, add oats, dates, apricots and salt. Stir in tahini, honey and vanilla until blended.

**3.** Press mixture into prepared pan and refrigerate for at least 30 minutes, until firm. Using foil liner, lift mixture from pan and invert onto a cutting board; peel off foil and cut into 16 bars.

# Multigrain Breakfast Bars

*Oats and quinoa are perfect foods for the beginning of the day: high in protein, they also contain essential fats and are rich in minerals, including zinc, calcium, magnesium and iron. Vitamin C assists in the absorption of iron, so add some orange juice in a travel mug for an ideal meal on the go.*

## Storage Tip

Wrap bars individually and refrigerate for up to 2 weeks.

- Preheat oven to 350°F (180°C)
- Large rimmed baking sheet, lined with parchment paper
- Food processor
- 9-inch (23 cm) square metal baking pan, lined with foil (see tip, page 67)

| | | |
|---|---|---|
| 1½ cups | large-flake (old-fashioned) rolled oats (certified GF, if needed) | 375 mL |
| 1 cup | quinoa, rinsed | 250 mL |
| ½ cup | chopped pecans or walnuts | 125 mL |
| ½ cup | brown rice syrup or liquid honey | 125 mL |
| ¾ cup | pitted soft dates (such as Medjool), chopped | 175 mL |
| ¼ cup | ground flax seeds (flaxseed meal) | 60 mL |
| 1 tsp | ground cinnamon | 5 mL |
| ⅛ tsp | fine sea salt | 0.5 mL |
| ½ cup | dried cranberries | 125 mL |
| ½ cup | chopped dried apricots | 125 mL |

1. Spread oats, quinoa and pecans on prepared baking sheet. Bake in preheated oven for 7 to 8 minutes or until fragrant and light golden.
2. In a small saucepan, warm brown rice syrup over medium-low heat.
3. In food processor, pulse oat mixture, warmed syrup, dates, flax seeds, cinnamon and salt until mixture begins to hold together as a dough.
4. Scrape mixture into a medium bowl. Break up any clumps of dates and, if needed, chop any large date chunks. Stir in cranberries and apricots.
5. Transfer mixture to prepared pan and press flat with a square of waxed paper. Freeze for 30 minutes. Using foil liner, lift mixture from pan and invert onto a cutting board; peel off foil and cut into 16 bars.

# Cocoa Quinoa Breakfast Squares

**Makes
9 squares**

*The intense flavor of cocoa powder and natural sweetness of plump dates coalesce with quinoa for a power-packed breakfast. Wrap the cooled squares in parchment or plastic wrap for a perfectly portable, make-ahead breakfast.*

## Storage Tip

Store the cooled quinoa squares tightly covered or in an airtight container in the refrigerator for up to 3 days. Serve cold or room temperature.

- **Preheat oven to 350°F (180°C)**
- **Blender or food processor**
- **8-inch (20 cm) square metal baking pan, lined with foil (see tip, page 67) and sprayed with nonstick cooking spray**

| | | |
|---|---|---|
| 1 cup | pitted soft dates (such as Medjool) | 250 mL |
| 1/3 cup | unsweetened cocoa powder (not Dutch process) | 75 mL |
| 1/4 tsp | fine sea salt | 1 mL |
| 2 cups | milk or plain non-dairy milk (such as soy, rice, almond or hemp) | 500 mL |
| 1 tsp | vanilla extract (GF, if needed) | 5 mL |
| 3 cups | hot cooked quinoa (see page 10) | 750 mL |
| 1/2 cup | ground flax seeds (flaxseed meal) | 125 mL |

1. In blender, combine dates, cocoa, salt, milk and vanilla; purée until smooth.
2. Transfer date mixture to a large bowl and stir in quinoa and flax seeds. Spread evenly in prepared pan.
3. Bake in preheated oven for 55 to 60 minutes or until firmly set. Let cool completely in pan on a wire rack. Using foil liner, lift mixture from pan onto a cutting board; peel off foil and cut into 9 squares.

# Seasonal Fruit Parfaits

**Makes
2 servings**

*With its ample doses of honey-sweetened quinoa, luxurious Greek yogurt and fresh fruit, this easy, elegant breakfast will knock pancakes off their pedestal.*

- **2 parfait glasses**

| | | |
|---|---|---|
| 1 cup | cooked quinoa (see page 10), chilled | 250 mL |
| 1/8 tsp | fine sea salt | 0.5 mL |
| 3 tbsp | liquid honey or pure maple syrup, divided | 45 mL |
| 1 cup | plain Greek yogurt | 250 mL |
| 1 1/2 cups | assorted diced seasonal fruit or berries | 375 mL |

1. In a small bowl, combine quinoa, salt and 2 tbsp (30 mL) of the honey.
2. Spoon half the yogurt into each parfait glass. Top each with half the quinoa mixture and half the fruit. Drizzle with the remaining honey.

# Quinoa Crunch

Here, quinoa is transformed into a crispy-sweet topping that's heavenly sprinkled on yogurt, cereal or muffins, mixed into trail mix or simply eaten out of hand.

## Tip

An equal amount of pure maple syrup, brown rice syrup or agave nectar may be used in place of the honey.

- **Preheat oven to 375°F (190°C)**
- **Rimmed baking sheet, lined with parchment paper**

| | | |
|---|---|---|
| 1 cup | quinoa, rinsed | 250 mL |
| 1 tbsp | vegetable oil | 15 mL |
| 1 tbsp | liquid honey | 15 mL |
| 1/8 tsp | fine sea salt | 0.5 mL |

1. In a small bowl, combine quinoa, oil, honey and salt. Spread in a single layer on prepared baking sheet.
2. Bake in preheated oven for 11 to 13 minutes, stirring occasionally, until quinoa is crisp. Transfer to a large plate and let cool completely.
3. Transfer quinoa crunch to an airtight container and store at room temperature for up to 1 month.

# Mango Carrot Quinoa Smoothie

**Makes 2 servings**

Begin the day by drinking your vegetables. This sunshiny blend of mango, carrot and quinoa — with a kick of ginger to boot — has more than enough zing to launch you into your day.

- **Blender**

| | | |
|---|---|---|
| 1 cup | frozen mango chunks | 250 mL |
| 3 tbsp | quinoa flakes or flour | 45 mL |
| 3/4 tsp | ground ginger | 3 mL |
| 1 cup | carrot juice | 250 mL |
| 1/2 cup | plain yogurt | 125 mL |
| 1 tbsp | liquid honey or agave nectar | 15 mL |

1. In blender, purée mango, quinoa flakes, ginger, carrot juice, yogurt and honey until smooth. Pour into two glasses and serve immediately.

## Variation

For a non-dairy alternative, substitute plain cultured soy or rice yogurt for the yogurt.

# Raspberry Vanilla Quinoa Shake

**Makes
2 servings**

*This shake derives its
deep flavor and rosy color
from raspberries, blended
with apple juice for
additional sweetness and
yogurt and quinoa flakes
for creaminess.*

- **Blender**

| | | |
|---|---|---|
| 1½ cups | frozen raspberries | 375 mL |
| 3 tbsp | quinoa flakes or flour | 45 mL |
| 1 cup | plain yogurt | 250 mL |
| ⅔ cup | unsweetened apple juice | 150 mL |
| 1 tsp | vanilla extract (GF, if needed) | 5 mL |

**1.** In blender, purée raspberries, quinoa flakes, yogurt, apple juice and vanilla until smooth. Pour into two glasses and serve immediately.

# Mixed Berry Quinoa Shake

**Makes
2 servings**

### Tip
For a non-dairy alternative, substitute plain cultured soy or rice yogurt for the yogurt.

- **Blender**

| | | |
|---|---|---|
| 1½ cups | mixed frozen berries | 375 mL |
| ½ cup | sliced frozen ripe banana | 125 mL |
| 3 tbsp | quinoa flakes or flour | 45 mL |
| ¾ cup | plain yogurt | 175 mL |
| ¾ cup | orange juice | 175 mL |

**1.** In blender, purée berries, banana, quinoa flakes, yogurt and orange juice until smooth. Pour into two glasses and serve immediately.

# Green Quinoa Smoothie

**Makes
2 servings**

*Eschew the drive-through
once and for all: this is
what real fast food is all
about. Ready in minutes,
this refreshing, nutrient-
dense elixir will satisfy
and energize you all
morning long.*

- **Blender**

| | | |
|---|---|---|
| 2 cups | loosely packed spinach leaves or trimmed kale leaves | 500 mL |
| 1 cup | green grapes | 250 mL |
| ¾ cup | sliced frozen ripe banana | 175 mL |
| ½ cup | chopped kiwifruit | 125 mL |
| 3 tbsp | quinoa flakes or flour | 45 mL |
| 1 cup | orange juice | 250 mL |

**1.** In blender, purée spinach, grapes, banana, kiwi, quinoa flakes and orange juice until smooth. Pour into two glasses and serve immediately.

# Pumpkin Pie Smoothie

**Makes 2 to 3 servings**

*Chock full of antioxidants, fiber and vitamin A, pumpkin rivals quinoa for top superfood status. Here, it stars in a sweet, creamy smoothie, offering delicious proof that it deserves a place in your pantry year-round.*

● **Blender**

| | | |
|---|---|---|
| 1 cup | sliced frozen ripe banana | 250 mL |
| 3 tbsp | quinoa flakes or flour | 45 mL |
| ½ tsp | pumpkin pie spice or ground cinnamon | 2 mL |
| 1⅓ cups | milk or plain non-dairy milk (such as soy, almond, rice or hemp) | 325 mL |
| ¾ cup | pumpkin purée (not pie filling) | 175 mL |
| ½ cup | ice cubes | 125 mL |
| 2 tbsp | pure maple syrup or liquid honey | 30 mL |
| 1 tsp | vanilla extract (GF, if needed) | 5 mL |

**1.** In blender, purée banana, quinoa flakes, pumpkin pie spice, milk, pumpkin, ice cubes, maple syrup and vanilla until smooth. Pour into glasses and serve immediately.

# Banana Date Quinoa Smoothie

**Makes 2 servings**

*Naturally sweetened with dates and banana, this creamy concoction may fool you into thinking you're sipping a thick ice cream shake.*

● **Blender**

| | | |
|---|---|---|
| 1 cup | sliced frozen ripe banana | 250 mL |
| ¼ cup | pitted Medjool or other soft dates, roughly chopped | 60 mL |
| ¼ cup | quinoa flakes or flour | 60 mL |
| ¼ tsp | ground cinnamon | 1 mL |
| 1½ cups | buttermilk | 375 mL |

**1.** In blender, purée banana, dates, quinoa flakes, cinnamon and buttermilk until smooth. Pour into two glasses and serve immediately.

## Variation

For a non-dairy alternative, replace the buttermilk with 1 cup (250 mL) plain cultured soy or rice yogurt plus ½ cup (125 mL) plain non-dairy milk (such as soy, almond, rice or hemp).

# Appetizers and Snacks

# Endive Filled with Cranberry Quinoa Crunch

**Makes 2 dozen appetizers**

It would be hard to overstate just how well the ingredients come together in this beautiful appetizer. The textural contrast — crunchy quinoa and crisp endive, apple and cabbage — is enhanced by a surprisingly complex dressing containing sweet, spicy and smoky elements.

| | | |
|---|---|---|
| 3 tbsp | quinoa, rinsed | 45 mL |
| ¼ tsp | chipotle chile powder or smoked paprika (hot or sweet) | 1 mL |
| 1 tbsp | cider vinegar | 15 mL |
| 1 tbsp | olive oil mayonnaise or tofu mayonnaise | 15 mL |
| 1 tbsp | plain Greek yogurt | 15 mL |
| 1 tsp | pure maple syrup or liquid honey | 5 mL |
| 1 | tart-sweet apple (such as Braeburn or Gala), peeled and chopped | 1 |
| 1 cup | finely chopped purple cabbage | 250 mL |
| ¼ cup | dried cranberries, chopped | 60 mL |
| | Fine sea salt and freshly cracked black pepper | |
| 24 | Belgian endive leaves (about 2 small heads) | 24 |

1. Heat a skillet over medium-high heat. Toast quinoa, stirring occasionally, for 3 to 4 minutes or until golden brown and just beginning to pop. Transfer to a medium bowl and let cool.

2. In a small bowl, whisk together chipotle chile powder, vinegar, mayonnaise, yogurt and maple syrup.

3. To the quinoa, add apple, cabbage and cranberries. Add dressing, gently tossing to coat. Season to taste with salt and pepper. Cover and refrigerate for 30 minutes.

4. Arrange endive leaves on a platter. Spoon about 2 tbsp (30 mL) quinoa mixture into the base of each leaf.

# Mushrooms Stuffed with Spinach, Quinoa and Blue Cheese

**Makes about 20 appetizers**

*Spinach and mushrooms go hand in hand, especially when quinoa and blue cheese are added to the mix.*

## Tip

When selecting mushrooms, choose those with a fresh, smooth appearance, free from major blemishes and with a dry surface. Once home, keep mushrooms refrigerated; they're best when used within a few days after purchase. When ready to use, gently wipe mushrooms with a damp cloth or soft brush to remove dirt particles. Alternatively, rinse mushrooms quickly with cold water, then immediately pat dry with paper towels.

- **Preheat oven to 350°F (180°C)**
- **Rimmed baking sheet, lined with parchment paper**

| | | |
|---|---|---|
| 2 tsp | extra virgin olive oil | 10 mL |
| 1 lb | medium-large cremini mushrooms (about 20), stems removed and finely chopped, caps left intact | 500 g |
| 1 cup | chopped onions | 250 mL |
| | Fine sea salt and freshly cracked black pepper | |
| ¾ cup | cooked quinoa (see page 10), cooled | 175 mL |
| 1 | package (10 oz/300 g) frozen chopped spinach, thawed and squeezed dry | 1 |
| 3 oz | blue cheese, crumbled | 90 g |
| ¼ tsp | ground nutmeg | 1 mL |

1. In a large skillet, heat oil over medium-high heat. Add mushroom stems, onions, and salt and pepper to taste; cook, stirring occasionally, for 8 to 10 minutes or until vegetables are softened. Transfer to a large bowl and let cool.

2. To the onion mixture, add quinoa, spinach, cheese and nutmeg, stirring until combined.

3. Arrange mushroom caps, hollow side up, in a single layer on prepared baking sheet. Divide spinach mixture evenly among mushrooms, mounding it in the center of each.

4. Bake in preheated oven for 18 to 22 minutes or until mushrooms are browned. Let cool on pan on a wire rack for 5 minutes before serving.

# Piquillo Peppers with Quinoa, Goat Cheese and Herb Filling

*Talk about an appetizer with swagger. The bold flavors start with tangy goat cheese. Then come layers of flavor from the fresh herbs, lemon, quinoa and piquillos.*

## Tip

Piquillos are small, sweet, fire-roasted red peppers imported from Spain. They are available online and at specialty food stores, and are well worth seeking out for their tenderness and subtle, smoky heat.

- **Pastry bag fitted with a ¼-inch (1 cm) tip**

| | | |
|---|---|---|
| 8 oz | creamy goat cheese, softened | 250 g |
| 1 cup | cooked black, red or white quinoa (see page 10), cooled | 250 mL |
| ½ cup | packed fresh mint leaves, chopped | 125 mL |
| 4 tbsp | minced fresh chives, divided | 60 mL |
| 2 tsp | finely grated lemon zest | 10 mL |
| 2 tbsp | freshly squeezed lemon juice | 30 mL |
| | Fine sea salt and freshly cracked black pepper | |
| 1 | jar (7 oz/198 mL) piquillo peppers (about 16 peppers), drained and patted dry | 1 |

1. In a medium bowl, combine cheese, quinoa, mint, 3 tbsp (45 mL) of the chives, lemon zest and lemon juice. Season to taste with salt and pepper.

2. Transfer cheese mixture to pastry bag and gently pipe filling into peppers. Place on a serving plate and sprinkle with the remaining chives. Serve immediately, or cover and refrigerate for up to 1 hour.

# Quinoa Jalapeño Poppers

**Makes 1 dozen appetizers**

## Tips

If you prefer a less spicy appetizer, remove the ribs from inside the jalapeños before stuffing them. To make them even less spicy, rinse the jalapeños under cold water after removing the ribs; pat dry before stuffing.

For the best flavor, do not use fat-free cream cheese.

- Preheat oven to 450°F (230°C)
- Small rimmed baking sheet, lined with parchment paper or foil

| | | |
|---|---|---|
| 4 oz | cream cheese (light or regular), softened | 125 g |
| ½ cup | cooked quinoa (see page 10), cooled | 125 mL |
| ½ cup | shredded extra-sharp (extra-old) Cheddar cheese | 125 mL |
| | Fine sea salt and freshly ground black pepper | |
| 6 | large jalapeño peppers, halved lengthwise and seeded | 6 |

1. In a small bowl, combine cream cheese, quinoa and Cheddar. Season to taste with salt and pepper.
2. Using a small spoon, fill each jalapeño half with about 1 tbsp (15 mL) cheese mixture. Place on prepared sheet.
3. Bake in preheated oven for 9 to 12 minutes or until cheese is browned and bubbly.

# Apricots Stuffed with Pistachio Mint Quinoa

**Makes 2 dozen appetizers**

*Caution: will disappear before your eyes. These quinoa-stuffed apricots always please a crowd and require minimal prep time.*

## Tip

The stuffed apricots may be prepared up to 24 hours ahead. Refrigerate in an airtight container. Bring to room temperature before serving.

- Small food processor

| | | |
|---|---|---|
| 1 | clove garlic, roughly chopped | 1 |
| ¼ cup | cooked quinoa (see page 10), cooled | 60 mL |
| 2 tbsp | lightly salted roasted pistachios or almonds | 30 mL |
| 1 tbsp | chopped fresh mint | 15 mL |
| 2 tbsp | crumbled feta cheese | 30 mL |
| ½ tsp | finely grated lime zest | 2 mL |
| 1 tbsp | freshly squeezed lime juice | 15 mL |
| | Freshly cracked black pepper | |
| 24 | soft dried apricots or plump pitted dates | 24 |

1. In food processor, combine garlic, quinoa, pistachios, mint, cheese, lime zest and lime juice; pulse until finely chopped. Season to taste with pepper.
2. Slice apricots on one side to form a pocket. Stuff apricots with quinoa mixture, dividing evenly.

# Cherry Tomatoes Stuffed with Avocado, Quinoa and Bacon

*These luscious little bites
have layers of flavor and
a tangy bite from the
blue cheese. They can be
prepared up to 2 hours
ahead of time, making
them perfect nibbles for a
fuss-free get-together.*

## Tips

Other varieties of cheese,
such as freshly grated
Parmesan or crumbled
goat or feta cheese, may
be used in place of the
blue cheese.

Hass avocados (sometimes
called Haas avocados) are
dark-skinned avocados
with a nutty, buttery flesh
and a longer shelf life than
other varieties, making
them the most popular
avocado in North America.
To determine whether a
Hass avocado is ripe, look
for purple-black skin and
gently press the top — a
ripe one will give slightly.

| | | |
|---|---|---:|
| 4 cups | cherry tomatoes (about 2 pint containers) | 1 L |
| 1 | firm-ripe Hass avocado | 1 |
| 1 tbsp | freshly squeezed lemon juice | 15 mL |
| 3 | slices bacon, cooked crisp, cooled and finely chopped | 3 |
| ¾ cup | cooked black or white quinoa (see page 10), cooled | 175 mL |
| ⅓ cup | finely chopped green onions | 75 mL |
| 2 tbsp | crumbled blue cheese | 30 mL |
| | Fine sea salt and freshly cracked black pepper | |

1. Using a sharp knife, cut a small slice from the top of each tomato. Using a small spoon or melon baller, scoop out and discard pulp. Place tomatoes, cut side down, on paper towels and let drain for 15 minutes.

2. Meanwhile, in a small bowl, mash avocado and lemon juice. Stir in bacon, quinoa, green onions and cheese. Season to taste with salt and pepper.

3. Spoon quinoa mixture into tomato shells, dividing evenly. Place on a serving platter, cover with plastic wrap and refrigerate for 1 hour before serving.

## Variation

For vegan appetizers, omit the bacon and blue cheese. Add ⅓ cup (75 mL) smoked almonds, finely chopped, to the quinoa mixture in step 2.

# Figs Stuffed with Sesame, Mint and Quinoa

*A flavorful trio — tart dried cranberries, quinoa and cool mint — combines with lush fresh figs in this creative appetizer.*

## Tips

The quinoa filling can be made up to 4 hours ahead. Cover and refrigerate until ready to use.

Other fruits, such as halved apricots or pitted Medjool dates, may be used in place of the figs.

| | | |
|---|---|---:|
| ½ tsp | ground coriander | 2 mL |
| 1 tbsp | freshly squeezed lemon juice | 15 mL |
| 1 tbsp | extra virgin olive oil | 15 mL |
| 2 tsp | liquid honey or agave nectar | 10 mL |
| 1½ cups | cooked quinoa (see page 10), cooled | 375 mL |
| ½ cup | packed fresh mint leaves, chopped | 125 mL |
| ⅓ cup | dried cranberries or tart cherries, chopped | 75 mL |
| 3 tbsp | toasted sesame seeds | 45 mL |
| | Fine sea salt and freshly cracked black pepper | |
| 12 | figs, stems trimmed off | 12 |

1. In a large bowl, whisk together coriander, lemon juice, oil and honey. Add quinoa, mint, cranberries and sesame seeds, tossing to combine. Season to taste with salt and pepper.

2. Cut figs in half lengthwise and scoop out some of the flesh onto a cutting board. Roughly chop flesh and stir into quinoa mixture. Place fig halves on a platter and heap with quinoa mixture.

# Herbed Quinoa Deviled Eggs

**Makes
8 appetizers**

*Quinoa contributes a
delicate sesame flavor
and a toothsome texture
to traditional deviled
eggs. Mayonnaise is a
common component in
deviled egg fillings, but
replacing it with Greek
yogurt lightens this into
a healthy snack and adds
another layer of flavor.*

| | | |
|---|---|---|
| 4 | large eggs | 4 |
| | Cold water | |
| | Ice water | |
| ½ cup | cooked quinoa (see page 10), cooled | 125 mL |
| 1½ tbsp | finely chopped fresh basil, parsley or dill | 22 mL |
| 3 tbsp | plain Greek yogurt | 45 mL |
| 1 tsp | Dijon mustard | 5 mL |
| | Fine sea salt and freshly cracked black pepper | |

1. Place eggs in a medium saucepan and add enough cold water to cover by 1 inch (2.5 cm). Bring to a boil over medium-high heat. Remove from heat, cover and let stand for 13 minutes. Drain and transfer eggs to a bowl of ice water. Let stand until cool.

2. Peel eggs and cut in half lengthwise. Transfer yolks to a medium bowl and mash with a fork until smooth. Stir in quinoa, basil, yogurt and mustard. Season to taste with salt and pepper.

3. Place egg whites, hollow side up, on a serving plate. Spoon yolk mixture into egg whites, dividing evenly. Cover and refrigerate for at least 15 minutes, until filling is set, or for up to 24 hours.

## Variation

*Southern Deviled Eggs:* Omit the basil and add 1 tbsp (15 mL) sweet pickle relish to the egg yolk mixture. Garnish tops of eggs with ¼ tsp (1 mL) sweet paprika.

# Egg and Quinoa Prosciutto Cups

### Makes 1 dozen appetizers

*Here, crisp prosciutto shells — a snap to make with the help of a mini muffin pan — cradle a delicate quiche-like quinoa filling.*

- **Preheat oven to 400°F (200°C)**
- **12-cup mini muffin pan, sprayed with nonstick cooking spray**

| | | |
|---|---|---|
| 6 | thin slices prosciutto, fat trimmed, halved crosswise | 6 |
| 3 | large eggs | 3 |
| ¼ cup | plain Greek yogurt | 60 mL |
| ⅓ cup | cooked quinoa (see page 10), cooled | 75 mL |
| 1 tbsp | freshly grated Parmesan cheese | 15 mL |
| 1 tbsp | minced fresh chives | 15 mL |
| | Fine sea salt and freshly ground black pepper | |

1. Press a piece of prosciutto into each prepared muffin cup.
2. In a medium bowl, whisk together eggs and yogurt until blended. Stir in quinoa, cheese and chives. Season to taste with salt and pepper. Divide mixture equally among muffin cups.
3. Bake in preheated oven for 10 to 12 minutes or until filling is just set. Let cool in pan on a wire rack for 15 minutes. Serve warm, let cool to room temperature or refrigerate until cold, for up to 8 hours.

# California Quinoa Temaki

*Delicately nutty quinoa is a great carrier of flavors, like the fresh vegetables, rich avocado and seaweed in these fresh temaki rolls — the perfect way to eat salad out of hand.*

## Tips

Seasoned rice vinegar has added sweeteners and salt. If you only have unseasoned rice vinegar, combine 1½ tsp (7 mL) rice vinegar, ½ tsp (2 mL) brown rice syrup, agave nectar or light brown sugar, and a pinch of salt; use in place of the seasoned rice vinegar.

Dry your hands thoroughly before working with the nori; even slightly damp hands can make it soggy.

| | | |
|---|---|---|
| 1 cup | cooked quinoa (see page 10), cooled | 250 mL |
| 2 tbsp | toasted sesame seeds | 30 mL |
| 2 tsp | seasoned rice vinegar, divided | 10 mL |
| 1 | small firm-ripe Hass avocado, diced | 1 |
| 2 | sheets toasted nori, halved | 2 |
| 1 | small red bell pepper, cut into thin strips | 1 |
| ½ cup | shredded or julienned carrots | 125 mL |
| ½ cup | quinoa sprouts (see page 13) or radish sprouts | 125 mL |
| | Wasabi paste and pickled ginger (optional) | |

1. In a small bowl, combine quinoa, sesame seeds and 1½ tsp (7 mL) of the vinegar.

2. Sprinkle avocado with remaining vinegar to prevent browning.

3. On a work surface, place a half-sheet of nori with a long side toward you, shiny side down. Spoon ¼ cup (60 mL) of the quinoa onto the lower right corner. Pat out quinoa to cover the right side of the nori at a diagonal (leaving the upper right corner uncovered). Top quinoa with one-quarter of the avocado, red pepper, carrots and sprouts.

4. Fold the upper right corner down over the quinoa and fillings. Bring the lower left corner over and around the covered fillings to form a cone. Place on a plate, with the end of the sheet tucked under the cone; the moisture from the quinoa and filling will cause the roll to self-seal. Repeat with the remaining nori and fillings.

5. Serve immediately, garnished with wasabi paste and pickled ginger, if desired. Or cover with plastic wrap and refrigerate for up to 8 hours; garnish just before serving.

# Quinoa and Vegetable Summer Rolls

*Summer rolls are quintessential Asian appetizers: easy to eat out of hand and perfect for pairing with a variety of beverages. Here, they get a spa makeover with vibrant vegetables and nutty quinoa as the filling. Lime juice, garlic and hot pepper flakes add great kick to the dipping sauce.*

## Dipping Sauce

| | | |
|---|---|---|
| 1 | clove garlic, thinly sliced | 1 |
| 1/4 tsp | hot pepper flakes | 1 mL |
| 1/4 cup | tamari or soy sauce (GF, if needed) | 60 mL |
| 3 tbsp | liquid honey or agave nectar | 45 mL |
| 3 tbsp | freshly squeezed lime juice | 45 mL |

## Summer Rolls

| | | |
|---|---|---|
| 1½ cups | cooked quinoa (see page 10), cooled | 375 mL |
| 8 | 8½-inch (21 cm) round rice paper wrappers | 8 |
| 2 | beets, peeled and julienned | 1 |
| 1 | large carrot, julienned | 1 |
| 1 | large red bell pepper, julienned | 1 |
| 1½ cups | quinoa sprouts (see page 13), radish sprouts or alfalfa sprouts | 375 mL |
| 1 cup | packed fresh basil leaves | 250 mL |

1. *Dipping sauce:* In a small bowl, whisk together garlic, hot pepper flakes, tamari, honey and lime juice.
2. *Summer rolls:* In a small bowl, combine quinoa and 1 tbsp (15 mL) of the dipping sauce.
3. In a large bowl of hot water, soak 1 wrapper for 60 to 90 seconds or until pliable. Transfer to a work surface. Near the bottom of the wrapper, place one-eighth of the quinoa mixture, beets, carrot, red pepper, quinoa sprouts and basil in a line, leaving ½ inch (1 cm) at either end. Fold the ends in and roll tightly to enclose filling; place on a plate. Repeat with the remaining ingredients.
4. Cover loosely and refrigerate for at least 30 minutes, until chilled, or for up to 2 hours. Cut rolls in half on the diagonal and serve with the remaining dipping sauce.

# Swiss Chard Quinoa Rolls

**Makes 8 rolls**

*Workaday Swiss chard leaves are transformed into elegant spring rolls stuffed with gorgeous ingredients from the garden. A tamari and lime dipping sauce makes an easy accompaniment.*

**Dipping Sauce**

| | | |
|---|---|---|
| 1/4 tsp | ground ginger | 1 mL |
| 1/4 cup | tamari or soy sauce (GF, if needed) | 60 mL |
| 2 tbsp | freshly squeezed lime juice | 30 mL |
| 1 tbsp | brown rice syrup or liquid honey | 15 mL |
| 2 tsp | toasted sesame oil | 10 mL |

**Rolls**

| | | |
|---|---|---|
| 3/4 cup | cooked quinoa (see page 10), cooled | 175 mL |
| 1/2 cup | packed fresh basil leaves, chopped | 125 mL |
| 8 | Swiss chard leaves, tough stems removed | 8 |
| 2/3 cup | shredded carrots | 150 mL |
| 2/3 cup | shredded peeled beet (about 1 medium) | 150 mL |
| 3/4 cup | quinoa sprouts (see page 13) or sunflower sprouts | 175 mL |

1. *Dipping sauce:* In a small bowl, whisk together ginger, tamari, lime juice, brown rice syrup and oil.
2. *Rolls:* In another small bowl, combine quinoa, basil and 1 tbsp (15 mL) of the sauce.
3. Place chard leaves on a work surface. Fill each with one-eighth of the quinoa mixture, carrots, beet and quinoa sprouts. Roll leaves around filling, tucking in edges, and place seam side down on a plate. Serve immediately, with the remaining dipping sauce, or cover loosely and refrigerate for up to 4 hours.

# Citrus Shrimp Lettuce Wraps

*Sure, brightly colored
vegetables are packed
with nutrition, but so is
lettuce: it's high in fiber,
vitamins A, B$_6$, C and K,
chromium, manganese
and more. Here, it gets
the high-flavor treatment
with an easily assembled
filling of shrimp, quinoa,
oranges and fresh mint.*

## Tips

If you can only find 10-oz
(287 mL) cans of mandarin
oranges, use 1$\frac{1}{2}$ cans.

For a simpler assembly,
serve as lettuce cups
instead of wraps. Place the
lettuce leaves on a platter,
rounded side down, and
spoon filling ingredients
and chili sauce into each.
Fold in sides slightly, like a
soft taco, to eat.

| | | |
|---|---|---|
| 1 | can (15 oz/425 mL) mandarin oranges packed in juice, drained and juice reserved | 1 |
| | Water | |
| 1 cup | quinoa, rinsed | 250 mL |
| 2 tsp | finely grated lime zest | 10 mL |
| 1 tbsp | freshly squeezed lime juice | 15 mL |
| | Fine sea salt and freshly ground black pepper | |
| 12 | Bibb or butter lettuce leaves | 12 |
| 1 | red bell pepper, cut into thin strips | 1 |
| 12 oz | cooked medium shrimp, peeled and deveined | 375 g |
| $\frac{1}{3}$ cup | packed fresh mint leaves | 75 mL |
| 3 tbsp | Thai sweet chili sauce | 45 mL |

1. Pour mandarin orange juice into a glass measuring cup and add enough water to equal 2 cups (500 mL).

2. In a medium saucepan, combine quinoa and orange juice mixture. Bring to a boil over medium-high heat. Reduce heat to low, cover and simmer for 12 to 15 minutes or until liquid is absorbed. Remove from heat and let stand, covered, for 5 minutes; fluff with a fork. Stir in lime zest and lime juice. Season to taste with salt and pepper. Let cool.

3. Place lettuce leaves on a work surface. Spoon quinoa mixture into the center of each leaf, dividing evenly. Top with mandarin oranges, red pepper, shrimp and mint. Drizzle with chili sauce. Roll leaves around filling, tucking in edges, and place seam side down on a plate.

# Crustless Mini Quinoa Quiches

**Makes 2 dozen mini quiches**

*The quinoa in these irresistible mini quiches imparts an unexpected boost of earthy flavor. Fragrant basil provides a fresh zing, accented by pungent garlic and nutty Parmesan cheese.*

## Tip

Larger quiches can be made by using a 12-cup regular muffin pan. Bake for 23 to 28 minutes.

- **Preheat oven to 350°F (180°C)**
- **Blender or food processor**
- **Two 12-cup mini muffin pans, sprayed with nonstick cooking spray**

| | | |
|---|---|---|
| 2 | cloves garlic, roughly chopped | 2 |
| ¼ tsp | fine sea salt | 1 mL |
| ⅛ tsp | freshly ground black pepper | 0.5 mL |
| 4 | large eggs | 4 |
| 1 cup | cottage cheese | 250 mL |
| 1 cup | cooked quinoa (see page 10), cooled | 250 mL |
| ⅔ cup | drained roasted red bell peppers, chopped | 150 mL |
| ¼ cup | packed fresh basil leaves, chopped | 60 mL |
| ¼ cup | freshly grated Parmesan cheese | 60 mL |

1. In blender, combine garlic, salt, pepper, eggs and cottage cheese; purée until smooth.
2. Transfer purée to a medium bowl and stir in quinoa, roasted peppers, basil and Parmesan.
3. Divide quinoa mixture equally among prepared muffin cups.
4. Bake in preheated oven for 18 to 23 minutes or until tops are golden brown. Let cool in pan on a wire rack for 5 minutes. Run a knife around each quiche and gently lift out of pan, then transfer to the rack to cool. Serve warm or let cool completely.

# Chipotle Cheese Quinoa Minis

**Makes
2 dozen minis**

*Enriched with cheese
and spiked with the
smoky heat of chipotle
chiles, these pleasingly
rich-tasting (but still
nutritious) quinoa bites
make a big flavor impact
with minimal effort.*

## Tip

The quinoa minis can
be assembled through
step 2 up to 4 hours ahead.
Cover and refrigerate. Bake
as directed when ready
to serve.

- **Preheat oven to 350°F (180°C)**
- **Two 12-cup mini muffin pans, sprayed with nonstick cooking spray**

| | | |
|---|---|---|
| 1 tsp | ground cumin | 5 mL |
| ¼ tsp | fine sea salt | 1 mL |
| 2 | large eggs | 2 |
| ⅓ cup | cottage cheese (regular or reduced-fat) | 75 mL |
| 1½ cups | cooked quinoa (see page 10), cooled | 375 mL |
| ½ cup | shredded white or extra-sharp (extra-old) Cheddar cheese | 125 mL |
| 1 cup | chipotle salsa | 250 mL |

1. In a medium bowl, whisk together cumin, salt, eggs and cottage cheese. Stir in quinoa, Cheddar and salsa.
2. Divide quinoa mixture equally among prepared muffin cups.
3. Bake in preheated oven for 15 to 20 minutes or until tops are golden brown. Let cool in pan on a wire rack for 3 minutes. Run a knife around each mini and gently lift out of pan, then transfer to the rack to cool. Serve warm or let cool completely.

# Lemon-Thyme Shrimp and Quinoa Minis

**Makes 18 minis**

*These pretty finger foods get their fullness of flavor from a crisp quinoa flake and Parmesan base topped with a creamy shrimp and cheese filling enlivened by lemon zest, thyme and chives.*

## Tips

The shrimp filling can be made up to 1 day ahead. Cover and refrigerate until ready to use.

The minis can be completely assembled and baked up to 2 hours ahead. Let cool, cover and refrigerate. Before serving, arrange on a baking sheet and warm in a 350°F (180°C) oven for 6 to 8 minutes.

- Preheat oven to 350°F (180°C)
- Two 12-cup mini muffin pans, 18 cups sprayed with nonstick cooking spray

| | | |
|---|---|---|
| 4 oz | cream cheese (light or regular), softened | 125 g |
| 1 | large egg | 1 |
| 1/3 cup | freshly grated Parmesan cheese, divided | 75 mL |
| 3 tbsp | chopped fresh chives, divided | 45 mL |
| 1 tsp | finely grated lemon zest | 5 mL |
| 1 tsp | dried thyme | 5 mL |
| 1/4 cup | plain Greek yogurt | 60 mL |
| 8 oz | cooked deveined peeled shrimp, chopped | 250 g |
| | Fine sea salt and freshly ground black pepper | |
| 3/4 cup | quinoa flakes | 175 mL |
| 2 tbsp | unsalted butter, melted | 30 mL |

1. In a medium bowl, using an electric mixer on medium speed, beat cream cheese until smooth. Beat in egg and half the Parmesan. Beat in 1 tbsp (15 mL) of the chives, lemon zest, thyme and yogurt. Gently stir in shrimp. Season with salt and pepper.

2. In a small bowl, combine the remaining Parmesan, quinoa flakes and 1 tbsp (15 mL) chives. Drizzle with butter, tossing to coat.

3. Press 2 tsp (10 mL) quinoa flakes mixture into bottom of each prepared muffin cup. Top with shrimp mixture, dividing evenly (about 1 tbsp/15 mL per cup). Sprinkle the remaining quinoa flakes mixture over top.

4. Bake in preheated oven for 25 to 30 minutes or until golden. Let cool in pan on a wire rack for 5 minutes. Run a knife around each mini and gently lift out of pan. Serve warm, sprinkled with the remaining chives.

# Quinoa Blini with Smoked Salmon

*Tangy yogurt and herbal dill perfectly complement lush smoked salmon in the easy topping for this sophisticated appetizer. It deliciously sets off the earthy flavor of the quinoa blini beneath.*

## Tip

The blini can be prepared up to 24 hours ahead. Let cool, cover and refrigerate. Before serving, arrange on a baking sheet and warm in a 350°F (180°C) oven for 5 to 7 minutes.

### Blini

| | | |
|---|---|---|
| ¾ cup | quinoa flour | 175 mL |
| 1 tsp | natural cane sugar or granulated sugar | 5 mL |
| ½ tsp | baking powder (GF, if needed) | 2 mL |
| ¼ tsp | baking soda | 1 mL |
| ¼ tsp | fine sea salt | 1 mL |
| 2 | large eggs | 2 |
| ⅔ cup | buttermilk | 150 mL |
| 1 tbsp | unsalted butter, melted | 15 mL |
| | Nonstick cooking spray | |

### Topping

| | | |
|---|---|---|
| 4 tsp | chopped fresh dill or chives, divided | 20 mL |
| ⅛ tsp | fine sea salt | 0.5 mL |
| ⅛ tsp | freshly cracked black pepper | 0.5 mL |
| ½ cup | plain Greek yogurt (regular or reduced-fat) | 125 mL |
| 4 oz | thinly sliced smoked salmon, cut into small pieces | 125 g |

1. *Blini:* In a medium bowl, whisk together quinoa flour, sugar, baking powder, baking soda and salt.
2. In a small bowl, whisk together eggs, buttermilk and butter until blended. Add the egg mixture to the flour mixture and stir until just blended.
3. Heat a large skillet over medium heat. Lightly spray with cooking spray. For each blini, spoon about 1½ tbsp (22 mL) batter into skillet, creating 4 to 5 blini per batch. Cook for 1 to 2 minutes or until bubbles appear on top. Turn blini over and cook for 1 minute or until golden brown. Using a spatula, transfer blini to a wire rack and let cool. Repeat with the remaining batter, spraying skillet and adjusting heat as necessary between batches.
4. *Topping:* In a small bowl, whisk together 1 tsp (5 mL) of the dill, salt, pepper and yogurt.
5. Arrange cooled blini on a platter. Spoon a small dollop of yogurt mixture in the center of each blini. Top with salmon and sprinkle with the remaining dill.

# Green Onion, Sesame and Quinoa Pancakes

*Green onions retain their vivid color and flavor in this easy appetizer, bringing garden freshness to the table no matter what the season. Quinoa flour and toasted sesame seeds — along with a dose of toasted sesame oil — lend just the right amount of contrast.*

## Tip

If you prefer to eat the pancakes hot, transfer them to a heatproof platter as they are cooked and keep them warm in a 200°F (100°C) oven.

| | | |
|---|---|---|
| 1 tbsp | toasted sesame oil | 15 mL |
| 2 cups | chopped green onions (about 2 bunches ) | 500 mL |
| ¾ cup | quinoa flour | 175 mL |
| 3 tbsp | toasted sesame seeds | 45 mL |
| ½ tsp | fine sea salt | 2 mL |
| ¼ tsp | freshly cracked black pepper | 1 mL |
| 2 | large eggs, lightly beaten | 2 |
| ¾ cup | milk | 175 mL |
| 2 cups | cooked quinoa (see page 10), cooled | 500 mL |
| | Vegetable oil | |
| | Hoisin sauce (optional; GF, if needed) | |

1. In a large nonstick skillet, heat sesame oil over medium-high heat. Add green onions and cook, stirring, for 4 to 5 minutes or until softened. Transfer to a large bowl and wipe out skillet.

2. To the green onions, add quinoa flour, sesame seeds, salt, pepper, eggs and milk, whisking until blended. Gently stir in quinoa.

3. Add 2 tsp (10 mL) vegetable oil to skillet and heat over medium heat. For each pancake, drop about ¼ cup (60 mL) batter into skillet and flatten slightly. Cook for 2 to 3 minutes per side or until golden. Transfer to a plate lined with paper towels. Repeat with the remaining batter, adding more oil and adjusting heat as necessary between batches. Serve warm or at room temperature, with hoisin sauce, if desired.

# Summer Corn and Quinoa Griddle Cakes

**Makes 18 cakes**

*A bite-size celebration of New World crops, these griddle cakes capture the golden sweetness of corn cut from the cob and elevate the flavor with the fragrant foundation of quinoa.*

| | | |
|---|---|---|
| ⅔ cup | quinoa flour | 150 mL |
| 1 tsp | fine sea salt | 5 mL |
| ¼ tsp | freshly cracked black pepper | 1 mL |
| 3 | large eggs, lightly beaten | 3 |
| 1 | small red bell pepper, chopped | 1 |
| 1½ cups | fresh or thawed frozen corn kernels | 375 mL |
| 1 cup | cooked quinoa (see page 10), cooled | 250 mL |
| ½ cup | packed fresh basil leaves, chopped | 125 mL |
| | Olive oil | |

1. In a medium bowl, whisk together quinoa flour, salt, pepper and eggs. Gently stir in red pepper, corn, quinoa and basil.

2. In a large nonstick skillet, heat 2 tsp (10 mL) oil over medium heat. For each griddle cake, drop about ¼ cup (60 mL) batter into skillet and flatten slightly. Cook for 2 to 3 minutes per side or until browned. Transfer to a plate lined with paper towels. Repeat with the remaining batter, adding more oil and adjusting heat as necessary between batches. Serve warm or at room temperature.

# Zucchini Quinoa Fritters

**Makes
1 dozen fritters**

*Fried zucchini is a
favorite appetizer, but
watch what happens
when it's coupled with
quinoa flour in a delicate
fritter. Fragrant, floral
basil — the scent of
summer — is a terrific
complement to the
tender, light flavor of the
zucchini, but you can
use other herbs from
the garden or an equal
amount of thinly sliced
green onions.*

| | | |
|---|---|---:|
| 1 lb | zucchini (about 2 medium), coarsely shredded | 500 g |
| 1 tsp | fine sea salt | 5 mL |
| 1 | large egg | 1 |
| ½ cup | packed fresh basil leaves, chopped | 125 mL |
| ½ cup | quinoa flour | 125 mL |
| ¼ tsp | freshly cracked black pepper | 1 mL |
| | Olive oil | |
| | Fine sea salt | |
| ½ cup | plain Greek yogurt | 125 mL |

1. Place zucchini in a colander set in the sink and sprinkle with salt. Let drain for 10 minutes, then press out as much liquid as possible.

2. In a large bowl, whisk egg. Stir in zucchini, basil, quinoa flour and pepper until blended.

3. In a large nonstick skillet, heat 2 tsp (10 mL) oil over medium heat. For each fritter, drop about ¼ cup (60 mL) batter into skillet and flatten slightly. Cook for 2 to 3 minutes per side or until browned. Transfer to a plate lined with paper towels and sprinkle with salt. Repeat with the remaining batter, adding more oil and adjusting heat as necessary between batches. Serve immediately, with yogurt.

# Ricotta and Sun-Dried Tomato Fritters

**Makes 18 fritters**

*The charm of quinoa increases exponentially when it's paired with creamy ricotta in a delectable fritter. Fresh parsley and sweet-savory sun-dried tomatoes round everything out.*

## Tip

Chilling the ricotta mixture blends the flavors and helps the fritters hold together.

| | | |
|---|---|---|
| 3 | large eggs | 3 |
| 2 | cloves garlic, minced | 2 |
| 2 cups | cooked quinoa (see page 10), cooled | 500 mL |
| 1/2 cup | panko or dry bread crumbs (GF, if needed) | 125 mL |
| 1/2 cup | freshly grated Parmesan cheese | 125 mL |
| 1 cup | ricotta cheese | 250 mL |
| 1 tsp | finely grated lemon zest | 5 mL |
| 1/2 cup | drained oil-packed sun-dried tomatoes, finely chopped | 125 mL |
| 2 tbsp | chopped fresh flat-leaf (Italian) parsley | 30 mL |
| | Fine sea salt and freshly cracked black pepper | |
| | Olive oil | |

1. In a large bowl, whisk eggs. Stir in garlic, quinoa, panko, Parmesan, ricotta and lemon zest until blended. Gently stir in tomatoes and parsley. Cover and refrigerate for 1 hour.

2. In a large nonstick skillet, heat 2 tsp (10 mL) oil over medium heat. For each fritter, drop about 1/4 cup (60 mL) batter into skillet and flatten slightly. Cook for 2 to 3 minutes per side or until browned. Transfer to a plate lined with paper towels. Repeat with the remaining batter, adding more oil and adjusting heat as necessary between batches. Serve warm or at room temperature.

# South Indian Lentil Cakes with Mint Raita

*Similar to falafel, these hearty cakes are equally delicious eaten as appetizers or piled into a wrap with lettuce, tomato and a generous spoonful of the raita.*

## Tip

Lentils are members of the protein-rich legume family. They are high in fiber and complex carbohydrates and relatively low in fat. They offer a substantial amount of vitamins A and B, as well as calcium, and are a particularly good source of iron and phosphorous.

| | | |
|---|---|---|
| 1 cup | dried green or brown lentils | 250 mL |
| ½ cup | quinoa, rinsed | 125 mL |
| 2 | cloves garlic, roughly chopped | 2 |
| 2 cups | packed fresh baby spinach | 500 mL |
| 1 cup | frozen petite peas, thawed | 250 mL |
| 1 cup | packed fresh cilantro leaves | 250 mL |
| ½ cup | chopped green onions | 125 mL |
| 1 tsp | ground ginger | 5 mL |
| 1 tsp | ground cumin | 5 mL |
| 1 tsp | fine sea salt | 5 mL |
| 1 tsp | freshly ground black pepper | 5 mL |
| | Vegetable oil | |
| ½ cup | shredded seeded peeled cucumber | 125 mL |
| 1 tbsp | chopped fresh mint | 15 mL |
| 1 cup | plain yogurt | 250 mL |
| | Fine sea salt and freshly ground black pepper | |

1. In a medium bowl, combine lentils and quinoa. Add enough water to cover by 3 inches (7.5 cm). Let stand at room temperature for 4 hours. Drain, reserving ¼ cup (60 mL) soaking water.

2. Transfer lentil mixture to food processor and process until chopped. Add garlic, spinach, peas, cilantro, green onions, ginger, cumin, salt and pepper. Process until a grainy paste forms, adding some of the reserved soaking water if needed.

3. In a large nonstick skillet, heat 2 tsp (10 mL) oil over medium-high heat. For each cake, drop about ¼ cup (60 mL) batter into skillet and flatten with a spatula to ¼-inch (1 cm) thickness. Reduce heat to medium and cook for 4 to 5 minutes per side or until golden. Transfer to a plate lined with paper towels. Repeat with the remaining batter, adding more oil as necessary and reheating pan to medium-high heat, then reducing to medium for each batch.

4. In a small bowl, combine cucumber, mint and yogurt. Season to taste with salt and pepper.

5. Serve lentil cakes warm or at room temperature, with mint raita.

# Mini Crab Quinoa Cakes

**Makes
2 dozen cakes**

*Earthy quinoa is the
perfect foil for lemony
crab. This sophisticated
starter is deceptively easy
to make, and the layered
flavors will impress
your guests.*

| | | |
|---|---|---|
| ½ tsp | fine sea salt | 2 mL |
| ¼ tsp | freshly cracked black pepper | 1 mL |
| ¼ cup | olive oil mayonnaise | 60 mL |
| 2 tbsp | Dijon mustard | 30 mL |
| 1 tsp | finely grated lemon zest | 5 mL |
| 1½ tbsp | freshly squeezed lemon juice | 22 mL |
| 1 cup | cooked quinoa (see page 10), cooled | 250 mL |
| ¾ cup | panko or dry bread crumbs (GF, if needed) | 175 mL |
| ½ cup | drained roasted red bell peppers, chopped | 125 mL |
| ¼ cup | finely chopped green onions | 60 mL |
| 2 | large egg whites, lightly beaten | 2 |
| 1 lb | cooked lump crabmeat, drained | 500 g |
| | Olive oil | |

1. In a large bowl, whisk together salt, pepper, mayonnaise, mustard, lemon zest and lemon juice. Stir in quinoa, panko, roasted peppers, green onions and egg whites. Gently fold in crab, being careful not to break it up much.

2. Divide crab mixture into 24 equal portions. Form each portion into a ½-inch (1 cm) thick patty and place on a plate. Cover loosely and refrigerate for at least 30 minutes, until chilled, or for up to 4 hours.

3. In a large nonstick skillet, heat 2 tsp (10 mL) oil over medium heat. Add 6 patties and cook for 2 to 3 minutes per side or until golden. Transfer to a plate lined with paper towels. Repeat with the remaining patties, adding more oil and adjusting heat as necessary between batches. Serve warm.

# Shrimp Cakes with Cilantro Yogurt Sauce

**Makes
2 dozen cakes**

*Here, a simple sauce
made from Greek yogurt,
cilantro and jalapeño
enhances Indian-spiced
shrimp and quinoa cakes
to great effect.*

• **Food processor**

### Cilantro Yogurt Sauce

| | | |
|---|---|---|
| 1 cup | packed fresh cilantro leaves, chopped | 250 mL |
| 2 tsp | minced seeded jalapeño pepper | 10 mL |
| 1 cup | plain yogurt | 250 mL |
| | Fine sea salt and freshly ground black pepper | |

### Shrimp and Quinoa Cakes

| | | |
|---|---|---|
| 1 lb | medium shrimp, peeled and deveined | 500 g |
| 2½ cups | cooked quinoa (see page 10), cooled | 625 mL |
| 1 cup | chopped green onions (about 1 bunch) | 250 mL |
| 2 tsp | garam masala | 10 mL |
| | Vegetable oil | |

1. *Sauce:* In a small bowl, whisk together cilantro, jalapeño and yogurt. Season to taste with salt and pepper. Cover and refrigerate until ready to serve.
2. *Cakes:* In food processor, combine shrimp, quinoa, green onions and garam masala; pulse until texture is coarse. Season with salt and pepper.
3. Divide shrimp mixture into 24 equal portions. Form each portion into a ½-inch (1 cm) thick patty.
4. In a large nonstick skillet, heat 2 tsp (10 mL) oil over medium heat. Add 6 patties and cook for 2 to 3 minutes per side or until golden. Transfer to a plate lined with paper towels. Repeat with the remaining patties, adding more oil and adjusting heat as necessary between batches. Serve warm, with yogurt sauce.

# Herbed Quinoa and Cranberry Rissoles

**Makes 1 dozen rissoles**

*"Rissole" comes from the French word* rissoler, *meaning "to brown," and typically refers to a small baked or fried croquette made from minced meat or fish. Quinoa, cranberries and artichoke hearts star in this sweet-savory interpretation.*

| | | |
|---|---|---|
| 2 cups | cooked quinoa (see page 10), cooled | 500 mL |
| 1/2 cup | finely chopped red onion | 125 mL |
| 1/2 cup | dried cranberries, roughly chopped | 125 mL |
| 1/2 cup | drained marinated artichoke hearts, coarsely chopped | 125 mL |
| 1/2 cup | chopped toasted pecans | 125 mL |
| 2 tsp | chopped fresh rosemary | 10 mL |
| | Fine sea salt and freshly cracked black pepper | |
| 1 cup | quinoa flakes or panko | 250 mL |
| 3 | large eggs, lightly beaten | 3 |
| 6 tsp | olive oil, divided | 30 mL |
| 3/4 cup | chunky cranberry sauce | 175 mL |
| 2 tbsp | minced fresh chives (optional) | 30 mL |

1. In a large bowl, combine quinoa, red onion, cranberries, artichoke hearts, pecans and rosemary. Season generously with salt and pepper. Gently stir in quinoa flakes and eggs.

2. Using a 1/4-cup (60 mL) measure, form quinoa mixture into twelve 2-inch (5 cm) wide patties. Place on a small baking sheet, cover and refrigerate for at least 30 minutes, until chilled, or for up to 24 hours.

3. In a large nonstick skillet, heat 2 tsp (10 mL) of the oil over medium heat. Add 4 patties, flattening them slightly with a spatula, and cook for 3 to 4 minutes per side or until golden brown and crispy. Repeat with the remaining oil and patties, adjusting heat as necessary between batches.

4. Serve each patty topped with 1 tbsp (15 mL) cranberry sauce and a sprinkle of chives (if using).

## Variations

Substitute chopped toasted walnuts for the pecans.

Replace the cranberries with dried cherries or chopped dried apricots.

# Quinoa Gougères

*The perfect party hors d'oeuvres, these gluten-free gougères have the crisp golden exterior and cloudlike interior you expect, but with a subtle nuance of sesame from the quinoa flour.*

## Tips

To check that the gougères are done, slit one open with a small, sharp knife; the center should be slightly eggy and moist, but not wet.

The gougères can be made up to 3 hours ahead. Let cool completely on rack. Let stand at room temperature or place in an airtight container. Warm on a baking sheet in a 350°F (180°C) oven for 5 to 10 minutes.

- **Preheat oven to 400°F (200°C)**
- **2 large rimmed baking sheets, lined with parchment paper**

| | | |
|---|---|---|
| ½ cup | water | 125 mL |
| ½ cup | milk | 125 mL |
| 3 tbsp | unsalted butter, cut into pieces | 45 mL |
| ¾ tsp | fine sea salt | 3 mL |
| 1 cup | quinoa flour | 250 mL |
| 4 | large eggs | 4 |
| 1 cup | shredded Gruyère cheese | 250 mL |
| ¼ tsp | freshly cracked black pepper | 1 mL |

1. In a medium saucepan, combine water, milk, butter and salt. Bring to a boil over medium-high heat, stirring until butter is melted. Add quinoa flour, stirring vigorously with a wooden spoon until flour absorbs liquid and comes together in a ball. Continue stirring vigorously for 1 minute or until dough no longer appears sticky. Remove from heat, scrape into a large bowl and let cool for 3 minutes.

2. Using an electric mixer on medium speed, beat in eggs, one at a time, making sure each egg is fully incorporated into the dough before adding another. Stir in cheese and pepper.

3. Using a 1-tbsp (15 mL) cookie scoop or a kitchen tablespoon, drop rounded portions of dough about 3 inches (7.5 cm) apart on prepared baking sheets. Gently press down any peaks of dough.

4. Bake in upper and lower thirds of preheated oven for 12 minutes. Reverse positions of pans and bake for 14 to 18 minutes or until golden brown. Transfer gougères to a wire rack. Serve hot or warm.

## Variation

Other grated or shredded cheeses, such as Cheddar, Gouda or Parmesan, may be used in place of the Gruyère.

# Blue Cheese and Pecan Coins

*Here's a perfect make-ahead appetizer for your next get-together. Each bite delivers a pleasing range of tastes: subtle sweetness from the pecans and quinoa flour, saltiness from the blue cheese and smokiness from the paprika. You'll be hard-pressed to find more appealing nibbles.*

## Storage Tip

Store coins in an airtight container at room temperature for up to 4 days.

- Food processor
- 2 large rimmed baking sheets, lined with parchment paper

| | | |
|---|---|---|
| 1 cup | toasted pecan halves, divided | 250 mL |
| ¾ cup | quinoa flour | 175 mL |
| ½ tsp | fine sea salt | 2 mL |
| ¼ tsp | hot smoked paprika or freshly cracked black pepper | 1 mL |
| ¼ tsp | baking soda | 1 mL |
| 2 tbsp | cold unsalted butter, cut into pieces | 30 mL |
| 4 oz | blue cheese, crumbled | 125 g |

1. In food processor, finely grind ½ cup (125 mL) of the pecans. Add quinoa flour, salt, paprika and baking soda; pulse to combine. Add butter and pulse until mixture resembles coarse meal. Add cheese and pulse 6 to 8 times or until dough comes together.

2. Transfer dough to a work surface lightly floured with quinoa flour. Divide dough in half. Form each half into a 4-inch (10 cm) long log.

3. Chop the remaining pecans and sprinkle them over a clean work surface. Roll logs in chopped pecans, gently pressing to adhere. Tightly wrap each log in plastic wrap and refrigerate for at least 3 hours, until chilled, or for up to 24 hours.

4. Preheat oven to 350°F (180°C).

5. Slice each log into 15 coins about ¼ inch (1 cm) thick. Place 1 inch (2.5 cm) apart on prepared baking sheets.

6. Bake in upper and lower thirds of preheated oven for 6 minutes. Reverse positions of pans and bake for 6 to 9 minutes or until centers are firm to the touch. Let cool in pans on a wire rack for 1 minute, then transfer to the rack to cool.

# Baked Quinoa Arancini

**Makes 18 balls**

*This delicious quinoa spin on a favorite Italian appetizer is destined to be a hit. Crisped in the oven instead of deep-fried, the arancini maintain a healthy profile despite their crisp exteriors and gooey, cheesy middles.*

- **Large rimmed baking sheet, lined with parchment paper**

| | | |
|---|---|---|
| 2 | large eggs | 2 |
| 2 cups | cooked quinoa (see page 10), cooled | 500 mL |
| 1/2 cup | freshly grated Romano or Parmesan cheese | 125 mL |
| | Fine sea salt and freshly cracked black pepper | |
| 3/4 cup | panko or dry bread crumbs (GF, if needed) | 175 mL |
| 4 oz | mozzarella cheese, cut into 18 cubes, each about 1/2 inch (1 cm) | 125 g |
| | Nonstick cooking spray (preferably olive oil) | |
| 1 cup | marinara sauce, warmed | 250 mL |

1. In a medium bowl, whisk eggs. Stir in quinoa and Romano. Season with salt and pepper. Cover and refrigerate for 1 hour.

2. Place panko in a shallow dish. Scoop 1 tbsp (15 mL) quinoa mixture into your palm. Place a cube of mozzarella in the middle, then top with another 1 tbsp (15 mL) quinoa mixture. Form into a ball, completely enclosing cheese. Roll ball in panko. Place on prepared baking sheet, spacing balls 1 inch (2.5 cm) apart. Repeat with remaining quinoa mixture and mozzarella. Cover and refrigerate for 30 minutes.

3. Preheat oven to 425°F (220°C).

4. Generously spray quinoa balls with cooking spray.

5. Bake in preheated oven for 20 to 25 minutes or until golden brown. Serve with warm marinara sauce.

# California Caviar

**Makes about
3⅓ cups
(825 mL)**

*The legendary Texan cook Helen Corbitt invented a simple, delicious black-eyed pea salad in 1940. Even though I now live in Texas, I hail from California, so I decided it was high time for a vegetarian California Caviar. Serve as a dip or a spread.*

## Tip

Leftovers are delicious as a vegetarian filling for burritos and omelets.

| | | |
|---|---|---|
| 1 | clove garlic, minced | 1 |
| ¾ tsp | chipotle chile powder | 3 mL |
| 1 tbsp | extra virgin olive oil | 15 mL |
| 1 tsp | finely grated lime zest | 5 mL |
| 1 tbsp | freshly squeezed lime juice | 15 mL |
| 1 tsp | agave nectar or liquid honey | 5 mL |
| 2½ cups | cooked black quinoa (see page 10), cooled | 625 mL |
| ½ cup | finely chopped red bell pepper | 125 mL |
| ¼ cup | finely chopped red onion | 60 mL |
| | Fine sea salt and freshly ground black pepper | |
| ½ cup | packed fresh cilantro leaves, minced | 125 mL |
| 3 tbsp | toasted sesame seeds | 45 mL |

1. In a large bowl, whisk together garlic, chipotle chile powder, oil, lime zest, lime juice and agave nectar. Add quinoa, red pepper and red onion, tossing to combine. Generously season with salt and pepper. Cover and refrigerate for at least 4 hours, until chilled, or overnight. Just before serving, stir in cilantro and sesame seeds.

# Quinoa Muhammara

**Makes about
2⅓ cups
(575 mL)**

*Spicy and mildly sweet, muhammara is a quintessential Middle Eastern appetizer.*

## Tip

This spread may also be served as a dip.

## Storage Tip

Store in an airtight container in the refrigerator for up to 3 days.

● **Food processor**

| | | |
|---|---|---|
| 3 | cloves garlic, minced | 3 |
| 1 | jar (12 oz/341 mL) roasted red bell peppers, drained | 1 |
| ¾ cup | cooked quinoa (see page 10), cooled | 175 mL |
| ⅓ cup | chopped toasted walnuts | 75 mL |
| 1 tsp | ground cumin | 5 mL |
| ¼ tsp | cayenne pepper | 1 mL |
| 2 tbsp | extra virgin olive oil | 30 mL |
| 1 tbsp | freshly squeezed lemon juice | 15 mL |
| 2 tsp | liquid honey, agave nectar or brown rice syrup | 10 mL |

1. In food processor, combine garlic, roasted peppers, quinoa, walnuts, cumin, cayenne, oil, lemon juice and honey; process until smooth. Transfer to a serving dish.

# Bolivian Guacamole

*Avocados and earthy
quinoa — two Bolivian
superfoods — join forces
in this spin on guacamole.
The emerald dip looks
especially gorgeous when
made with black or
red quinoa.*

| | | |
|---|---|---|
| 3 | firm-ripe Hass avocados, diced | 3 |
| ½ cup | cooked red, black or white quinoa (see page 10), cooled | 125 mL |
| ½ cup | packed fresh cilantro leaves, chopped | 125 mL |
| ¼ tsp | ground cumin | 1 mL |
| Pinch | chipotle chile powder or cayenne pepper | Pinch |
| 2 tbsp | freshly squeezed lime juice | 30 mL |
| | Fine sea salt | |

**1.** In a medium bowl, using a fork, combine avocados, quinoa, cilantro, cumin, chipotle chile powder and lime juice. Gently mash until guacamole is well blended but still slightly chunky. Season to taste with salt.

# Middle Eastern Eggplant Dip

*Melt-in-your-mouth
roasted eggplant gets a
stealthy boost of protein
from quinoa in this
impressive snack. Roasted
peppers and lemon juice
brighten all.*

**Tip**

This dip may also be
served as a spread.

**Storage Tip**

Store in an airtight
container in the
refrigerator for up to
3 days.

- **Preheat oven to 450°F (230°C)**
- **Large rimmed baking sheet, sprayed with nonstick cooking spray (preferably olive oil)**
- **Food processor**

| | | |
|---|---|---|
| 1 | large eggplant (about 1 lb/500 g), trimmed and halved lengthwise | 1 |
| ½ cup | loosely packed fresh parsley leaves, chopped, divided | 125 mL |
| 2 | cloves garlic, roughly chopped | 2 |
| 1 cup | cooked quinoa (see page 10), cooled | 250 mL |
| ¾ cup | drained roasted red bell peppers | 175 mL |
| ¼ cup | tahini | 60 mL |
| 1 tbsp | freshly squeezed lemon juice | 15 mL |

**1.** Place eggplant cut side down on prepared baking sheet. Prick all over with a fork. Bake in preheated oven for 40 to 45 minutes or until soft and collapsed. Let cool completely in pan.

**2.** Scoop eggplant flesh into food processor, discarding skin. Set aside 1 tbsp (15 mL) of the parsley. Add the remaining parsley, garlic, quinoa, roasted peppers, tahini and lemon juice to the food processor and process until smooth. Transfer dip to a serving dish and garnish with the reserved parsley.

# Warm Artichoke Quinoa Dip

*Here, quinoa teams up
with artichokes and
fontina cheese in an
irresistible dip.*

## Tips

For the best flavor, do not
use fat-free cream cheese.

The cooked quinoa can be
hot, cooled or chilled —
whatever you have
on hand.

The dip can be assembled
through step 2 up to
24 hours ahead. Cover
and refrigerate. Bake as
directed when ready
to serve.

- **Preheat oven to 400°F (200°C)**
- **4-cup (1 L) baking dish, sprayed with nonstick cooking spray**

| | | |
|---|---|---:|
| 2 tsp | olive oil | 10 mL |
| 1 cup | finely chopped onion | 250 mL |
| 2 | cloves garlic, minced | 2 |
| 1 tsp | dried thyme | 5 mL |
| 1 | can (14 oz/398 mL) artichoke hearts, drained and coarsely chopped | 1 |
| ¼ cup | dry white wine | 60 mL |
| 4 oz | cream cheese (light or regular), softened | 125 g |
| 1 cup | cooked quinoa (see page 10) | 250 mL |
| ⅓ cup | fresh flat-leaf (Italian) parsley, chopped | 75 mL |
| 4 oz | fontina cheese, diced, divided | 125 g |
| | Pita wedges or pita chips | |

1. In a large skillet, heat oil over medium-high heat. Add onion and cook, stirring, for 5 to 6 minutes or until softened. Add garlic and thyme; cook, stirring, for 30 seconds. Add artichokes and wine; cook, stirring, for 5 to 6 minutes or until liquid evaporates.

2. Remove skillet from heat and stir in cream cheese until blended. Fold in quinoa, parsley and three-quarters of the fontina. Transfer to prepared baking dish and sprinkle with the remaining fontina.

3. Bake in preheated oven for 25 to 30 minutes or until golden and bubbly. Serve warm, with pita wedges.

# Bubbly Layered Quinoa Dip

*Baked cheese dips are too often loaded with calories but flat in flavor. Big flavor is the operative force here: think chipotles, olives, Greek yogurt, herbs and sharp Cheddar. Quinoa makes the dish sing, complementing the other south-of-the-border ingredients.*

## Tip

The cooked quinoa can be hot, cooled or chilled — whatever you have on hand.

- **Preheat oven to 350°F (180°C)**
- **8- or 9-inch (20 or 23 cm) square glass baking dish, sprayed with nonstick cooking spray**

| | | |
|---|---|---|
| 1 | can (15 oz/425 mL) fat-free or vegetarian refried beans | 1 |
| 1½ cups | cooked quinoa (see page 10) | 375 mL |
| 2½ tsp | ground cumin | 12 mL |
| 1½ cups | chipotle salsa, divided | 375 mL |
| 1 cup | frozen corn kernels, thawed | 250 mL |
| ⅓ cup | chopped green onions | 75 mL |
| ¼ cup | chopped ripe black olives | 60 mL |
| 1 cup | shredded sharp (old) white Cheddar cheese | 250 mL |
| 1 cup | plain Greek yogurt | 250 mL |
| 1½ tbsp | freshly squeezed lime juice | 22 mL |
| ¼ cup | packed fresh cilantro leaves, chopped | 60 mL |
| | Baked tortilla chips | |

1. In a large bowl, combine beans, quinoa, cumin and ½ cup (250 mL) of the salsa. Spread evenly in prepared baking dish. Spread the remaining salsa evenly on top.
2. In a small bowl, combine corn, green onions and olives. Spoon evenly over salsa. Sprinkle with cheese.
3. Bake in preheated oven for 18 to 22 minutes or until bubbly. Let cool for 10 minutes.
4. In a small bowl, combine yogurt and lime juice. Spread evenly over cheese. Sprinkle with cilantro. Serve with tortilla chips.

# Eight-Layer Tex-Mex Dip

*I grew up eating a
variation of this fantastic
dip in the '80s. While
incredibly delicious,
it was also incredibly
rich and high in fat and
calories. I've given the
family favorite a modern
spin by adding an eighth
layer — quinoa — and
streamlining the existing
layers. It's better than
ever and is practically a
meal in itself.*

## Tip

Hass avocados (sometimes
called Haas avocados) are
dark-skinned avocados
with a nutty, buttery flesh
and a longer shelf life than
other varieties, making
them the most popular
avocado in North America.
To determine whether a
Hass avocado is ripe, look
for purple-black skin and
gently press the top — a
ripe one will give slightly.

- **8-inch (20 cm) glass pie plate**

| | | |
|---|---|---|
| 1 | can (15 oz/425 mL) fat-free or vegetarian refried beans | 1 |
| 2 tbsp | freshly squeezed lime juice, divided | 30 mL |
| | Fine sea salt and freshly ground black pepper | |
| ¾ cup | plain Greek yogurt | 175 mL |
| 1⅓ cups | cooked quinoa (see page 10), cooled | 325 mL |
| ½ cup | packed fresh cilantro leaves, chopped | 125 mL |
| 1 tsp | ground cumin | 5 mL |
| 1 cup | chipotle salsa | 250 mL |
| 1 | firm-ripe Hass avocado, diced small | 1 |
| 1 cup | shredded romaine lettuce | 250 mL |
| ½ cup | shredded extra-sharp (extra-old) Cheddar cheese | 125 mL |
| ½ cup | thinly sliced green onions | 125 mL |
| | Baked tortilla chips | |

1. In a medium bowl, combine beans and half the lime juice. Season to taste with salt and pepper. Spread in pie plate. Spread yogurt evenly on top.
2. In a small bowl, combine quinoa, cilantro, cumin and the remaining lime juice. Season to taste with salt and pepper. Spoon over yogurt layer. Add layers of salsa, avocado, lettuce, cheese and green onions. Cover and refrigerate for at least 30 minutes, until chilled, or for up to 2 hours. Serve with tortilla chips.

# Garlicky White Bean Spread

**Makes about
2 cups (500 mL)**

**Tip**

If using a 19-oz (540 mL) can of beans, drain and measure out 1⅔ cups (400 mL) beans.

This spread may also be served as a dip.

**Storage Tip**

Store in an airtight container in the refrigerator for up to 3 days.

• **Food processor**

| | | |
|---|---|---|
| 3 | cloves garlic, minced | 3 |
| 1 | can (14 to 15 oz/398 to 425 mL) cannellini (white kidney) beans, drained and rinsed | 1 |
| ⅔ cup | cooked quinoa (see page 10), cooled | 150 mL |
| 1 tbsp | dried Italian seasoning | 15 mL |
| ½ tsp | fine sea salt | 2 mL |
| ¼ cup | freshly squeezed lemon juice | 60 mL |
| 1 tbsp | extra virgin olive oil | 15 mL |
| ¼ cup | packed fresh flat-leaf (Italian) parsley, chopped | 60 mL |

1. In food processor, combine garlic, beans, quinoa, Italian seasoning, salt, lemon juice and oil; process until smooth. Transfer to a serving dish and stir in parsley.

# Black Bean and Quinoa Salsa

**Makes about
4 cups (1 L)**

*This salsa has a surprisingly complex flavor.*

**Tip**

If using a 19-oz (540 mL) can of beans, drain and measure out 1⅔ cups (400 mL) beans.

For a spicier salsa, leave in the jalapeño seeds.

**Storage Tip**

Store in an airtight container in the refrigerator for up to 2 days. Fold in the avocado just before serving.

| | | |
|---|---|---|
| 1 | can (14 to 15 oz/398 to 425 mL) black beans, drained and rinsed | 1 |
| 1 cup | cooked quinoa (see page 10), cooled | 250 mL |
| 1 cup | diced tomatoes | 250 mL |
| ¾ cup | cooked fresh or thawed frozen corn kernels | 175 mL |
| ¼ cup | packed fresh cilantro leaves, chopped | 60 mL |
| 1 tbsp | minced seeded jalapeño pepper | 15 mL |
| 2 tsp | ground cumin | 10 mL |
| 3 tbsp | freshly squeezed lime juice | 45 mL |
| 1 | firm-ripe Hass avocado, diced | 1 |

1. In a medium bowl, combine beans, quinoa, tomatoes, corn, cilantro, jalapeño, cumin and lime juice. Gently fold in avocado. Cover and refrigerate for 30 minutes to blend the flavors.

# Pineapple and Quinoa Salsa

**Makes about
2½ cups
(625 mL)**

**Tip**

For the best results, make this salsa at least 30 minutes ahead to let the flavors mingle.

**Storage Tip**

Store in an airtight container in the refrigerator for up to 2 days.

| | | |
|---|---|---|
| 1 | small jalapeño pepper, seeded and minced | 1 |
| 1½ cups | diced fresh pineapple | 375 mL |
| ¾ cup | cooked black quinoa (see page 10), cooled | 175 mL |
| ¾ cup | packed fresh cilantro leaves, chopped | 175 mL |
| ¼ cup | finely chopped red onion | 60 mL |
| ⅛ tsp | fine sea salt | 0.5 mL |
| 1 tsp | finely grated lime zest | 5 mL |
| 2 tbsp | freshly squeezed lime juice | 30 mL |

**1.** In a medium bowl, combine jalapeño, pineapple, quinoa, cilantro, red onion, salt, lime zest and lime juice.

# Avocado, Orange and Quinoa Salsa

**Makes 3 cups
(750 mL)**

*A foundation of sunny oranges and nutty quinoa is the perfect destination for those perfectly firm-ripe avocados sitting on your counter.*

**Tip**

If you can only find 10-oz (287 mL) cans of mandarin oranges, use 1½ cans.

| | | |
|---|---|---|
| 2 | small firm-ripe Hass avocados, diced | 2 |
| 1 | can (15 oz/425 mL) mandarin oranges packed in juice, drained and coarsely chopped | 1 |
| 1 cup | cooked black, red or white quinoa (see page 10), cooled | 250 mL |
| ⅓ cup | finely chopped red onion | 75 mL |
| ⅓ cup | packed fresh cilantro leaves, chopped | 75 mL |
| ¼ tsp | chipotle chile powder or cayenne pepper | 1 mL |
| 1 tbsp | freshly squeezed lime juice | 15 mL |
| | Fine sea salt | |

**1.** In a large bowl, combine avocados, mandarin oranges, quinoa, red onion, cilantro, chipotle chile powder and lime juice, tossing gently. Season to taste with salt. Cover and refrigerate for at least 30 minutes, until chilled, or for up to 2 hours.

# Quinoa Caponata

*The subtle, nuanced
flavors of quinoa lay the
foundation for a new
twist on caponata. Ample
amounts of eggplant
are rendered silky
and satisfying, while
tomatoes, capers and
fresh basil add a healthy
dose of Mediterranean
sunshine, brightening the
flavor and color.*

## Storage Tip

Store in an airtight
container in the
refrigerator for up to
3 days. Stir in the basil and
sprinkle with pine nuts just
before serving.

| | | |
|---|---|---|
| 1 tbsp | olive oil | 15 mL |
| 1 | large eggplant, trimmed and cut into ½-inch (1 cm) cubes | 1 |
| 1¼ cups | chopped onions | 300 mL |
| 5 | cloves garlic, minced | 5 |
| 1 | can (14 to 15 oz/398 to 425 mL) diced tomatoes, with juice | 1 |
| ⅓ cup | quinoa, rinsed | 75 mL |
| 2 tsp | dried Italian seasoning | 10 mL |
| ½ cup | dry white wine or water | 125 mL |
| 2 tbsp | balsamic vinegar | 30 mL |
| 2 tbsp | drained capers | 30 mL |
| | Fine sea salt and freshly cracked black pepper | |
| ¾ cup | packed fresh basil, thinly sliced | 175 mL |
| ¼ cup | toasted pine nuts | 60 mL |

1. In a large skillet, heat oil over medium-high heat. Add eggplant, onions and garlic; cook, stirring, for 12 to 15 minutes or until eggplant is soft and browned.
2. Stir in tomatoes with juice, quinoa, Italian seasoning, wine, vinegar and capers. Reduce heat to low, cover and simmer, stirring occasionally, for 15 to 18 minutes or until vegetables and quinoa are very tender. Season to taste with salt and pepper. Stir in basil.
3. Transfer caponata to a serving bowl. Serve warm, at room temperature or chilled, sprinkled with pine nuts.

# Parmesan Quinoa Crisps

*Crackers often get
short shrift as vehicles
for a slice of cheese.
But with Parmesan
incorporated into the
dough, these nibbles can
hold their own. Because
they're made without
preservatives, these
delicate crisps taste best
when freshly baked. Serve
them as a healthy snack
or as an accompaniment
with cocktails.*

## Storage Tip

Layer crisps between
sheets of waxed paper in
an airtight container and
store at room temperature
for up to 2 days. If
necessary, crisp on a
baking sheet in a 350°F
(180°C) oven.

- **Food processor**
- **18- by 13-inch (45 by 33 cm) rimmed baking sheet, lined with parchment paper**

| | | |
|---|---|---|
| 1¼ cups | quinoa, rinsed | 300 mL |
| 2¾ cups | water | 675 mL |
| ¾ cup | freshly grated Parmesan cheese | 175 mL |
| | Fine sea salt and freshly ground black pepper | |

1. In a medium saucepan, combine quinoa and water. Bring to a boil over medium-high heat. Reduce heat to low, cover and simmer for 15 to 20 minutes or until water is absorbed and quinoa is very soft and somewhat mushy. Transfer to a large bowl and let cool completely.

2. In food processor, process cooled quinoa until smooth. Scrape into a large bowl and stir in cheese. Season to taste with salt and pepper.

3. Preheat oven to 450°F (230°C).

4. Scoop half the quinoa mixture into a mound on prepared baking sheet. Cover with plastic wrap, then press or roll out very thin, covering most of the baking sheet.

5. Bake for 10 to 12 minutes or until mixture appears dry, golden and crisp. Carefully transfer parchment to a cutting board and, using a sharp knife, score quinoa mixture into 4 pieces. Transfer parchment to a wire rack and let crisps cool completely.

6. Line baking sheet with another sheet of parchment paper. Repeat steps 4 and 5 with the remaining quinoa mixture.

# Tamari Quinoa, Nut and Seed Mix

**Makes about 3½ cups (875 mL)**

*A handful of these golden nuts, quinoa flakes and green pumpkin seeds is just the nibble you need to tame your appetite between meals. Tamari adds depth of flavor to the mix.*

## Storage Tip

Store in an airtight container at room temperature for up to 2 weeks.

- **Large rimmed baking sheet, lined with parchment paper or foil**

| | | |
|---|---|---|
| 1 tbsp | toasted sesame oil | 15 mL |
| ⅔ cup | quinoa flakes | 150 mL |
| ¾ cup | lightly salted roasted green pumpkin seeds (pepitas) | 175 mL |
| ¾ cup | lightly salted roasted peanuts | 175 mL |
| ¾ cup | lightly salted roasted almonds | 175 mL |
| ¾ cup | toasted pecan halves | 175 mL |
| ¼ tsp | wasabi powder or cayenne pepper | 1 mL |
| 1½ tbsp | tamari or soy sauce (GF, if needed) | 22 mL |
| 1 tbsp | freshly squeezed lime juice | 15 mL |

1. In a large skillet, heat oil over medium heat. Add quinoa flakes and cook, stirring, for 1 to 2 minutes or until golden. Add pumpkin seeds, peanuts, almonds, pecans, wasabi powder, tamari and lime juice; cook, stirring, for 2 to 3 minutes or until dry.

2. Spread mixture on prepared baking sheet and let cool.

# Almond Quinoa Power Bars

**Makes 8 bars**

*Together with walnuts and almond butter, quinoa flakes give these bars a major punch of protein power.*

## Tip

Any other toasted or roasted nuts or seeds can be substituted for the almonds.

## Storage Tip

See page 115.

- **8-inch (20 cm) square metal baking pan, lined with foil and sprayed with nonstick cooking spray**

| | | |
|---|---|---|
| ½ cup | brown rice syrup or liquid honey | 125 mL |
| ⅓ cup | unsweetened natural almond butter | 75 mL |
| ¾ tsp | almond extract (GF, if needed) | 3 mL |
| 2 cups | quinoa flakes | 500 mL |
| ½ cup | coarsely chopped lightly salted roasted almonds | 125 mL |

1. In a large bowl, whisk together brown rice syrup, almond butter and almond extract until well blended. Stir in quinoa flakes and almonds until just combined.

2. Using your hands, a spatula or a large piece of waxed paper, press quinoa mixture firmly into prepared pan. Refrigerate for 30 minutes. Using foil liner, lift mixture from pan and invert onto a cutting board. Peel off foil and cut into 8 bars.

# Sugar-Free Quinoa Granola Bars

**Makes 8 bars**

*When you've had your fill of overly sweet granola bars from the grocery store, turn to this recipe. Naturally sweetened with dates and super-ripe bananas, and bolstered with protein-rich quinoa flakes, these bars will satisfy and energize you in the most delicious way.*

## Tips

Lining a pan with foil is easy. Begin by turning the pan upside down. Tear off a piece of foil longer than the pan, then mold the foil over the pan. Remove the foil and set it aside. Flip the pan over and gently fit the shaped foil into the pan, allowing the foil to hang over the sides (the overhang ends will work as "handles" when the contents of the pan are removed).

Mash the bananas very thoroughly so that no large chunks remain.

- **Preheat oven to 350°F (180°C)**
- **8-inch (20 cm) square metal baking dish, lined with foil (see tip, at left) and sprayed with nonstick cooking spray**

| | | |
|---|---|---|
| ½ tsp | fine sea salt | 2 mL |
| ¼ tsp | ground cardamom or cinnamon | 1 mL |
| 1 cup | mashed very ripe bananas | 250 mL |
| 2 tbsp | coconut oil, warmed, or vegetable oil | 30 mL |
| 2 tsp | vanilla extract (GF, if needed) | 10 mL |
| 2 cups | quinoa flakes | 500 mL |
| ½ cup | chopped pitted Medjool dates | 125 mL |
| ½ cup | chopped toasted nuts (such as walnuts, hazelnuts or pecans) | 125 mL |

1. In a large bowl, combine salt, cardamom, bananas, oil and vanilla. Stir in quinoa flakes, dates and nuts. Using your hands, a spatula or a large piece of waxed paper, press mixture firmly into prepared pan.

2. Bake in preheated oven for 25 to 30 minutes or until golden and edges appear crisp. Let cool completely in pan on a wire rack. Using foil liner, lift mixture from pan and invert onto a cutting board. Peel off foil and cut into 8 bars.

# Maple Quinoa Granola Bars

**Makes 24 bars**

*Loaded with flavor and plenty of crunchy goodness, these bars will soon become your favorite form of portable energy. Vary them any which way: with spices, dried fruits, nuts or different sweeteners.*

## Tip

Measure the oil in a glass measuring cup, then measure the maple syrup in the same cup; the residue from the oil will allow the syrup to slide right out without sticking.

## Storage Tip

Store cooled granola bars in an airtight container at room temperature for up to 1 week. Or wrap them in plastic wrap, then foil, completely enclosing them, and freeze for up to 6 months. Let thaw at room temperature for 1 hour before serving.

- **Preheat oven to 350°F (180°C)**
- **Large baking sheet, lined with parchment paper**
- **13- by 9-inch (33 by 23 cm) metal baking pan, lined with foil (see tip, page 111) and sprayed with nonstick cooking spray**

| | | |
|---|---|---|
| 3 cups | quick-cooking rolled oats (certified GF, if needed) | 750 mL |
| 1 cup | quinoa, rinsed | 250 mL |
| ½ tsp | ground cinnamon | 2 mL |
| ½ tsp | fine sea salt | 2 mL |
| ⅓ cup | vegetable oil | 75 mL |
| ⅔ cup | pure maple syrup | 150 mL |
| 2 tsp | vanilla extract (GF, if needed) | 10 mL |

1. Spread oats and quinoa on prepared baking sheet. Bake in preheated oven for 10 to 12 minutes, stirring once or twice, until golden brown. Remove from oven, leaving oven on, and let cool in pan for 5 minutes.

2. In a large bowl, whisk together cinnamon, salt, oil, maple syrup and vanilla. Stir in cooled oats mixture. Spread mixture in prepared pan.

3. Bake for 25 to 30 minutes or until golden brown. Let cool in pan on a wire rack for 5 minutes. Using foil liner, lift mixture from pan and invert onto a cutting board. While still warm, peel off foil and cut into 24 bars. Let cool completely.

# Chewy Coconut Quinoa Bars

**Makes 15 bars**

*How could something that tastes so good also be good for you? Eating is believing.*

## Tips

Any other variety of natural nut or seed butter, such as peanut, sunflower seed or cashew butter, may be used in place of the almond butter.

If the bars crumble while you're cutting them, refrigerate for 15 to 30 minutes, until they are more firm.

## Storage Tip

Store cooled bars in an airtight container at room temperature for up to 5 days. Or wrap them in plastic wrap, then foil, completely enclosing them, and freeze for up to 6 months. Let thaw at room temperature for 1 hour before serving.

- **Preheat oven to 350°F (180°C)**
- **8-inch (20 cm) square metal baking pan, lined with foil (see tip, page 111) and sprayed with nonstick cooking spray**

| | | |
|---|---|---|
| 2 cups | quinoa flakes | 500 mL |
| 2 cups | unsweetened flaked coconut | 500 mL |
| 1 tsp | ground ginger | 5 mL |
| ½ tsp | fine sea salt | 2 mL |
| ¾ cup | liquid honey or brown rice syrup | 175 mL |
| 6 tbsp | coconut oil, warmed, or vegetable oil | 90 mL |
| ⅓ cup | unsweetened natural almond butter | 75 mL |

1. In a large bowl, combine quinoa flakes, coconut, ginger and salt.
2. In a medium bowl, whisk together honey, oil and almond butter until blended.
3. Add the honey mixture to the quinoa mixture and stir until evenly coated. Using your hands, a spatula or a large piece of waxed paper, press mixture firmly into prepared pan.
4. Bake in preheated oven for 30 to 40 minutes or until browned at the edges but still slightly soft at the center. Let cool completely in pan on a wire rack. Using foil liner, lift mixture from pan and invert onto a cutting board. Peel off foil and cut into 15 bars.

# Multi-Seed Energy Bars

*You've never had an energy bar quite like this one: a medley of seeds — quinoa, sunflower and sesame — coalesce in a crisp-chewy base. Stow one away for a mid-morning energy boost.*

## Tips

Any dried fruit, or a combination of dried fruits, may be used. Try raisins, cranberries, blueberries, cherries and/or chopped apricots.

If you're not following a gluten-free diet, try other puffed grain cereals, such as wheat or barley, in place of the puffed rice.

## Storage Tip

Store cooled bars in an airtight container at room temperature for up to 5 days. Or wrap them in plastic wrap, then foil, completely enclosing them, and freeze for up to 6 months. Let thaw at room temperature for 1 hour before serving.

- **Preheat oven to 350°F (180°C)**
- **Large rimmed baking sheet**
- **8-inch (20 cm) square metal baking pan, lined with foil (see tip, page 111) and sprayed with nonstick cooking spray**

| | | |
|---|---|---|
| 1 cup | quinoa flakes | 250 mL |
| 1/2 cup | sunflower seeds | 125 mL |
| 3 tbsp | toasted sesame seeds | 45 mL |
| 1 cup | unsweetened puffed rice or millet cereal | 250 mL |
| 1 cup | chopped dried fruit | 250 mL |
| 1/4 cup | natural cane sugar or packed dark brown sugar | 60 mL |
| 1/4 tsp | fine sea salt | 1 mL |
| 1/3 cup | tahini or sunflower seed butter | 75 mL |
| 1/4 cup | pure maple syrup or brown rice syrup | 60 mL |
| 1 tsp | vanilla extract (GF, if needed) | 5 mL |

1. Spread quinoa flakes, sunflower seeds and sesame seeds on prepared baking sheet. Bake in preheated oven for 8 to 10 minutes, shaking halfway through, until golden and fragrant.
2. Transfer quinoa mixture to a large bowl and stir in cereal and fruit.
3. In a small saucepan, combine sugar, salt, tahini and maple syrup. Heat over medium-low heat, stirring constantly, for 2 to 4 minutes or until sugar is dissolved and mixture is bubbly. Stir in vanilla.
4. Immediately pour tahini mixture over quinoa mixture, stirring with a spatula until quinoa mixture is coated.
5. Using your hands, a spatula or a large piece of waxed paper, press quinoa mixture firmly into prepared pan. Refrigerate for 30 minutes or until firm. Using foil liner, lift mixture from pan and invert onto a cutting board. Peel off foil and cut into 12 bars.

# Toasted Quinoa Energy Bars

*These bars taste like the best candy you've never had before — reason enough to invest in a food processor.*

## Storage Tip

Store bars in an airtight container at room temperature for up to 1 week or in the refrigerator for up to 3 weeks. Or wrap them in plastic wrap, then foil, completely enclosing them, and freeze for up to 6 months. Let thaw at room temperature for 1 hour before serving.

- **Food processor**
- **8- by 4-inch (20 by 10 cm) metal loaf pan, lined with foil (see tip, page 111) and sprayed with nonstick cooking spray**

| | | |
|---|---|---|
| 1 cup | quinoa, rinsed | 250 mL |
| ¾ cup | packed pitted Medjool dates | 175 mL |
| ¾ cup | dried cranberries or dried cherries | 175 mL |
| ¼ tsp | ground cinnamon | 1 mL |

1. Heat a large skillet over medium-high heat. Toast quinoa, stirring occasionally, for 3 to 4 minutes or until golden brown and just beginning to pop. Transfer to a large bowl and let cool.

2. In food processor, pulse dates and cranberries until mixture resembles a thick paste. Transfer to a medium bowl.

3. In the same food processor (no need to clean it), pulse cooled quinoa 3 to 4 times or until roughly chopped. Add to fruit paste, along with cinnamon. Using your fingers or a wooden spoon, combine well.

4. Using your hands, a spatula or a large piece of waxed paper, press quinoa mixture firmly into prepared pan. Refrigerate for 15 minutes. Using foil liner, lift mixture from pan and invert onto a cutting board. Peel off foil and cut into 6 bars.

## Variations

*Apricot Energy Bars:* Reduce the dates to ½ cup (125 mL) and replace the cranberries with 1 cup (250 mL) packed soft dried apricots.

Form the quinoa mixture into 1-inch (2.5 cm) balls instead of making bars.

# Dried Fruit and Quinoa Power Bars

## Makes 12 bars

*Forgo the cloying chocolate and peanut butter power bars in favor of these lemony apricot bars. A combination of tofu and quinoa ensures that they still have all the protein power you need.*

## Tip

Any dried fruit, or a combination of dried fruits, may be used. Try raisins, cranberries, blueberries, cherries and/ or chopped apricots.

## Storage Tip

Store bars in an airtight container in the refrigerator for up to 1 week. Or wrap them in plastic wrap, then foil, completely enclosing them, and freeze for up to 6 months. Let thaw at room temperature for 1 hour before serving.

- Preheat oven to 350°F (180°C)
- Food processor
- 8-inch (20 cm) square metal baking pan, lined with foil (see tip, page 111) and sprayed with nonstick cooking spray

| | | |
|---|---|---|
| 1½ cups | quinoa flakes | 375 mL |
| 2 tbsp | quinoa flour | 30 mL |
| ½ tsp | fine sea salt | 2 mL |
| 1 | large egg | 1 |
| ½ cup | drained soft silken tofu | 125 mL |
| ½ cup | agave nectar or liquid honey | 125 mL |
| 3 tbsp | coconut oil, warmed, or vegetable oil | 45 mL |
| 1 tbsp | finely grated lemon zest | 15 mL |
| 1 tbsp | freshly squeezed lemon juice | 15 mL |
| ½ cup | chopped toasted walnuts | 125 mL |
| 1½ cups | unsweetened puffed grain cereal | 375 mL |
| 1 cup | chopped dried fruit | 250 mL |

1. Heat a large skillet over medium-high heat. Toast quinoa flakes, stirring constantly, for 3 to 4 minutes or until golden brown. Transfer to a large bowl and let cool.

2. In food processor, combine quinoa flour, salt, egg, tofu, agave nectar, oil, lemon zest and lemon juice; pulse until smooth.

3. To the quinoa flakes, add walnuts, cereal and fruit. Stir in tofu mixture until well blended. Spread evenly in prepared pan.

4. Bake in preheated oven for 35 to 40 minutes or until golden and set at the center. Let cool completely in pan on a wire rack. Using foil liner, lift mixture from pan and invert onto a cutting board. Peel off foil and cut into 12 bars.

# Tart Cherry Quinoa Power Bars

**Makes 12 bars**

*Decked out with quinoa, coconut, almonds and dried cherries, these bars will spoil you for all other power bars. Not too sweet, they make a great pre- or post-workout snack, or an energizing breakfast on the run.*

## Tip

Other dried fruits, such as cranberries, blueberries or chopped apricots, may be used in place of the cherries.

## Storage Tip

Store bars in an airtight container at room temperature for up to 1 week or in the refrigerator for up to 3 weeks. Or wrap them in plastic wrap, then foil, completely enclosing them, and freeze for up to 6 months. Let thaw at room temperature for 1 hour before serving.

- **Preheat oven to 350°F (180°C)**
- **Large rimmed baking sheet**
- **8-inch (20 cm) square metal baking pan, lined with foil (see tip, page 111) and sprayed with nonstick cooking spray**

| | | |
|---|---|---|
| 2 cups | large-flake (old-fashioned) rolled oats (certified GF, if needed) | 500 mL |
| 2/3 cup | sliced almonds | 150 mL |
| 1/2 cup | quinoa, rinsed and patted dry | 125 mL |
| 1/2 cup | unsweetened flaked coconut | 125 mL |
| 3/4 cup | dried tart cherries, finely chopped | 175 mL |
| 1/2 cup | brown rice syrup, golden cane syrup or pure maple syrup | 125 mL |
| 2 tbsp | coconut oil or olive oil | 30 mL |
| 1/2 tsp | fine sea salt | 2 mL |
| 1 tsp | almond extract (GF, if needed) | 5 mL |

1. Spread oats, almonds, quinoa and coconut on prepared baking sheet. Bake in preheated oven for 8 to 10 minutes, shaking halfway through, until golden and fragrant. Transfer to a large bowl and stir in cherries. Reduce oven temperature to 325°F (160°C).

2. In a medium saucepan, combine brown rice syrup, oil and salt. Cook over medium heat, stirring constantly, for 4 to 5 minutes or until bubbling. Remove from heat and stir in almond extract.

3. Immediately pour syrup mixture over oat mixture and stir with a spatula until coated. Using your hands, a spatula or a large piece of waxed paper, press oat mixture firmly into prepared pan.

4. Bake for 10 minutes or until golden and aromatic. Let cool completely in pan on a wire rack. Using foil liner, lift mixture from pan and invert onto a cutting board. Peel off foil and cut into 12 bars.

# Chocolate Quinoa Energy Bites

**Makes
2 dozen bars**

*I predict you will make
these on-the-go energy
bites again and again.
Kids love them too, so be
sure to keep a separate
stash just for yourself.*

## Tip

If you prefer, you can
use unsweetened carob
powder in place of the
cocoa powder.

## Storage Tip

Store bars in an airtight
container in the
refrigerator for up to
1 week. Or wrap them
in plastic wrap, then foil,
completely enclosing
them, and freeze for up
to 6 months. Let thaw
at room temperature for
1 hour before serving.

- **Food processor**
- **9-inch (23 cm) square metal baking pan, lined with foil (see tip, page 111)**

| | | |
|---|---|---|
| 1¼ cups | raw cashews | 300 mL |
| ⅔ cup | quinoa flakes | 150 mL |
| 1 cup | unsweetened flaked coconut | 250 mL |
| ½ cup | unsweetened cocoa powder (not Dutch process) | 125 mL |
| ½ tsp | fine sea salt | 2 mL |
| ½ cup | agave nectar, brown rice syrup or liquid honey | 125 mL |
| 2 tsp | vanilla extract (GF, if needed) | 10 mL |

1. In food processor, combine cashews, quinoa flakes and coconut; pulse until finely chopped. Add cocoa powder, salt, agave nectar and vanilla; pulse until mixture forms a dough.

2. Using your hands, a spatula or a large piece of waxed paper, press dough into prepared pan. Refrigerate for 1 hour or until firm. Using foil liner, lift dough from pan and invert onto a cutting board. Peel off foil and cut into 24 bars.

# Sunflower Quinoa Snack Squares

*One of my earliest recipe-making memories comes from preschool, where I stirred up a batch of peanut butter and oat "candies." Here, I've given the same essential combination a modern spin with sunflower seed butter, quinoa flakes and dried apricots and cranberries.*

## Tips

Substitute 2 cups (500 mL) large-flake (old-fashioned) rolled oats (certified GF, if needed) for half the quinoa flakes.

Use this recipe as a template: use any variety of natural nut or seed butter (such as peanut, cashew, almond or tahini), seeds or nuts and dried fruit of your choice.

## Storage Tip

Store squares in an airtight container at room temperature for up to 1 week or in the refrigerator for up to 3 weeks. Or wrap them in plastic wrap, then foil, completely enclosing them, and freeze for up to 6 months. Let thaw at room temperature for 1 hour before serving.

- **8-inch (20 cm) square metal or glass baking dish, lined with foil (see tip, page 111) and sprayed with nonstick cooking spray**

| | | |
|---|---|---|
| 1 tsp | fine sea salt | 5 mL |
| 1 cup | sunflower seed butter | 250 mL |
| ½ cup | agave nectar, liquid honey or brown rice syrup | 125 mL |
| 2 tsp | vanilla extract (GF, if needed) | 10 mL |
| 4 cups | quinoa flakes | 1 L |
| 1 cup | lightly salted roasted sunflower seeds | 250 mL |
| ¾ cup | chopped dried apricots | 175 mL |
| ½ cup | dried cranberries | 125 mL |

1. In a large bowl, combine salt, sunflower seed butter, agave nectar and vanilla until blended. Stir in quinoa flakes, sunflower seeds, apricots and cranberries until well combined.

2. Using your hands, a spatula or large piece of waxed paper, press quinoa mixture firmly into prepared pan. Refrigerate for 30 minutes or until firm. Using foil liner, lift mixture from pan and invert onto a cutting board. Peel off foil and cut into 16 squares.

# Quinoa Cashew Power Balls

**Makes 16 balls**

*The bag of quinoa in your pantry may have been purchased to contribute to good health, but you'll want to make these delicately sweet power balls for their great taste. Cashews add to the richness and subtle sweetness.*

## Tip

Look for roasted cashews lightly seasoned with sea salt.

## Storage Tip

Store cooled power balls in an airtight container at room temperature for up to 3 days. Or wrap them in plastic wrap, then foil, completely enclosing them, and freeze for up to 6 months. Let thaw at room temperature for 2 to 3 hours before serving.

- **Food processor**
- **Rimmed baking sheet, lined with parchment paper**

| | | |
|---|---|---|
| ⅔ cup | quinoa, rinsed | 150 mL |
| 1⅓ cups | water | 325 mL |
| 1½ cups | lightly salted roasted cashews | 375 mL |
| 1 tsp | ground cinnamon | 5 mL |
| 3 tbsp | dark (cooking) molasses or pure maple syrup | 45 mL |
| 1 tsp | vanilla extract (GF, if needed) | 5 mL |

1. In a large saucepan, combine quinoa and water. Bring to a boil over medium-high heat. Reduce heat to low, cover and simmer for 12 to 15 minutes or until water is absorbed. Remove from heat and let stand, covered, for 5 minutes; fluff with a fork. Spread quinoa on an unlined baking sheet and refrigerate until completely cooled.

2. Preheat oven to 375°F (190°C).

3. In food processor, pulse cashews until finely chopped. Add cooled quinoa, cinnamon, molasses and vanilla; pulse until mixture forms a dough.

4. Form dough into 16 balls of equal size. Place 1 inch (2.5 cm) apart on prepared baking sheet.

5. Bake in preheated oven for 20 to 25 minutes or until golden brown. Let cool in pan on a wire rack for 10 minutes, then transfer to the rack to cool.

# PB&J Quinoa Power Balls

*Peanuts and dried
blueberries share
more than an affinity
for each other in this
delicious snack: they
both contain a naturally
occurring compound
called resveratrol, which,
according to recent
studies, appears to reduce
fat stores in the human
body. Each of these power
balls tastes like a candy
truffle version of a peanut
butter and jelly sandwich,
with the chopped dried
blueberries as the "jam."*

## Tips

Look for roasted peanuts
lightly seasoned with
sea salt.

Other dried fruits, such
as cranberries, cherries or
chopped apricots, may
be used in place of the
blueberries.

## Storage Tip

Store power balls in an
airtight container in the
refrigerator for up to
1 week. Or wrap them
in plastic wrap, then foil,
completely enclosing
them, and freeze for up
to 6 months. Let thaw
at room temperature for
1 hour before serving.

- **Food processor**

| | | |
|---|---|---|
| 1½ cups | quinoa flakes, divided | 375 mL |
| 1 cup | lightly salted roasted peanuts | 250 mL |
| ¼ cup | ground flax seeds (flaxseed meal) | 60 mL |
| ⅔ cup | dried blueberries | 150 mL |
| Pinch | fine sea salt | Pinch |
| ½ cup | unsweetened natural peanut butter | 125 mL |
| 3 tbsp | brown rice syrup or liquid honey | 45 mL |
| 1 tsp | vanilla extract (GF, if needed) | 5 mL |

1. In food processor, combine 1 cup (250 mL) of the quinoa flakes, peanuts and flax seeds; pulse until finely chopped. Add blueberries, salt, peanut butter, brown rice syrup and vanilla; pulse until mixture forms a dough.

2. Place the remaining quinoa flakes in a shallow dish. Form dough into 24 balls of equal size. Roll balls in quinoa flakes until evenly coated. Transfer to an airtight container and refrigerate for 1 hour.

# Cheddar Poppy Seed Quinoa Balls

**Makes 30 balls**

*Snack time just got a little more exciting. Tangy with Cheddar cheese and delicately crunchy from poppy seeds on the inside and quinoa flakes on the outside, these little bites keep your fingers reaching for another, and another, and ... well, you know how it goes. Enjoy!*

## Tip

The quinoa balls can be formed and rolled in quinoa flakes up to 24 hours ahead. Cover and refrigerate. Bake as directed when ready to serve.

• **2 large rimmed baking sheets, lined with foil and sprayed with nonstick cooking spray**

| | | |
|---|---|---|
| ²⁄₃ cup | quinoa, rinsed | 150 mL |
| 1¹⁄₃ cups | ready-to-use vegetable or chicken broth (GF, if needed) | 325 mL |
| 1 cup | shredded white Cheddar cheese | 250 mL |
| 3 tbsp | poppy seeds | 45 mL |
| ³⁄₄ cup | quinoa flakes | 175 mL |

1. In a medium saucepan, combine quinoa and broth. Bring to a boil over medium-high heat. Reduce heat to low, cover and simmer for 12 to 15 minutes or until broth is absorbed. Remove from heat and let stand, covered, for 5 minutes; fluff with a fork. Add cheese and poppy seeds, stirring until cheese is melted. Let cool for 30 minutes.

2. Preheat oven to 425°F (220°C).

3. Place quinoa flakes in a shallow dish. Form quinoa mixture into 1-inch (2.5 cm) balls. Roll balls in quinoa flakes until evenly coated. Place 2 inches (5 cm) apart on prepared baking sheet.

4. Bake in upper and lower thirds of preheated oven for 5 minutes. Reverse positions of pans and bake for 5 to 7 minutes or until golden brown and just set when lightly touched with fingertips. Serve warm or transfer balls to a wire rack and let cool to room temperature.

## Variations

Substitute toasted sesame seeds or roasted hemp seeds for the poppy seeds.

If you're not following a gluten-free diet, an equal amount of panko (Japanese bread crumbs) can be used in place of the quinoa flakes.

# Soups, Stews and Chilis

# Hungarian Sweet-and-Sour Quinoa Soup

*In this redesigned interpretation of a Hungarian classic, softened beets and cabbage join earthy quinoa, and natural cane sugar gives the hot paprika broth a subtle undercurrent of sweetness.*

## Storage Tip

Store the cooled soup in an airtight container in the refrigerator for up to 3 days or in the freezer for up to 6 months. Thaw overnight in the refrigerator or in the microwave using the Defrost function. Warm soup in a medium saucepan over medium-low heat.

| | | |
|---|---|---|
| 1 tbsp | olive oil | 15 mL |
| 2 cups | chopped onions | 500 mL |
| 1½ cups | diced carrots | 375 mL |
| 3 | cloves garlic, minced | 3 |
| 2 tsp | caraway seeds, crushed | 10 mL |
| 1½ tsp | hot smoked paprika | 7 mL |
| 6 cups | shredded coleslaw mix (shredded cabbage and carrots) | 1.5 L |
| 4 cups | diced peeled trimmed beets (about 6 medium) | 1 L |
| ¼ cup | tomato paste (GF, if needed) | 60 mL |
| 3 tbsp | natural cane sugar or packed dark brown sugar | 45 mL |
| 10 cups | ready-to-use reduced-sodium vegetable or chicken broth (GF, if needed) | 2.5 L |
| 2 tbsp | cider vinegar or red wine vinegar | 30 mL |
| 1 cup | quinoa, rinsed | 250 mL |
| | Fine sea salt and freshly cracked black pepper | |
| 1 cup | plain Greek yogurt | 250 mL |
| ¼ cup | chopped fresh chives | 60 mL |

1. In a large pot, heat oil over medium-high heat. Add onions and carrots; cook, stirring, for 6 to 8 minutes or until softened. Add garlic, caraway seeds and paprika; cook, stirring, for 1 minute. Add coleslaw mix, beets and tomato paste; cook, stirring, for 10 minutes.

2. Stir in sugar, broth and vinegar; bring to a boil. Reduce heat to low, cover and simmer for 75 minutes. Stir in quinoa, cover and simmer, stirring occasionally, for 15 to 20 minutes or until quinoa is tender. Season to taste with salt and pepper. Serve dolloped with yogurt and sprinkled with chives.

# Gingered Beet and Quinoa Soup

*This gorgeous scarlet soup offers a striking presentation and a beautiful expression of flavors. A dollop of thick yogurt and a flurry of fresh mint add panache.*

## Tip

If you prefer a silken texture, you can purée the finished soup. Working in batches, transfer soup to food processor or blender (or use immersion blender in pot) and purée until smooth. Return soup to pot (if necessary) and heat over low heat, uncovered, for 4 to 5 minutes or until warm.

## Storage Tip

Store the cooled soup in an airtight container in the refrigerator for up to 2 days or in the freezer for up to 6 months. Thaw overnight in the refrigerator or in the microwave using the Defrost function. Warm soup in a medium saucepan over medium-low heat.

| | | |
|---|---|---|
| 4 cups | diced peeled beets | 1 L |
| 6 cups | ready-to-use reduced-sodium vegetable or chicken broth, divided | 1.5 L |
| 1 tbsp | extra virgin olive oil | 15 mL |
| 2 cups | chopped onions | 500 mL |
| 1½ tbsp | ground ginger | 22 mL |
| ⅔ cup | quinoa, rinsed | 150 mL |
| | Fine sea salt and freshly ground black pepper | |
| ½ cup | plain Greek yogurt | 125 mL |
| ⅓ cup | packed fresh mint leaves, chopped | 75 mL |

1. In a medium microwave-safe bowl, combine beets and 2 cups (500 mL) of the broth. Cover loosely and microwave on High for 15 minutes or until beets are tender. Set aside.

2. Meanwhile, in a large pot, heat oil over medium-high heat. Add onions and cook, stirring, for 6 to 8 minutes or until softened. Add ginger and cook, stirring, for 30 seconds.

3. Stir in beet mixture, quinoa and the remaining broth; bring to a boil. Reduce heat to low, cover and simmer for 15 to 20 minutes or until quinoa is tender. Season to taste with salt and pepper. Serve dolloped with yogurt and sprinkled with mint.

# Quinoa and Bok Choy Soup

*Lightly simmered bok choy, with its almost bitter leaves and sweet, succulent stems, offers a fine balance of flavor and texture in this easily assembled soup. Ginger, tamari and toasted sesame oil enrich the quick mushroom broth; quinoa makes the soup hearty enough for a main dish.*

## Storage Tip

Store the cooled soup in an airtight container in the refrigerator for up to 2 days. Warm in a pot over medium-low heat.

| | | |
|---|---|---|
| 3 | cloves garlic, minced | 3 |
| 1 tbsp | ground ginger | 15 mL |
| 1 cup | red or white quinoa, rinsed | 250 mL |
| 7 cups | ready-to-use reduced-sodium chicken or vegetable broth (GF, if needed) | 1.75 L |
| 2 tbsp | tamari or soy sauce (GF, if needed) | 30 mL |
| 2 tbsp | unseasoned rice vinegar | 30 mL |
| 1 tbsp | toasted sesame oil | 15 mL |
| 1 lb | shiitake or cremini mushrooms, stems removed, if necessary, sliced | 500 g |
| 6 cups | sliced bok choy | 1.5 L |
| ¾ cup | thinly sliced green onions | 175 mL |
| | Fine sea salt and freshly ground black pepper | |

1. In a large pot, combine garlic, ginger, quinoa, broth, tamari, vinegar and oil. Bring to a boil over medium-high heat. Reduce heat to low, cover and simmer for 15 minutes or until quinoa is tender.

2. Stir in mushrooms and simmer, uncovered, stirring occasionally, for 5 minutes or until mushrooms are tender. Stir in bok choy and green onions; simmer for 3 to 4 minutes or until bok choy is wilted. Season to taste with salt and pepper.

# Broccoli Rabe and Quinoa Peasant Soup

*I'd gladly eat this soup any day, even if it wasn't packed with nutrition. But packed with nutrition it is, from the antioxidants and vitamins A and C of the broccoli rabe to the protein in the beans to the lycopene in the tomatoes.*

## Tip

Broccoli rabe can carry a lot of hidden dirt, so be sure to rinse it thoroughly before adding it to the soup. After cutting broccoli rabe as indicated, place it in a large bowl of cold water and agitate it to loosen the dirt. Lift broccoli rabe from the bowl, leaving dirt and silt behind. Repeat if necessary.

## Storage Tip

Store the cooled soup in an airtight container in the refrigerator for up to 3 days or in the freezer for up to 6 months. Thaw overnight in the refrigerator or in the microwave using the Defrost function. Warm soup in a medium saucepan over medium-low heat.

| | | |
|---|---|---|
| 1 tbsp | olive oil | 15 mL |
| 1½ cups | chopped onions | 375 mL |
| 4 | cloves garlic, minced | 4 |
| 2 tsp | dried basil | 10 mL |
| ⅔ cup | quinoa, rinsed | 150 mL |
| ½ cup | Marsala or sherry | 125 mL |
| 1 | can (28 oz/796 mL) crushed tomatoes | 1 |
| 4 cups | ready-to-use reduced-sodium vegetable or chicken broth (GF, if needed) | 1 L |
| 3 tbsp | tomato paste (GF, if needed) | 45 mL |
| 2 | cans (each 14 to 19 oz/398 to 540 mL) white beans, drained and rinsed | 2 |
| 1 lb | broccoli rabe (1 bunch), cut crosswise into 1-inch (2.5 cm) pieces | 500 g |
| | Fine sea salt and freshly ground black pepper | |
| ½ cup | freshly grated Parmesan cheese | 125 mL |

1. In a large pot, heat oil over medium-high heat. Add onions and cook, stirring, for 5 to 6 minutes or until softened. Add garlic and basil; cook, stirring, for 30 seconds. Add quinoa and Marsala; cook, stirring, for 1 minute.

2. Stir in tomatoes, broth and tomato paste; bring to a boil. Reduce heat to low, cover and simmer, stirring occasionally, for 15 minutes or until quinoa is tender.

3. In a small bowl, coarsely mash half the beans with a fork. Stir mashed beans, whole beans and broccoli rabe into the soup. Cover and simmer, stirring occasionally, for 4 to 5 minutes or until quinoa and broccoli rabe are tender. Season to taste with salt and pepper. Serve sprinkled with cheese.

# Irish Cabbage Quinoa Soup

*Cabbage soup may be a traditional offering for St. Patrick's Day, but it doesn't have to be bland and predictable. Here, more delicate savoy cabbage is used in place of regular cabbage, quinoa and Canadian bacon add richness without heaviness, and ready-to-use broth is laced with butter, onions and caraway. This is a guaranteed crowd-pleaser, whether the crowd is family or a last-minute gathering of friends.*

## Tips

When puréeing soup in a food processor or blender, fill the bowl no more than halfway full at a time.

An immersion blender may be used to partially purée the soup (instead of transferring one-third of it to a food processor). Pulse the immersion blender in the soup 5 to 6 times.

## Storage Tip

Store the cooled soup in an airtight container in the refrigerator for up to 1 day. Warm in a medium saucepan over medium-low heat.

- **Food processor or blender**

| | | |
|---|---|---|
| 4 tsp | unsalted butter, divided | 20 mL |
| 1½ cups | chopped onions | 375 mL |
| 1½ tsp | caraway seeds, crushed | 7 mL |
| ½ tsp | freshly ground black pepper | 2 mL |
| ¾ cup | quinoa, rinsed | 175 mL |
| 6 cups | ready-to-use reduced-sodium chicken broth (GF, if needed) | 1.5 L |
| 6 cups | thinly sliced savoy cabbage (about ¾ head) | 1.5 L |
| 4 oz | sliced Canadian (back) bacon, coarsely chopped | 125 g |
| | Fine sea salt and freshly ground black pepper | |

1. In a large pot, melt half the butter over medium-high heat. Add onions, caraway seeds and pepper; cook, stirring occasionally, for 5 to 6 minutes or until onions are softened.

2. Stir in quinoa and broth; bring to a boil. Reduce heat to low, cover and simmer, stirring occasionally, for 15 minutes. Stir in cabbage, cover and simmer, stirring once or twice, for 4 to 5 minutes or until cabbage is wilted and quinoa is tender.

3. Transfer one-third of the soup to food processor and purée until smooth. Return puréed soup to pot and stir in bacon. Simmer, uncovered, stirring occasionally, for 2 to 3 minutes to warm through. Season to taste with salt and pepper.

# Holishke Quinoa Soup

*Holishkes are stuffed cabbage rolls served on Succoth, a joyous seven-day autumn harvest festival (a kind of Jewish Thanksgiving). The stuffing serves as a symbol of abundance. Here, the celebratory dish is transformed into a rich and robust soup, with quinoa in place of the more traditional rice. The result is every bit as festive.*

## Storage Tip

Store the cooled soup in an airtight container in the refrigerator for up to 1 day. Warm in a medium saucepan over medium-low heat.

| | | |
|---|---|---|
| 1 tbsp | olive oil | 15 mL |
| 2 cups | chopped onions | 500 mL |
| 2 cups | chopped carrots | 500 mL |
| 4 | cloves garlic, minced | 4 |
| 1 tbsp | dried dillweed | 15 mL |
| 2 tsp | hot smoked paprika | 10 mL |
| 1½ tsp | ground cinnamon | 7 mL |
| 1 tsp | ground allspice | 5 mL |
| 1 cup | quinoa, rinsed | 250 mL |
| 1 | can (28 oz/796 mL) crushed tomatoes | 1 |
| 8 cups | ready-to-use reduced-sodium chicken or vegetable broth (GF, if needed) | 2 L |
| ½ cup | tomato paste (GF, if needed) | 125 mL |
| 8 cups | sliced savoy cabbage (about 1 small head) | 2 L |
| ½ cup | packed fresh flat-leaf (Italian) parsley leaves, chopped | 125 mL |
| | Fine sea salt and freshly cracked black pepper | |

1. In a large pot, heat oil over medium-high heat. Add onions and carrots; cook, stirring, for 6 to 8 minutes or until softened. Add garlic, dill, paprika, cinnamon and allspice; cook, stirring, for 1 minute.

2. Stir in quinoa, tomatoes, broth and tomato paste; bring to a boil. Reduce heat to low, cover and simmer, stirring occasionally, for 15 minutes. Stir in cabbage, cover and simmer, stirring once or twice, for 4 to 5 minutes or until cabbage is wilted and quinoa is tender. Stir in parsley. Season to taste with salt and pepper.

# Moroccan Carrot Quinoa Soup

*Inspired by North African ingredients and flavors, this gorgeous orange soup is perfectly outfitted for spring with a bright blend of carrots and lemon, and final flourishes of yogurt and fresh mint for zing.*

## Tip

When puréeing soup in a food processor or blender, fill the bowl no more than halfway full at a time.

## Storage Tip

Store the cooled soup in an airtight container in the refrigerator for up to 2 days or in the freezer for up to 6 months. Thaw overnight in the refrigerator or in the microwave using the Defrost function. Warm soup in a medium saucepan over medium-low heat.

### • Food processor, blender or immersion blender

| | | |
|---|---|---|
| 1 tbsp | extra virgin olive oil | 15 mL |
| 1½ cups | chopped onions | 375 mL |
| 1¼ lbs | carrots, chopped (about 3 cups/750 mL) | 625 g |
| ½ cup | quinoa flakes or quinoa flour | 125 mL |
| 2 tsp | ground cumin | 10 mL |
| 1 tsp | ground cinnamon | 5 mL |
| 4 cups | ready-to-use reduced-sodium chicken or vegetable broth (GF, if needed) | 1 L |
| 2 tbsp | freshly squeezed lemon juice | 30 mL |
| 1 tbsp | liquid honey | 15 mL |
| | Fine sea salt and freshly ground black pepper | |
| ½ cup | plain yogurt | 125 mL |
| ⅓ cup | packed fresh mint or cilantro leaves, minced | 75 mL |

1. In a large pot, heat oil over medium-high heat. Add onions and cook, stirring, for 5 to 6 minutes or until softened.

2. Stir in carrots, quinoa flakes, cumin, cinnamon and broth; bring to a boil. Reduce heat and simmer, stirring occasionally, for 25 to 30 minutes or until carrots are very soft.

3. Working in batches, transfer soup to food processor (or use immersion blender in pot) and purée until smooth. Return soup to pot (if necessary) and whisk in lemon juice and honey. Warm over medium heat, stirring, for 1 minute. Season to taste with salt and pepper. Serve dolloped with yogurt and sprinkled with mint.

# Roasted Cauliflower Quinoa Soup

**Makes 8 servings**

*Roasting cauliflower brings out its best by caramelizing its edges and playing up its nuttiness. The nuttiness quotient is increased with the addition of quinoa, while fresh lime juice and cumin add just the right sharp-savory notes.*

## Tip

When puréeing soup in a food processor or blender, fill the bowl no more than halfway full at a time.

## Storage Tip

Store the cooled soup in an airtight container in the refrigerator for up to 2 days or in the freezer for up to 6 months. Thaw overnight in the refrigerator or in the microwave using the Defrost function. Warm soup in a medium saucepan over medium-low heat.

- **Preheat oven to 450°F (230°C)**
- **Large rimmed baking sheet, lined with foil and sprayed with nonstick cooking spray**
- **Blender**

| | | |
|---|---|---|
| 6 cups | cauliflower florets (about 1 large head) | 1.5 L |
| 4 tsp | vegetable oil, divided | 20 mL |
| | Fine sea salt | |
| 2 cups | chopped onions | 500 mL |
| ½ cup | quinoa flakes | 125 mL |
| 2 tsp | ground cumin | 10 mL |
| 6 cups | water | 1.5 L |
| 1½ tbsp | freshly squeezed lime juice | 22 mL |
| | Freshly ground black pepper | |
| ⅓ cup | packed fresh cilantro leaves, roughly chopped | 75 mL |

1. On prepared baking sheet, toss cauliflower with half the oil and 2 tsp (10 mL) salt. Spread in a single layer. Roast in preheated oven for 35 to 45 minutes, stirring occasionally, until golden brown and tender.

2. Meanwhile, in a large pot, heat the remaining oil over medium-high heat. Add onions and cook, stirring, for 6 to 8 minutes or until softened.

3. Stir in roasted cauliflower, quinoa flakes, cumin, 2 tsp (10 mL) salt and water; bring to a boil. Reduce heat and simmer, stirring occasionally, for 20 minutes or until cauliflower is very soft.

4. Working in batches, transfer soup to food processor (or use immersion blender in pot) and purée until smooth. Return soup to pot (if necessary) and whisk in lime juice. Warm over medium heat, stirring, for 1 minute. Season to taste with salt and pepper. Serve sprinkled with cilantro.

# Smoky Corn and Quinoa Chowder

**Makes 6 servings**

*Here's a soup with year-round appeal — it seems to suit every season, and because the ingredients come from the pantry and freezer, it's convenient anytime: quick and simple enough for weeknights, but impressive as a first course at the Thanksgiving table, too.*

## Tips

When puréeing soup in a food processor or blender, fill the bowl no more than halfway full at a time.

An immersion blender may be used to partially purée the soup (instead of transferring one-third of it to a food processor). Pulse the immersion blender in the soup 5 to 6 times.

## Storage Tip

Store the cooled soup in an airtight container in the refrigerator for up to 2 days or in the freezer for up to 6 months. Thaw overnight in the refrigerator or in the microwave using the Defrost function. Warm soup in a medium saucepan over medium-low heat.

- **Food processor or blender**

| | | |
|---|---|---|
| 2 | slices bacon, chopped | 2 |
| 4 | green onions, thinly sliced, green and white parts separated | 4 |
| 2 | cloves garlic, minced | 2 |
| 1 tsp | ground cumin | 5 mL |
| ¾ tsp | hot smoked paprika | 3 mL |
| 5 cups | fresh or frozen corn kernels | 1.25 L |
| ⅔ cup | quinoa flakes or quinoa flour | 150 mL |
| 6 cups | ready-to-use reduced-sodium vegetable or chicken broth (GF, if needed) | 1.5 L |
| | Fine sea salt and freshly cracked black pepper | |

1. In a large pot, cook bacon over medium-high heat until crisp. Using a slotted spoon, transfer bacon to a plate lined with paper towels.

2. Add white portions of green onions to the fat remaining in the pan; cook, stirring, for 2 to 3 minutes or until softened. Add garlic, cumin and paprika; cook, stirring, for 30 seconds.

3. Stir in corn, quinoa flakes and broth; bring to a boil. Reduce heat and simmer, stirring occasionally, for 15 minutes.

4. Working in batches, transfer half the soup to food processor and purée until smooth. Return puréed soup to pot and season to taste with salt and pepper. Simmer, stirring occasionally, for 2 to 3 minutes to warm through. Serve sprinkled with bacon and green parts of green onions.

# Mushroom and Quinoa Soup

*I'm something of a
mushroom fiend — throw
a few into a dish and
I'll very likely eat it.
But I'm also discerning
and can give this easy
soup unqualified high
marks. It's a departure
from creamy mushroom
soup. Instead, the
mushrooms are simmered
in a Marsala-laced broth
and complemented by
the delicate nuances
of quinoa.*

## Storage Tip

Store the cooled soup in
an airtight container in
the refrigerator for up to
2 days or in the freezer
for up to 6 months.
Thaw overnight in the
refrigerator or in the
microwave using the
Defrost function. Warm
soup in a medium
saucepan over medium-
low heat.

| | | |
|---|---|---:|
| 1 tbsp | extra virgin olive oil | 15 mL |
| 1 lb | cremini or button mushrooms, chopped | 500 g |
| 2 cups | chopped onions | 500 mL |
| 1½ cups | chopped carrots | 375 mL |
| 1½ cups | chopped celery | 375 mL |
| 2 tsp | chopped fresh rosemary | 10 mL |
| 1¼ cups | quinoa, rinsed | 300 mL |
| 8 cups | ready-to-use reduced-sodium beef or vegetable broth (GF, if needed) | 2 L |
| ½ cup | Marsala or sherry | 125 mL |
| | Fine sea salt and freshly ground black pepper | |
| 3 tbsp | chopped fresh flat-leaf (Italian) parsley | 45 mL |

1. In a large pot, heat oil over medium-high heat. Add mushrooms, onions, carrots and celery; cook, stirring, for 6 to 8 minutes or until slightly softened. Reduce heat to medium-low and cook, stirring occasionally, for 15 to 20 minutes or until vegetables are browned.

2. Stir in quinoa, broth and Marsala. Increase heat to medium-high and bring to a boil, stirring often. Reduce heat to medium, cover, leaving lid ajar, and simmer, stirring occasionally, for 15 to 20 minutes or until quinoa is tender. Season to taste with salt and pepper. Stir in parsley.

# Spinach, Quinoa and Broccoli Bisque

*This gorgeous green soup is elegant enough for company, but also just right for an easy weeknight supper with grilled cheese sandwiches alongside. It's so velvety, it's hard to believe there's neither cream nor butter in this soup. Quinoa flakes are the secret, adding richness and complexity in one fell swoop.*

## Tips

For best results, use a vegetable peeler to peel the thick outer layer off the broccoli stems before chopping.

When puréeing soup in a food processor or blender, fill the bowl no more than halfway full at a time.

## Storage Tip

Store the cooled soup in an airtight container in the refrigerator for up to 2 days or in the freezer for up to 6 months. Thaw overnight in the refrigerator or in the microwave using the Defrost function. Warm soup in a medium saucepan over medium-low heat.

• **Food processor, blender or immersion blender**

| | | |
|---|---|---|
| 1 tbsp | olive oil | 15 mL |
| 1½ cups | chopped onions | 375 mL |
| 2 | cloves garlic, minced | 2 |
| 2½ tsp | dried basil | 12 mL |
| ¼ tsp | freshly ground black pepper | 1 mL |
| 1½ lbs | broccoli, coarsely chopped (florets and peeled stems) | 750 g |
| ½ cup | quinoa flakes or quinoa flour | 125 mL |
| 6 cups | ready-to-use reduced-sodium vegetable or chicken broth (GF, if needed) | 1.5 L |
| 1½ cups | water | 375 mL |
| 6 cups | packed spinach leaves | 1.5 L |
| | Fine sea salt and freshly ground black pepper | |

1. In a large pot, heat oil over medium-high heat. Add onions and cook, stirring, for 5 to 6 minutes or until softened. Add garlic, basil and pepper; cook, stirring, for 30 seconds.

2. Stir in broccoli, quinoa flakes, broth and water; bring to a boil. Reduce heat and simmer, stirring occasionally, for 15 minutes. Stir in spinach and simmer for 3 to 4 minutes or until broccoli is tender.

3. Working in batches, transfer soup to food processor (or use immersion blender in pot) and purée until smooth. Return soup to pot (if necessary). Warm over medium heat, stirring, for 1 minute. Season to taste with salt and pepper.

# Creamy Tomato Quinoa Soup

*When quinoa flakes are added to puréed soups, such as this creamy tomato concoction, they lend a silken creaminess, without dairy.*

## Tips

When puréeing soup in a food processor or blender, fill the bowl no more than halfway full at a time.

Canned tomatoes vary in their sweetness, so taste for sweetness in the finished soup — you may want to add a bit of honey or another sweetener to balance the acidity of the tomatoes.

## Storage Tip

Store the cooled soup in an airtight container in the refrigerator for up to 2 days or in the freezer for up to 6 months. Thaw overnight in the refrigerator or in the microwave using the Defrost function. Warm soup in a medium saucepan over medium-low heat.

• **Food processor, blender or immersion blender**

| | | |
|---|---|---|
| 1 tbsp | extra virgin olive oil | 15 mL |
| 1¼ cups | chopped onions | 300 mL |
| 2 tsp | dried basil | 10 mL |
| ⅛ tsp | cayenne pepper | 0.5 mL |
| ⅔ cup | quinoa flakes or quinoa flour | 150 mL |
| 1 | can (28 oz/796 mL) crushed tomatoes | 1 |
| 3 cups | ready-to-use reduced-sodium chicken or vegetable broth (GF, if needed) | 750 mL |
| ¼ cup | tomato paste (GF, if needed) | 60 mL |
| | Fine sea salt and freshly ground black pepper | |

1. In a large pot, heat oil over medium-high heat. Add onions and cook, stirring, for 5 to 6 minutes or until softened. Add basil and cayenne; cook, stirring, for 30 seconds.

2. Stir in quinoa flakes, tomatoes, broth and tomato paste; bring to a boil. Reduce heat and simmer, stirring occasionally, for about 20 minutes to blend the flavors.

3. Working in batches, transfer soup to food processor (or use immersion blender in pot) and purée until smooth. Return soup to pot (if necessary). Warm over medium heat, stirring, for 1 minute. Season to taste with salt and black pepper.

# Spicy Maple Pumpkin Soup

**Makes
8 servings**

*Buttermilk and a bit of
cayenne provide just the
right balance of tart and
spicy in this healthful,
satisfying soup, thickened
with quinoa flakes and
sweetened ever so slightly
with maple syrup.*

## Tip

If 15-oz (425 mL) cans
of pumpkin purée aren't
available, purchase two
28-oz (796 mL) cans and
measure out 3½ cups
(875 mL). Refrigerate extra
pumpkin in an airtight
container for up to 1 week.

## Storage Tip

Store the cooled soup in
an airtight container in
the refrigerator for up to
2 days or in the freezer
for up to 6 months.
Thaw overnight in the
refrigerator or in the
microwave using the
Defrost function. Warm
soup in a medium
saucepan over
medium-low heat.

| | | |
|---|---|---|
| ⅓ cup | quinoa flakes or quinoa flour | 75 mL |
| 2½ tsp | pumpkin pie spice | 12 mL |
| ¼ tsp | cayenne pepper | 1 mL |
| 2 | cans (each 15 oz/425 mL) pumpkin purée (not pie filling) | 2 |
| 5 cups | ready-to-use reduced-sodium chicken or vegetable broth (GF, if needed) | 1.25 L |
| 2 tbsp | pure maple syrup | 30 mL |
| 1 cup | buttermilk | 250 mL |
| | Fine sea salt and freshly cracked black pepper | |
| | Lightly salted roasted green pumpkin seeds (pepitas) (optional) | |

1. In a large pot, combine quinoa flakes, pumpkin pie spice, cayenne, pumpkin, broth and maple syrup. Bring to a boil over medium-high heat. Reduce heat and simmer, stirring occasionally, for 20 minutes.

2. Reduce heat to low and whisk in buttermilk. Simmer, stirring occasionally, for 5 minutes (do not let boil). Season to taste with salt and black pepper. Serve sprinkled with pepitas, if desired.

# Thai Curry Quinoa Soup

*Pumpkin and coconut
milk may sound like an
unusual combination
for a savory dish, but
the sweet squash-
coconut combination is
common in Southeast
Asian cuisines and
works seamlessly in this
streamlined soup. Quinoa
and Thai red curry paste
impart exotic notes,
and fresh lime juice and
cilantro provide bright
contrast to the rich
coconut broth.*

## Tip

If 15-oz (425 mL) cans of
pumpkin aren't available,
purchase one 28-oz
(796 mL) can and measure
out 1¾ cups (425 mL).
Refrigerate extra pumpkin
in an airtight container for
up to 1 week.

## Storage Tip

Store the cooled soup in
an airtight container in
the refrigerator for up to
2 days or in the freezer
for up to 6 months.
Thaw overnight in the
refrigerator or in the
microwave using the
Defrost function. Warm
soup in a medium
saucepan over
medium-low heat.

| | | |
|---|---|---|
| ⅔ cup | quinoa, rinsed | 150 mL |
| 2 tbsp | natural cane sugar or packed light brown sugar | 30 mL |
| 3 cups | ready-to-use reduced-sodium vegetable or chicken broth (GF, if needed) | 750 mL |
| 2 tbsp | Thai red curry paste | 30 mL |
| ½ cup | packed fresh cilantro leaves, chopped, divided | 125 mL |
| 1 | can (15 oz/425 mL) pumpkin purée (not pie filling) | 1 |
| 1 cup | light coconut milk | 250 mL |
| 1 tbsp | freshly squeezed lime juice | 15 mL |
| | Fine sea salt and freshly ground black pepper | |

1. In a large pot, whisk together quinoa, sugar, broth and curry paste. Bring to a boil over medium-low heat. Reduce heat and simmer, stirring occasionally, for 15 minutes or until quinoa is tender.
2. Whisk in half the cilantro, pumpkin, coconut milk and lime juice. Simmer, stirring once or twice, for 5 minutes. Season to taste with salt and pepper. Serve sprinkled with the remaining cilantro.

## Variation

For a heartier soup, add 2 cups (500 mL) shredded or diced cooked chicken breast or 12 oz (375 g) cooked small or medium shrimp along with the pumpkin and coconut.

# Swiss Chard, Sweet Potato and Quinoa Soup

**Makes 6 servings**

*Here, the distinctive, mellow sweetness of sweet potatoes is augmented by the subtle sesame flavor of quinoa and the grassy flavor of Swiss chard for a harmonious balance of flavors and textures.*

## Storage Tip

Store the cooled soup in an airtight container in the refrigerator for up to 2 days or in the freezer for up to 6 months. Thaw overnight in the refrigerator or in the microwave using the Defrost function. Warm soup in a medium saucepan over medium-low heat.

| | | |
|---|---|---|
| 2 tsp | extra virgin olive oil | 10 mL |
| 2 cups | chopped onions | 500 mL |
| 2 | large sweet potatoes (each about 1 lb/500 g), peeled and cut into 1/4-inch (0.5 cm) cubes | 2 |
| 3/4 cup | quinoa, rinsed | 175 mL |
| | Freshly ground black pepper | |
| 5 cups | ready-to-use reduced-sodium chicken or vegetable broth (GF, if needed) | 1.25 L |
| 6 cups | packed chopped Swiss chard, tough stems removed | 1.5 L |
| 2 tbsp | freshly squeezed lemon juice | 30 mL |
| | Fine sea salt | |
| 1/2 cup | basil pesto | 125 mL |

1. In a large pot, heat oil over medium-high heat. Add onions and cook, stirring, for 5 to 6 minutes or until softened.

2. Stir in sweet potatoes, quinoa, 3/4 tsp (3 mL) pepper and broth; bring to a boil. Reduce heat to low, cover, leaving lid ajar, and simmer, stirring occasionally, for 20 to 25 minutes or until sweet potatoes are very tender but not falling apart.

3. Stir in Swiss chard, cover and simmer for 5 minutes or until greens are wilted. Stir in lemon juice. Season to taste with salt and pepper.

4. Serve each bowl of soup with a dollop of pesto swirled in.

# Winter Squash Quinoa Bisque

## Storage Tip

Store the cooled soup in an airtight container in the refrigerator for up to 2 days or in the freezer for up to 6 months. Thaw overnight in the refrigerator or in the microwave using the Defrost function. Warm soup in a medium saucepan over medium-low heat.

| | | |
|---|---|---|
| 1 tbsp | unsalted butter | 15 mL |
| 1¼ cups | minced onions | 300 mL |
| ½ cup | quinoa flakes or quinoa flour | 125 mL |
| 1½ tsp | dried thyme | 7 mL |
| 2 | packages (each 12 oz/375 g) frozen winter squash purée, thawed | 2 |
| 4 cups | ready-to-use reduced-sodium chicken or vegetable broth (GF, if needed) | 1 L |
| | Fine sea salt and freshly ground black pepper | |
| 3 tbsp | minced fresh chives (optional) | 45 mL |

1. In a large pot, melt butter over medium-high heat. Add onions and cook, stirring, for 5 to 6 minutes or until softened.
2. Stir in quinoa flakes, thyme, squash and broth; bring to a boil. Reduce heat to low, cover and simmer, stirring occasionally, for 25 to 30 minutes or until thickened. Season to taste with salt and pepper. Serve sprinkled with chives, if desired.

### Variation

Use 3 cups (750 mL) canned pumpkin purée (not pie filling) in place of the frozen winter squash purée.

# Big Batch Vegetable Quinoa Soup

*Here, an assortment of vegetables is transformed into an easy, versatile, yet boast-worthy soup. And because you can use frozen or fresh vegetables, it's a soup to be enjoyed year-round.*

| | | |
|---|---|---|
| 8 cups | assorted fresh or frozen vegetables | 2 L |
| 2 cups | chopped onions | 500 mL |
| 1 cup | quinoa, rinsed | 250 mL |
| 1 tbsp | dried Italian seasoning | 15 mL |
| 1 | can (28 oz/796 mL) diced tomatoes, with juice | 1 |
| 8 cups | ready-to-use reduced-sodium vegetable or chicken broth (GF, if needed) | 2 L |
| | Fine sea salt and freshly ground black pepper | |

1. In a large pot, combine assorted vegetables, onions, quinoa, Italian seasoning, tomatoes with juice and broth. Bring to a boil over medium-high heat. Reduce heat to low, cover and simmer, stirring occasionally, for 25 minutes or until vegetables and quinoa are to low tender. Season to taste with salt and pepper.

# Quinoa Soupe au Pistou

*Soup au pistou is a hearty
vegetable soup with a
good measure of pistou
(the French version of
pesto) stirred in right
before serving. I've taken
some liberties here by
using prepared (Italian)
basil pesto in place of the
pistou, but the results are
equally dazzling. When
the pesto is stirred in, the
soup turns a vibrant green
and becomes perfumed
with the intense, sweet
aroma of basil mixed with
garlic.*

## Storage Tip

Store the cooled soup in
an airtight container in
the refrigerator for up to
2 days or in the freezer
for up to 6 months.
Thaw overnight in the
refrigerator or in the
microwave using the
Defrost function. Warm
soup in a medium
saucepan over
medium-low heat.

| | | |
|---|---|---|
| 2 tsp | extra virgin olive oil | 10 mL |
| 1½ cups | chopped onions | 375 mL |
| | Freshly cracked black pepper | |
| 2 | zucchini, halved lengthwise and thinly sliced | 2 |
| 2 | cans (each 14 to 15 oz/398 to 425 mL) diced tomatoes, with juice | 2 |
| 6 cups | ready-to-use reduced-sodium vegetable or chicken broth (GF, if needed) | 1.5 L |
| 12 oz | green beans, trimmed and cut into thirds (about 1½ cups/375 mL) | 375 g |
| ½ cup | quinoa, rinsed | 125 mL |
| 1 | can (14 to 19 oz/398 to 540 mL) white beans, drained and rinsed | 1 |
| | Fine sea salt | |
| ½ cup | basil pesto | 125 mL |
| ⅓ cup | freshly grated Parmesan cheese | 75 mL |

1. In a large pot, heat oil over medium-high heat. Add onions and ¼ tsp (1 mL) pepper; cook, stirring, for 5 to 6 minutes or until softened.

2. Stir in zucchini, tomatoes with juice and broth; bring to a boil. Reduce heat and simmer, stirring occasionally, for 15 minutes. Stir in green beans, quinoa and white beans; simmer, stirring occasionally, for 15 to 20 minutes or until quinoa is tender. Season to taste with salt and pepper. Serve dolloped with pesto and sprinkled with cheese.

# Lemony Quinoa Primavera Soup

*Basic vegetable soup is fine, but a 30-minute vegetable soup made with quinoa and spring vegetables, enveloped in a lemon and herb broth and topped with nutty Parmesan cheese, gives an old favorite a fresh spring angle.*

## Storage Tip

Store the cooled soup in an airtight container in the refrigerator for up to 2 days or in the freezer for up to 6 months. Thaw overnight in the refrigerator or in the microwave using the Defrost function. Warm soup in a medium saucepan over medium-low heat.

| | | |
|---|---|---|
| 1 cup | quinoa, rinsed | 250 mL |
| 8 cups | ready-to-use reduced-sodium vegetable or chicken broth (GF, if needed) | 2 L |
| 1 tbsp | finely grated lemon zest | 15 mL |
| 1 lb | asparagus, trimmed and sliced diagonally into 1/4-inch (0.5 cm) pieces, tips intact | 500 g |
| 1 1/2 cups | frozen petite peas | 375 mL |
| 1/3 cup | minced fresh chives | 75 mL |
| 2 tbsp | freshly squeezed lemon juice | 30 mL |
| | Fine sea salt and freshly cracked black pepper | |
| 1/3 cup | freshly grated Parmesan cheese | 75 mL |

1. In a large pot, combine quinoa, broth and lemon zest. Bring to a boil over medium-high heat. Reduce heat to low, cover and simmer, stirring occasionally for 15 minutes.

2. Stir in asparagus and peas; simmer, uncovered, for 3 to 5 minutes or until quinoa and asparagus are tender. Stir in chives and lemon juice. Season to taste with salt and pepper. Serve sprinkled with cheese.

# Belgian Winter Vegetable Bisque

*This soup was inspired by stoemp, a Belgian dish of mashed potatoes with vegetables. As good as it is the day you make it, it is even better for lunch the day after.*

## Tip

When puréeing soup in a food processor or blender, fill the bowl no more than halfway full at a time.

## Storage Tip

Store the cooled soup in an airtight container in the refrigerator for up to 2 days or in the freezer for up to 6 months. Thaw overnight in the refrigerator or in the microwave using the Defrost function. Warm soup in a medium saucepan over medium-low heat.

- **Food processor, blender or immersion blender**

| | | |
|---|---|---|
| 1 tbsp | unsalted butter | 15 mL |
| 2½ cups | chopped onions | 625 mL |
| 1½ cups | chopped carrots | 375 mL |
| 1½ cups | chopped parsnips | 375 mL |
| 2 cups | diced peeled yellow-fleshed potatoes (such as Yukon gold) | 500 mL |
| ½ cup | quinoa flakes or quinoa flour | 125 mL |
| ½ tsp | ground nutmeg | 2 mL |
| 4 cups | ready-to-use reduced-sodium vegetable or chicken broth (GF, if needed) | 1 L |
| ½ cup | packed fresh flat-leaf (Italian) parsley, chopped | 125 mL |
| 1 | bottle (12 oz/341 mL) lager-style beer | 1 |
| | Fine sea salt and freshly ground black pepper | |

1. In a large pot, melt butter over medium-high heat. Add onions, carrots and parsnips; cook, stirring, for 7 to 9 minutes or until slightly softened.

2. Stir in potatoes, quinoa flakes, nutmeg and broth; bring to a boil. Reduce heat and simmer, stirring occasionally, for 25 to 30 minutes or until potatoes are very tender.

3. Working in batches, transfer soup to food processor (or use immersion blender in pot) and purée until smooth. Return soup to pot (if necessary) and whisk in parsley and beer. Simmer, stirring occasionally, for 10 minutes. Season to taste with salt and pepper.

# Country Captain Quinoa Soup

**Makes
6 servings**

*Country Captain is a classic Southern chicken stew long associated with Georgia. Some food historians contend that it made its way to Savannah — once an important port in the spice trade — via a British sea captain traveling from India. Although I've adapted it from a thick chicken stew to a vegetarian quinoa soup, I've kept many of the other traditional elements in place, including onions, garlic, bell peppers, curry, cayenne and a little sweetness from currants and brightness from tomatoes.*

## Storage Tip

Store the cooled soup in an airtight container in the refrigerator for up to 2 days or in the freezer for up to 6 months. Thaw overnight in the refrigerator or in the microwave using the Defrost function. Warm soup in a medium saucepan over medium-low heat.

| | | |
|---|---|---|
| 1 tbsp | olive oil | 15 mL |
| 2 cups | chopped onions | 500 mL |
| 1 | red bell pepper, chopped | 1 |
| 4 | cloves garlic, minced | 4 |
| 1½ tbsp | mild curry powder | 22 mL |
| 2 tsp | ground ginger | 10 mL |
| ¼ tsp | cayenne pepper | 1 mL |
| 1 | large tart apple (such as Granny Smith), peeled and chopped | 1 |
| 1 cup | quinoa, rinsed | 250 mL |
| 3 tbsp | dried currants or chopped raisins | 45 mL |
| 1 | can (28 oz/796 mL) diced tomatoes, with juice | 1 |
| 6 cups | ready-to-use reduced-sodium vegetable broth (GF, if needed) | 1.5 L |
| ½ cup | chopped fresh cilantro | 125 mL |
| | Fine sea salt and freshly ground black pepper | |
| ½ cup | plain yogurt | 125 mL |

1. In a large pot, heat oil over medium-high heat. Add onions and red pepper; cook, stirring, for 6 to 8 minutes or until softened. Add garlic, curry powder, ginger and cayenne; cook, stirring, for 30 seconds.

2. Stir in apple, quinoa, currants, tomatoes with juice and broth; bring to a boil. Reduce heat to low, cover and simmer, stirring occasionally, for 15 to 20 minutes or until quinoa is tender. Stir in cilantro. Season to taste with salt and black pepper. Serve dolloped with yogurt.

# Lentil and Quinoa Soup

*When a dark, chilly autumn afternoon portends the first freezing night of fall, I head to the kitchen and begin making a steaming pot of this soup for dinner.*

## Tip

When you're heating up leftovers of this soup, stir in a little water if it's too thick.

## Storage Tip

Store the cooled soup in an airtight container in the refrigerator for up to 2 days or in the freezer for up to 6 months. Thaw overnight in the refrigerator or in the microwave using the Defrost function. Warm soup in a medium saucepan over medium-low heat.

| | | |
|---|---|---|
| 4 | cloves garlic, minced | 4 |
| 2 cups | chopped onions | 500 mL |
| 2 cups | chopped carrots | 500 mL |
| 1 cup | chopped celery | 250 mL |
| 1½ cups | dried brown lentils, rinsed | 375 mL |
| 1 tbsp | dried Italian seasoning | 15 mL |
| 1 | can (28 oz/796 mL) crushed tomatoes | 1 |
| 8 cups | ready-to-use reduced-sodium chicken or vegetable broth (GF, if needed) | 2 L |
| 1 cup | quinoa, rinsed | 250 mL |
| 2 tbsp | balsamic vinegar | 30 mL |
| | Fine sea salt and freshly cracked black pepper | |

**1.** In a large pot, combine garlic, onions, carrots, celery, lentils, Italian seasoning, tomatoes and broth. Bring to a boil over medium-high heat. Reduce heat to low, cover and simmer, stirring occasionally, for 35 minutes.

**2.** Stir in quinoa, cover and simmer, stirring occasionally, for 15 to 20 minutes or until quinoa and lentils are tender. Stir in vinegar. Season to taste with salt and pepper.

# Indian-Spiced Split Pea and Quinoa Soup

*This stunning gold and red soup is positively addictive in the cold winter months: stick-to-the-ribs satisfying without being heavy, subtly spiced with coriander and bright with the finishing flavors of ginger, cilantro and yogurt. Each sip will bring the warmth of the Indian sun to mind.*

## Tip

Dried yellow lentils or green split peas may be used in place of the yellow split peas.

## Storage Tip

Store the cooled soup in an airtight container in the refrigerator for up to 3 days or in the freezer for up to 6 months. Thaw overnight in the refrigerator or in the microwave using the Defrost function. Warm soup in a medium saucepan over medium-low heat.

- **Food processor or blender**

### Soup

| | | |
|---|---|---|
| 1 tbsp | vegetable oil | 15 mL |
| 2 cups | chopped onions | 500 mL |
| 1½ cups | chopped carrots | 375 mL |
| 2 tsp | ground coriander | 10 mL |
| 1 cup | dried yellow split peas, rinsed | 250 mL |
| 7 cups | ready-to-use reduced-sodium chicken or vegetable broth (GF, if needed) | 1.75 L |
| ⅔ cup | red or white quinoa, rinsed | 150 mL |
| ¾ cup | water (approx.) | 175 mL |
| | Fine sea salt and freshly ground black pepper | |
| 1 cup | plain yogurt | 250 mL |

### Chutney

| | | |
|---|---|---|
| 1 | 1-inch (2.5 cm) piece gingerroot, roughly chopped | 1 |
| 1 cup | packed fresh cilantro leaves | 250 mL |
| 1 tbsp | freshly squeezed lime juice | 15 mL |
| 1 tbsp | toasted sesame oil | 15 mL |

1. *Soup:* In a large pot, heat oil over medium-high heat. Add onions, carrots and coriander; cook, stirring, for 6 to 8 minutes or until vegetables are softened.

2. Stir in peas and broth; bring to a boil. Reduce heat to low, cover and simmer, stirring occasionally, for 20 minutes. Stir in quinoa, cover and simmer for 15 to 20 minutes or until peas and quinoa are tender.

3. Transfer 2 cups (500 mL) of the soup solids to food processor. Add water and purée until smooth. Return purée to pot and simmer, uncovered, stirring often, for 5 minutes to blend the flavors, thinning soup with additional water if too thick. Season to taste with salt and pepper.

4. *Chutney:* In clean food processor, combine ginger, cilantro, lime juice and sesame oil; pulse until finely chopped.

5. Serve soup topped with chutney and dollops of yogurt.

# Black-Eyed Pea, Collard and Quinoa Soup

**Makes 8 servings**

*I like beans — a lot — but I love black-eyed peas. Also known as cow peas, they are thought to have originated in North Africa, where they have been eaten for centuries. Here, they pack a spicy broth with plenty of folate, while collard greens add vitamin A and onions contribute vitamin C.*

## Storage Tip

Store the cooled soup in an airtight container in the refrigerator for up to 2 days or in the freezer for up to 6 months. Thaw overnight in the refrigerator or in the microwave using the Defrost function. Warm soup in a medium saucepan over medium-low heat.

| | | |
|---|---|---|
| 2 tsp | vegetable oil | 10 mL |
| 2 cups | chopped onions | 500 mL |
| 1½ cups | chopped carrots | 375 mL |
| 1 cup | chopped celery | 250 mL |
| 1 tbsp | ground cumin | 15 mL |
| 2 tsp | dried thyme | 10 mL |
| ¼ tsp | cayenne pepper | 1 mL |
| 8 cups | chopped collard greens (tough stems and center ribs removed) | 2 L |
| ¾ cup | quinoa, rinsed | 175 mL |
| 8 cups | ready-to-use reduced-sodium chicken or vegetable broth (GF, if needed) | 2 L |
| 2 | cans (each 14 to 19 oz/398 to 540 mL) black-eyed peas, drained and rinsed | 2 |
| 1 tbsp | red wine vinegar or cider vinegar | 15 mL |
| | Fine sea salt and freshly ground black pepper | |

1. In a large pot, heat oil over medium-high heat. Add onions, carrots and celery; cook, stirring, for 6 to 8 minutes or until softened. Add cumin, thyme and cayenne; cook, stirring, for 30 seconds.

2. Stir in collard greens, quinoa and broth; bring to a boil. Reduce heat to low, cover and simmer, stirring occasionally, for 15 minutes. Stir in peas and vinegar; cover and simmer for 5 minutes or until quinoa is tender. Season to taste with salt and black pepper.

# Lemony Chickpea and Quinoa Soup

**Makes 6 servings**

*How could something so easy to make taste so complex? This little soup pulls it off, while packing in a slew of good-for-you ingredients, too.*

## Storage Tip

Store the cooled soup in an airtight container in the refrigerator for up to 2 days or in the freezer for up to 6 months. Thaw overnight in the refrigerator or in the microwave using the Defrost function. Warm soup in a medium saucepan over medium-low heat.

| | | |
|---|---|---|
| 2 tsp | extra virgin olive oil | 10 mL |
| 2 cups | chopped onions | 500 mL |
| 3 | cloves garlic, minced | 3 |
| 1 tbsp | dried Italian seasoning | 15 mL |
| ½ cup | quinoa, rinsed | 125 mL |
| 2 | cans (each 14 to 19 oz/398 to 540 mL) chickpeas, drained and rinsed | 2 |
| 8 cups | ready-to-use reduced-sodium chicken or vegetable broth (GF, if needed) | 2 L |
| 1 cup | packed fresh parsley leaves, chopped | 250 mL |
| 1 tsp | finely grated lemon zest | 5 mL |
| 3 tbsp | freshly squeezed lemon juice | 45 mL |
| | Fine sea salt and freshly ground black pepper | |
| ⅓ cup | freshly grated Parmesan cheese | 75 mL |

**1.** In a large pot, heat oil over medium-high heat. Add onions and cook, stirring, for 6 to 8 minutes or until softened. Add garlic and Italian seasoning; cook, stirring, for 1 minute.

**2.** Stir in quinoa, chickpeas and broth; bring to a boil. Reduce heat to medium-low, cover, leaving lid ajar, and simmer, stirring occasionally, for 15 to 20 minutes or until quinoa is tender. Stir in parsley, lemon zest and lemon juice. Season to taste with salt and pepper. Serve sprinkled with cheese.

# Quinoa Harira

*Hearty enough to satisfy
the biggest appetites, this
exotically spiced dish
is based on the North
African soup harira.
Harira is typically made
with rice, but in this
interpretation, quinoa
stands in as a modern
twist. The results are
spectacularly delicious,
especially on day two,
when the flavors have had
further chance to mingle.*

## Storage Tip

Store the cooled soup in
an airtight container in
the refrigerator for up to
2 days or in the freezer
for up to 6 months.
Thaw overnight in the
refrigerator or in the
microwave using the
Defrost function. Warm
soup in a medium
saucepan over
medium-low heat.

| | | |
|---|---|---|
| 1 tbsp | extra virgin olive oil | 15 mL |
| 2 cups | chopped onions | 500 mL |
| 1 tbsp | ground cumin | 15 mL |
| 2 tsp | ground ginger | 10 mL |
| ⅔ cup | dried brown lentils, rinsed | 150 mL |
| 1 | can (28 oz/796 mL) crushed tomatoes | 1 |
| 8 cups | ready-to-use reduced-sodium chicken or vegetable broth (GF, if needed) | 2 L |
| ⅔ cup | quinoa, rinsed | 150 mL |
| 1 | can (14 to 19 oz/398 to 540 mL) chickpeas, drained and rinsed | 1 |
| 1 cup | packed fresh cilantro leaves, chopped | 250 mL |
| 1 cup | packed fresh flat-leaf (Italian) parsley leaves, chopped | 250 mL |
| 1 tbsp | freshly squeezed lemon juice | 15 mL |
| | Fine sea salt and freshly ground black pepper | |

1. In a large pot, heat oil over medium-high heat. Add onions and cook, stirring, for 6 to 8 minutes or until softened. Add cumin and ginger; cook, stirring, for 30 seconds.
2. Stir in lentils, tomatoes and broth; bring to a boil. Reduce heat to low, cover, leaving lid ajar, and simmer for 30 minutes.
3. Stir in quinoa and chickpeas; cover, leaving lid ajar, and simmer, stirring occasionally, for 15 to 20 minutes or until lentils and quinoa are tender. Stir in cilantro, parsley and lemon juice. Season to taste with salt and pepper.

# Tortilla Quinoa Soup

*The flavors of Mexico
shine in this favorite
soup. With the addition
of some fresh, flavorful
toppings — tortilla chips,
avocado, cilantro and
yogurt — it's as beautiful
as it is darn good.*

## Storage Tip

Prepare soup through
step 2 and let cool. Store
in an airtight container in
the refrigerator for up to
2 days or in the freezer
for up to 6 months. Thaw
overnight in the refrigerator
or in the microwave
using the Defrost
function. Warm soup
in a medium saucepan
over medium-low heat.
Continue with step 3.

| | | |
|---|---|---:|
| 1 tbsp | olive oil | 15 mL |
| 1½ tbsp | chili powder | 22 mL |
| 1½ cups | frozen corn kernels | 375 mL |
| ⅔ cup | quinoa, rinsed | 150 mL |
| 2 | cans (each 10 oz/284 mL) diced tomatoes with chiles and garlic, with juice | 2 |
| 1 | can (14 to 19 oz/398 to 540 mL) black beans, drained and rinsed | 1 |
| 4 cups | ready-to-use reduced-sodium chicken or vegetable broth (GF, if needed) | 1 L |
| 2 cups | crushed tortilla chips, divided | 500 mL |
| 1 tbsp | freshly squeezed lime juice | 15 mL |
| | Fine sea salt and freshly ground black pepper | |
| ½ cup | packed fresh cilantro leaves | 125 mL |

**Suggested Accompaniments**

Plain Greek yogurt

Diced firm-ripe Hass avocado

Crumbled queso fresco

Thinly sliced radishes

1. In a large pot, heat oil over medium-high heat. Add chili powder and cook, stirring, for 30 to 60 seconds or until fragrant.

2. Stir in corn, quinoa, tomatoes with juice, beans and broth; bring to a boil. Reduce heat to low, cover and simmer, stirring occasionally, for 15 to 20 minutes or until quinoa is tender. Stir in 1 cup (250 mL) of the tortilla chips and simmer, uncovered, for 2 minutes or until softened. Stir in lime juice. Season to taste with salt and pepper.

3. Serve sprinkled with cilantro and the remaining chips, along with any of the suggested accompaniments, as desired.

# Jamaican Beans and Quinoa Soup

*Here's an incredibly easy soup interpretation of the accompaniment found at most Jamaican meals: rice and peas. Stepping in as understudies are red beans (a common option in place of pigeon peas) and quinoa, which create a new synergy in this cool-weather comfort-food dish.*

## Tip

To make the soup vegetarian, simply omit the bacon and use vegetable broth.

## Storage Tip

Store the cooled soup in an airtight container in the refrigerator for up to 3 days or in the freezer for up to 6 months. Thaw overnight in the refrigerator or in the microwave using the Defrost function. Warm soup in a medium saucepan over medium-low heat.

| | | |
|---|---|---|
| 2 | slices bacon, chopped | 2 |
| ¾ cup | quinoa, rinsed | 175 mL |
| 1 tsp | ground cumin | 5 mL |
| ½ tsp | ground allspice | 2 mL |
| 2 | cans (each 14 to 19 oz/398 to 540 mL) red beans, drained and rinsed | 2 |
| 4 cups | ready-to-use reduced-sodium chicken or vegetable broth (GF, if needed) | 1 L |
| 1½ cups | chunky hot salsa | 375 mL |
| ½ cup | packed fresh cilantro leaves, chopped | 125 mL |
| | Fine sea salt and freshly ground black pepper | |

1. In a large pot, cook bacon over medium-high heat, stirring, until crisp.
2. Stir in quinoa, cumin, allspice, beans, broth and salsa; bring to a boil. Reduce heat to low, cover and simmer for 15 to 20 minutes or until quinoa is tender. Stir in cilantro. Season to taste with salt and pepper.

## Variation

Reduce the broth to 3 cups (750 mL). Add 1 cup (250 mL) light coconut milk after the quinoa is cooked; simmer for 1 to 2 minutes to heat through.

# Quinoa e Fagioli

*Here, quinoa takes
the place of pasta in
an updated version of
pasta e fagioli. This
thick soup has "family
favorite" written all
over it. The simplicity
of the ingredients makes
it a dish that is fabulous
for a casual dinner at
home from early fall to
late winter.*

## Tip

If using the larger 19-oz
(540 mL) cans of beans,
you may want to add up
to ½ cup (125 mL) extra
broth to thin the soup.

## Storage Tip

Store the cooled soup in
an airtight container in
the refrigerator for up to
2 days or in the freezer
for up to 6 months.
Thaw overnight in the
refrigerator or in the
microwave using the
Defrost function. Warm
soup in a medium
saucepan over
medium-low heat.

| | | |
|---|---|---:|
| 1 tbsp | extra virgin olive oil | 15 mL |
| 2 cups | chopped onions | 500 mL |
| 1¼ cups | chopped celery | 300 mL |
| 1¼ cups | chopped carrots | 300 mL |
| 3 | cloves garlic, minced | 3 |
| 1 tbsp | dried Italian seasoning | 15 mL |
| 2 | cans (each 14 to 19 oz/398 to 540 mL) cannellini (white kidney) beans, drained and rinsed | 2 |
| ¾ cup | quinoa, rinsed | 175 mL |
| 1 | can (28 oz/796 mL) diced tomatoes, with juice | 1 |
| 6 cups | ready-to-use reduced-sodium chicken or vegetable broth (GF, if needed) | 1.5 L |
| | Fine sea salt and freshly ground black pepper | |
| ½ cup | packed fresh flat-leaf (Italian) parsley leaves, chopped | 125 mL |
| ¼ cup | freshly grated Parmesan cheese | 60 mL |

1. In a large pot, heat oil over medium-high heat. Add onions, celery and carrots; cook, stirring, for 6 to 8 minutes or until softened. Add garlic and Italian seasoning; cook, stirring, for 30 seconds.

2. In a small bowl, mash ½ cup (125 mL) of the beans with a fork. Stir mashed beans, whole beans, quinoa, tomatoes with juice and broth into the pot. Bring to a boil. Reduce heat to low, cover and simmer, stirring occasionally, for 15 to 20 minutes or until quinoa is tender. Remove from heat and let stand for 5 minutes. Stir in parsley. Season to taste with salt and pepper. Serve sprinkled with cheese.

# Kale and Quinoa Minestrone

**Makes 8 servings**

*Everyone needs a few recipes that meet the trifecta of busy weeknight meal requirements: easy, fast and fabulous. Add this soup, which is super-healthy to boot, to your pile.*

## Storage Tip

Store the cooled soup in an airtight container in the refrigerator for up to 2 days or in the freezer for up to 6 months. Thaw overnight in the refrigerator or in the microwave using the Defrost function. Warm soup in a medium saucepan over medium-low heat.

| 1 tbsp | extra virgin olive oil | 15 mL |
|---|---|---|
| 1½ cups | chopped onions | 375 mL |
| 1½ cups | chopped carrots | 375 mL |
| 1 cup | chopped celery | 250 mL |
| 4 | cloves garlic, minced | 4 |
| 8 cups | chopped kale (tough stems and center ribs removed) | 2 L |
| 1½ tbsp | dried Italian seasoning | 22 mL |
| ¾ cup | quinoa, rinsed | 175 mL |
| 1 | jar (26 oz/700 mL) marinara sauce | 1 |
| 8 cups | ready-to-use reduced-sodium vegetable or chicken broth (GF, if needed) | 2 L |
| 1 | can (14 to 19 oz/398 to 540 mL) white beans, drained and rinsed | 1 |
| | Fine sea salt and freshly ground black pepper | |

1. In a large pot, heat oil over medium-high heat. Add onions, carrots and celery; cook, stirring, for 6 to 8 minutes or until softened. Add garlic, kale and Italian seasoning; cook, stirring, for 1 minute.

2. Stir in quinoa, marinara sauce and broth; bring to a boil. Reduce heat, cover, leaving lid ajar, and simmer, stirring occasionally, for 20 minutes or until quinoa is tender.

3. In a small bowl, mash half the beans with a fork. Stir mashed beans and whole beans into the pot. Simmer, stirring occasionally, for 5 to 10 minutes or until soup is slightly thickened. Season to taste with salt and pepper.

# Tuscan White Bean Quinoa Soup

*Don't be misled by its plain-looking appearance: this newfangled version of Tuscan bean soup is thoroughly satisfying and delicious.*

## Storage Tip

Store the cooled soup in an airtight container in the refrigerator for up to 2 days or in the freezer for up to 6 months. Thaw overnight in the refrigerator or in the microwave using the Defrost function. Warm soup in a medium saucepan over medium-low heat.

| | | |
|---|---|---|
| 1 tbsp | extra virgin olive oil | 15 mL |
| 2 cups | chopped onions | 500 mL |
| 1½ cups | chopped carrots | 375 mL |
| 1½ cups | chopped celery | 375 mL |
| 4 | cloves garlic, minced | 4 |
| 1 tbsp | dried basil | 15 mL |
| ½ tsp | freshly cracked black pepper | 2 mL |
| 1 | can (14 to 15 oz/398 to 425 mL) diced tomatoes, with juice | 1 |
| 6 cups | ready-to-use reduced-sodium chicken or vegetable broth (GF, if needed) | 1.5 L |
| 2½ cups | water | 625 mL |
| 2 | cans (each 14 to 19 oz/398 to 540 mL) white beans, drained and rinsed | 2 |
| 1 cup | quinoa, rinsed | 250 mL |
| | Fine sea salt and freshly ground black pepper | |

1. In a large pot, heat oil over medium-high heat. Add onions, carrots and celery; cook, stirring, for 6 to 8 minutes or until softened. Add garlic and basil; cook, stirring, for 1 minute.

2. Stir in tomatoes with juice, broth and water; bring to a boil. Stir in beans. Reduce heat to low, cover and simmer, stirring occasionally, for 20 minutes.

3. Stir in quinoa. Cover and simmer, stirring occasionally, for 15 to 20 minutes or until quinoa is tender. Season to taste with salt and pepper.

# Edamame Succotash Soup

*I developed this soup in the depths of winter, when I was craving something soothing and hearty but fresh-tasting. The edamame cozies up to the sweet corn in a way that manages to be both new and familiar. Quinoa flakes take the place of cream to add a silky texture. And in case you were wondering, there is no cream in creamed corn (at least, not traditional or canned varieties).*

## Storage Tip

Store the cooled soup in an airtight container in the refrigerator for up to 2 days or in the freezer for up to 6 months. Thaw overnight in the refrigerator or in the microwave using the Defrost function. Warm soup in a medium saucepan over medium-low heat.

| | | |
|---|---|---|
| 2 | slices bacon, chopped | 2 |
| 1 | onion, chopped | 1 |
| 1½ cups | diced peeled yellow-fleshed potatoes (such as Yukon gold) | 375 mL |
| 2 tsp | dried basil | 10 mL |
| ½ tsp | freshly cracked black pepper | 2 mL |
| 5 cups | ready-to-use reduced-sodium vegetable or chicken broth (GF, if needed) | 1.25 L |
| 1½ cups | fresh or thawed frozen corn kernels | 375 mL |
| 1½ cups | frozen shelled edamame | 375 mL |
| ½ cup | quinoa flakes or quinoa flour | 125 mL |
| 1 | can (14 to 15 oz/398 to 425 mL) creamed corn | 1 |
| | Fine sea salt and freshly ground black pepper | |

1. In a large pot, cook bacon over medium-high heat, stirring, until crisp. Using a slotted spoon, transfer bacon to a plate lined with paper towels.

2. Add onion to the fat remaining in the pot and cook, stirring occasionally, for 5 to 6 minutes or until softened.

3. Stir in potatoes, basil, pepper and broth; bring to a boil. Reduce heat and simmer for 10 to 12 minutes or until potatoes are just tender. Stir in corn kernels, edamame, quinoa flakes and creamed corn; simmer for 7 to 9 minutes or until edamame are tender. Season to taste with salt and pepper. Serve sprinkled with bacon.

# Chinese Hot-and-Sour Quinoa Soup

*If you're looking for a fast yet flavorful soup full of the flavors of China, look no further. Quickly swirling the eggs with a chopstick as you add them to the hot broth causes them to form thin ribbons.*

## Storage Tip

Store the cooled soup in an airtight container in the refrigerator for up to 2 days. Warm in a medium saucepan over medium-low heat.

| | | |
|---|---|---:|
| 6 cups | ready-to-use reduced-sodium chicken or vegetable broth (GF, if needed) | 1.5 L |
| 2 tbsp | tamari or soy sauce (GF, if needed) | 30 mL |
| 2 tsp | ground ginger | 10 mL |
| 1 tsp | freshly ground black pepper | 5 mL |
| 8 oz | shiitake or button mushrooms, sliced | 250 g |
| ¾ cup | quinoa, rinsed | 175 mL |
| 2 tbsp | cornstarch | 30 mL |
| 3 tbsp | unseasoned rice vinegar or cider vinegar | 45 mL |
| 2 | large eggs, lightly beaten | 2 |
| 3 | green onions, thinly sliced | 3 |
| 1½ cups | diced drained soft or firm tofu (about 8 oz/250 g) | 375 mL |

1. In a large pot, combine broth, tamari, ginger and pepper. Bring to a boil over medium-high heat. Stir in mushrooms and quinoa. Reduce heat to low, cover and simmer, stirring occasionally, for 15 to 20 minutes or until quinoa is tender.

2. In a small bowl, whisk together cornstarch and vinegar. Stir into soup and simmer, stirring constantly, until thickened, about 1 minute.

3. Remove from heat and gradually pour in eggs, swirling in one direction with a chopstick or fork to create long strands. Stir in green onions and tofu. Cover and let stand for 2 minutes or until tofu is warmed through. Serve immediately.

# Miso Soup with Peas and Shiitakes

## Storage Tip

Store the cooled soup in an airtight container in the refrigerator for up to 2 days or in the freezer for up to 6 months. Thaw overnight in the refrigerator or in the microwave using the Defrost function. Warm soup in a medium saucepan over medium-low heat.

| | | |
|---|---|---|
| 8 oz | shiitake or button mushrooms, chopped | 250 g |
| 1 cup | red, black or white quinoa, rinsed | 250 mL |
| 6 cups | ready-to-use reduced-sodium chicken or vegetable broth (GF, if needed) | 1.5 L |
| 2 cups | sugar snap peas, thinly sliced on a diagonal | 500 mL |
| 3 tbsp | white or yellow miso | 45 mL |
| 1 tsp | unseasoned rice vinegar or cider vinegar | 5 mL |
| | Fine sea salt and freshly ground black pepper | |
| ½ cup | packed fresh basil leaves, thinly sliced into ribbons | 125 mL |

1. In a large pot, combine mushrooms, quinoa and broth. Bring to a boil over medium-high heat. Reduce heat to medium and cook, stirring occasionally, for 20 minutes.

2. Stir in peas, reduce heat and simmer, stirring, for 4 to 5 minutes or until just tender. Stir in miso and vinegar; simmer for 1 to 2 minutes to blend the flavors. Stir in basil. Season to taste with salt and pepper.

# Avgolemono Quinoa Soup

*Avgolemono is Greek for "egg-lemon" and is made with egg yolks and lemon juice mixed with broth, then heated until the mixture thickens but before it boils, so the egg doesn't curdle.*

## Storage Tip

Store the cooled soup in an airtight container in the refrigerator for up to 24 hours. Warm in a medium saucepan over medium-low heat.

| | | |
|---|---|---|
| ¾ cup | quinoa, rinsed | 175 mL |
| 8 cups | ready-to-use reduced-sodium chicken or vegetable broth (GF, if needed) | 2 L |
| 4 | large eggs, at room temperature | 4 |
| ⅓ cup | freshly squeezed lemon juice | 75 mL |
| ¼ cup | water | 60 mL |
| | Fine sea salt and freshly ground black pepper | |

1. In a medium saucepan, combine quinoa and broth. Bring to a boil over medium-high heat. Reduce heat to low, cover and simmer for 15 to 20 minutes or until quinoa is tender.

2. In a medium bowl, whisk together eggs, lemon juice and water. Gradually whisk in 1 cup (250 mL) of the hot broth. Gradually whisk egg mixture into the remaining quinoa mixture and simmer, stirring constantly, for 1 to 3 minutes or until steaming. Do not let boil. Season to taste with salt and pepper.

# Asparagus, Quinoa and Egg Soup

*A little butter, egg and fresh dill turn asparagus and quinoa into the best of friends in this salute-to-spring soup.*

## Tip

Once the eggs are added, be careful not to let the soup boil or the eggs may curdle.

## Storage Tip

Store the cooled soup in an airtight container in the refrigerator for up to 24 hours. Warm in a medium saucepan over medium-low heat.

| | | |
|---|---|---|
| 1 tbsp | unsalted butter | 15 mL |
| 2 cups | finely chopped onions | 500 mL |
| 1 cup | finely chopped celery | 250 mL |
| 1/2 cup | quinoa, rinsed | 125 mL |
| 6 cups | ready-to-use reduced-sodium vegetable or chicken broth (GF, if needed) | 1.5 L |
| 1 lb | asparagus, trimmed and cut into 1/4-inch (0.5 cm) pieces | 500 g |
| 2 | large eggs, at room temperature | 2 |
| 2 tbsp | minced fresh dill | 30 mL |
| 1/4 cup | freshly squeezed lemon juice | 60 mL |
| | Fine sea salt and freshly ground black pepper | |

1. In a large pot, melt butter over medium-high heat. Add onions and celery; cook, stirring, for 6 to 8 minutes or until softened.

2. Stir in quinoa and broth; bring to a boil. Reduce heat and simmer, stirring occasionally, for 14 minutes. Stir in asparagus and simmer, stirring once or twice, for 5 to 8 minutes or until quinoa is tender.

3. In a medium bowl, whisk eggs until well blended. Gradually whisk in about 2 cups (500 mL) of the hot soup. Gradually whisk egg mixture into the remaining soup and simmer, stirring constantly, for 2 to 3 minutes or until thickened. Do not let boil. Stir in dill and lemon juice. Season to taste with salt and pepper. Serve immediately.

# Pesci and Quinoa in Acqua Pazza

*Sophisticated and healthy, yet incredibly easy, this soup, whose name is Italian for "white fish in crazy water," brings the flavor of the Mediterranean to your table. The anchovy paste can be found in tubes where canned tuna is shelved. It's a convenient and frugal way to add tremendous flavor to soups such as this.*

## Tips

An equal amount of Asian fish sauce (GF, if needed) may be used in place of the anchovy paste.

For reasons of both convenience and frugality, consider using thawed frozen fish fillets in this recipe.

## Storage Tip

Store the cooled soup in an airtight container in the refrigerator for up to 24 hours. Warm in a medium saucepan over medium-low heat.

| | | |
|---|---|---|
| 1 tbsp | olive oil | 15 mL |
| 3 | cloves garlic, minced | 3 |
| 1 tbsp | Old Bay seasoning | 15 mL |
| 1 tsp | hot pepper flakes | 5 mL |
| 2 tsp | anchovy paste | 10 mL |
| ½ cup | dry white wine | 125 mL |
| ⅔ cup | quinoa, rinsed | 150 mL |
| 5 cups | ready-to-use reduced-sodium vegetable or chicken broth (GF, if needed) | 1.25 L |
| 1 cup | drained roasted red bell peppers, chopped | 250 mL |
| 3 tbsp | drained capers, roughly chopped | 45 mL |
| 1 lb | skinless cod, halibut or other white fish fillets, cut into 1-inch (2.5 cm) pieces | 500 g |
| 1 cup | packed fresh flat-leaf (Italian) parsley leaves, chopped | 250 mL |
| | Fine sea salt and freshly ground black pepper | |

1. In a large pot, heat oil over medium-high heat. Add garlic, Old Bay seasoning, hot pepper flakes and anchovy paste; cook, stirring, for 30 seconds. Add wine, scraping up any browned bits on bottom of pot.
2. Stir in quinoa and broth; bring to a boil. Reduce heat and simmer for 15 to 20 minutes or until quinoa is tender. Add roasted pepper and capers; return to a simmer.
3. Stir in cod, cover and simmer for about 5 minutes or until fish is opaque and flakes easily when tested with a fork. Stir in parsley. Season to taste with salt and black pepper.

# Manhattan Fish and Quinoa Chowder

*Unlike creamy New England chowder, Manhattan clam chowder (also known as Fulton Fish Market clam chowder) has clear broth, plus tomato for color and flavor. Food historians contend that the use of tomatoes in place of milk was initially the work of Portuguese immigrants in Rhode Island, as tomato-based stews were a traditional part of Portuguese cuisine. "Manhattan" chowder was a pejorative name given by scornful New Englanders to further distinguish the two types.*

## Storage Tip

Store the cooled soup in an airtight container in the refrigerator for up to 2 days or in the freezer for up to 6 months. Thaw overnight in the refrigerator or in the microwave using the Defrost function. Warm soup in a medium saucepan over medium-low heat.

| | | |
|---|---|---|
| 2 | slices bacon, chopped | 2 |
| 2 cups | chopped onions | 500 mL |
| 1½ cups | chopped carrots | 375 mL |
| ¾ cup | quinoa, rinsed | 175 mL |
| 1½ tsp | dried thyme | 7 mL |
| 2 | bottles (each 8 oz/227 mL) clam juice | 2 |
| 1 | can (28 oz/796 mL) crushed tomatoes | 1 |
| 2½ cups | water | 625 mL |
| ¼ cup | tomato paste (GF, if needed) | 60 mL |
| 1 lb | skinless tilapia fillets, cut into 2-inch (5 cm) pieces | 500 g |
| | Fine sea salt and freshly cracked black pepper | |

1. In a large pot, cook bacon over medium-high heat, stirring, until crisp. Add onions and carrots; cook, stirring occasionally, for 6 to 8 minutes or until softened.
2. Stir in quinoa, thyme, clam juice, tomatoes, water and tomato paste; bring to a boil. Reduce heat to low, cover and simmer, stirring occasionally, for 15 to 20 minutes or until quinoa is tender.
3. Add tilapia, cover and simmer for 2 to 3 minutes or until fish is opaque and flakes easily when tested with a fork. Season to taste with salt and pepper.

# Smoked Salmon Chowder

*Though easy enough for
a busy weeknight, this
soup is also a go-to dish
for entertaining: it has a
serious "wow" factor.*

## Tip

Be careful not to let the
soup boil once the milk
is added; keep the heat
low or the soup could
boil over.

## Storage Tip

Store the cooled soup
in an airtight container
in the refrigerator for up
to 24 hours. Warm in a
medium saucepan over
medium-low heat.

| | | |
|---|---|---:|
| 2 tsp | olive oil | 10 mL |
| 1½ cups | chopped onions | 375 mL |
| 1 cup | quinoa, rinsed | 250 mL |
| 3 cups | ready-to-use reduced-sodium chicken or vegetable broth (GF, if needed) | 750 mL |
| 3 cups | milk or plain non-dairy milk (such as soy, almond, rice or hemp) | 750 mL |
| 12 oz | skinless salmon fillet, cut into 1-inch (2.5 cm) pieces | 375 g |
| 4 oz | smoked salmon, finely chopped | 125 g |
| ¼ cup | chopped fresh dill | 60 mL |
| 2 tbsp | freshly squeezed lemon juice | 30 mL |
| | Fine sea salt and freshly ground black pepper | |

**1.** In a large pot, heat oil over medium-high heat. Add onions and cook, stirring, for 5 to 6 minutes or until softened.

**2.** Stir in quinoa and broth; bring to a boil. Reduce heat to low, cover and simmer, stirring occasionally, for 15 to 20 minutes or until quinoa is tender. Stir in milk and return to a simmer.

**3.** Stir in salmon fillet and smoked salmon; cover and simmer for 5 to 6 minutes or until salmon fillet is opaque and flakes easily when tested with a fork. Do not let boil. Stir in dill and lemon juice. Season to taste with salt and pepper.

# Shrimp and Quinoa Callaloo

*Also called pepper pot soup, this Jamaican dish has many guises and can be made with meats as well as fish and seafood. It dates back to the Arawak Indians, who prepared a stew that was kept going on the fire, with new ingredients added every day. I've kept this version simple, with shrimp, quinoa and a quick cooking time.*

## Storage Tip

Store the cooled soup in an airtight container in the refrigerator for up to 2 days. Warm in a medium saucepan over medium-low heat.

| | | |
|---|---|---|
| 1 | large sweet potato (about 1 lb/500 g), peeled and cut into 1/2-inch (1 cm) cubes | 1 |
| 2 cups | fresh or frozen sliced okra | 500 mL |
| 1 1/4 tsp | ground allspice | 6 mL |
| 3/4 tsp | dried thyme | 3 mL |
| 2 | cans (each 10 oz/284 mL) diced tomatoes with chiles, with juice | 2 |
| 5 cups | ready-to-use reduced-sodium vegetable or chicken broth (GF, if needed) | 1.25 L |
| 6 cups | chopped kale or collard greens (tough stems and center ribs removed) | 1.5 L |
| 2/3 cup | quinoa, rinsed | 150 mL |
| 12 oz | fresh or thawed frozen medium shrimp, peeled and deveined | 375 g |
| 1 cup | light coconut milk | 250 mL |
| 1 tbsp | freshly squeezed lime juice | 15 mL |
| | Fine sea salt and freshly ground black pepper | |

1. In a large pot, combine sweet potato, okra, allspice, thyme, tomatoes with juice and broth. Bring to a boil over medium-high heat. Reduce heat to low, cover and simmer for 10 minutes.

2. Stir in kale and quinoa; cover and simmer, stirring occasionally, for 15 to 20 minutes or until sweet potatoes, kale and quinoa are tender.

3. Stir in shrimp, coconut milk and lime juice; simmer, uncovered, for 3 to 5 minutes or until shrimp are pink, firm and opaque. Season to taste with salt and pepper.

# Easy Chicken Quinoa Soup

*An old-fashioned, ever-comforting favorite gets a newfangled twist, thanks to quinoa in place of the usual noodles or rice.*

## Storage Tip

Store the cooled soup in an airtight container in the refrigerator for up to 3 days or in the freezer for up to 6 months. Thaw overnight in the refrigerator or in the microwave using the Defrost function. Warm soup in a medium saucepan over medium-low heat.

| | | |
|---|---|---|
| 2 tsp | olive oil | 10 mL |
| 1 cup | chopped onions | 250 mL |
| 1 cup | chopped carrots | 250 mL |
| 1 cup | chopped celery | 250 mL |
| ½ tsp | freshly ground black pepper | 2 mL |
| 1 cup | quinoa, rinsed | 250 mL |
| 6 cups | ready-to-use reduced-sodium chicken or vegetable broth (GF, if needed) | 1.5 L |
| 2 cups | diced or shredded cooked chicken breast | 500 mL |
| | Fine sea salt and freshly ground black pepper | |
| 3 tbsp | chopped fresh flat-leaf (Italian) parsley | 45 mL |

1. In a large pot, heat oil over medium-high heat. Add onions, carrots, celery and pepper; cook, stirring, for 6 to 8 minutes or until vegetables are softened.
2. Stir in quinoa and broth; bring to a boil. Reduce heat to low, cover and simmer, stirring occasionally, for 15 to 20 minutes or until quinoa is tender.
3. Stir in chicken. Simmer, uncovered, for 5 minutes to heat through and blend the flavors. Season to taste with salt and pepper. Serve sprinkled with parsley.

# Florentine Chicken Quinoa Soup

*This beautiful soup is loaded with spinach, which earns the dish its name.*

## Storage Tip

Store the cooled soup in an airtight container in the refrigerator for up to 2 days. Warm in a medium saucepan over medium-low heat.

| | | |
|---|---|---|
| ⅔ cup | quinoa, rinsed | 150 mL |
| 1 | can (28 oz/796 mL) diced tomatoes, with juice | 1 |
| 4 cups | ready-to-use reduced-sodium chicken or vegetable broth (GF, if needed) | 1 L |
| 8 cups | packed baby spinach | 2 L |
| 2 cups | diced or shredded cooked chicken breast | 500 mL |
| ¼ cup | basil pesto | 60 mL |
| | Fine sea salt and freshly ground black pepper | |

1. In a medium saucepan, combine quinoa, tomatoes and broth. Bring to a boil over medium-high heat. Reduce heat to low, cover and simmer for 15 to 20 minutes or until quinoa is tender.
2. Stir in spinach, chicken and pesto; cover and simmer for 1 to 2 minutes or until chicken is hot and spinach is wilted. Season to taste with salt and pepper.

# Peruvian Chicken Sopa de Quinoa

*Variations of chicken and quinoa soup can be found throughout Peru, from street vendors and fine dining establishments alike. This version features several other New World ingredients: peanuts, potatoes, tomatoes and corn. The sum is a spectacular celebration of quinoa in a bowl.*

## Tip

If you have a peanut allergy, substitute another natural nut or seed butter, such as cashew, almond, sunflower or soybean.

## Storage Tip

Store the cooled soup in an airtight container in the refrigerator for up to 2 days or in the freezer for up to 6 months. Thaw overnight in the refrigerator or in the microwave using the Defrost function. Warm soup in a medium saucepan over medium-low heat.

| | | |
|---|---|---|
| 1 tbsp | unsalted butter | 15 mL |
| 1½ cups | chopped onions | 375 mL |
| 1½ cups | chopped carrots | 375 mL |
| 4 | cloves garlic, minced | 4 |
| 1 tbsp | ground cumin | 15 mL |
| 1 tsp | paprika | 5 mL |
| 1 | can (28 oz/796 mL) diced tomatoes, with juice | 1 |
| 6 cups | ready-to-use reduced-sodium chicken or vegetable broth (GF, if needed) | 1.5 L |
| ¼ cup | unsweetened natural peanut butter | 60 mL |
| 2 cups | diced peeled yellow-fleshed potatoes (such as Yukon gold) | 500 mL |
| 1½ cups | fresh or frozen corn kernels | 375 mL |
| ¾ cup | quinoa, rinsed | 175 mL |
| 2 cups | diced zucchini | 500 mL |
| 2 cups | shredded cooked chicken breast | 500 mL |
| 1 cup | packed fresh cilantro leaves, chopped | 250 mL |
| 2 tbsp | freshly squeezed lime juice | 30 mL |
| | Fine sea salt and freshly ground black pepper | |

1. In a large pot, melt butter over medium-high heat. Add onions and carrots; cook, stirring, for 6 to 8 minutes or until softened. Add garlic, cumin and paprika; cook, stirring, for 30 seconds.

2. Stir in tomatoes with juice, broth and peanut butter; bring to a boil. Stir in potatoes, corn and quinoa. Reduce heat to medium, cover, leaving lid ajar, and cook, stirring occasionally, for 15 minutes. Add zucchini and cook, stirring occasionally, for 10 to 15 minutes or until potatoes are very tender but not falling apart.

3. Stir in chicken, cilantro and lime juice; simmer for 5 minutes to heat through and blend the flavors. Season to taste with salt and pepper.

# Thai Chicken and Coconut Soup

*Why resort to takeout? This spicy coconut broth, brimming with quinoa and the flavors of Thailand, is a wonderful way to make chicken soup brand new.*

## Tip

An equal amount of mild or hot curry powder may be used in place of the curry paste. The flavor will be somewhat different and the spiciness will be more pronounced, but the result will be equally delicious.

| | | |
|---|---|---|
| 2 tsp | vegetable oil | 10 mL |
| 3 tbsp | minced gingerroot | 45 mL |
| 1 tbsp | Thai green curry paste | 15 mL |
| 5 cups | ready-to-use reduced-sodium chicken broth, divided | 1.25 L |
| 12 oz | boneless skinless chicken breasts (about 2 medium) | 375 g |
| 2/3 cup | quinoa, rinsed | 150 mL |
| 1 tbsp | natural cane sugar or packed light brown sugar | 15 mL |
| 1 tbsp | finely grated lime zest | 15 mL |
| 1½ cups | light coconut milk | 375 mL |
| ¼ cup | freshly squeezed lime juice | 60 mL |
| 2 tbsp | Asian fish sauce (GF, if needed) | 30 mL |
| | Fine sea salt and freshly ground black pepper | |
| ½ cup | packed fresh cilantro leaves | 125 mL |
| ½ cup | packed fresh basil leaves, thinly sliced | 125 mL |

1. In a large pot, heat oil over medium-high heat. Add ginger and curry paste; cook, stirring, for 30 seconds.

2. Stir in 2 cups (500 mL) of the broth and bring to a boil. Add chicken, reduce heat to medium-low, cover and simmer for 5 minutes or until chicken is no longer pink inside. Using tongs, transfer chicken to a cutting board and cut crosswise into thin strips.

3. Add quinoa, sugar, lime zest and the remaining broth to the pot. Increase heat to medium-high and bring to a boil. Reduce heat to low, cover and simmer for 15 to 20 minutes or until quinoa is tender.

4. Return chicken and any accumulated juices to the pot, along with coconut milk, lime juice and fish sauce. Simmer, uncovered, for 1 to 2 minutes. Season to taste with salt and pepper. Serve sprinkled with cilantro and basil.

## Variation

This soup is easily converted to a vegetarian dish: simply substitute vegetable broth for the chicken broth; 2 cups (500 mL) diced firm tofu for the chicken; and soy sauce (GF, if needed) for the fish sauce.

# Turkey Soup with Quinoa Dumplings

In this easy, versatile
recipe, leftover turkey is
transformed into a boast-
worthy soup. Tender
quinoa dumplings on
top will have everyone
running to the table.

## Tip

Before squeezing the
lemon juice for the soup,
note that you'll need
1 tbsp (15 mL) lemon zest
for the dumplings. It is
much easier to zest citrus
fruit before juicing it.

## Storage Tip

Store the cooled soup
in an airtight container
in the refrigerator for
up to 2 days. Warm in a
medium saucepan over
medium-low heat.

### Soup

| | | |
|---|---|---|
| 2 cups | thinly sliced carrots | 500 mL |
| 1¼ cups | thinly sliced celery | 300 mL |
| ½ tsp | dried thyme | 2 mL |
| 6 cups | ready-to-use reduced-sodium chicken broth (GF, if needed) | 1.5 L |
| 3 cups | diced or shredded cooked turkey or chicken breast | 750 mL |
| 2 tbsp | freshly squeezed lemon juice (see tip, at left) | 30 mL |
| | Fine sea salt and freshly ground black pepper | |

### Dumplings

| | | |
|---|---|---|
| ¾ cup | quinoa flour | 175 mL |
| ⅓ cup | yellow cornmeal | 75 mL |
| 1¼ tsp | baking powder (GF, if needed) | 6 mL |
| ½ tsp | fine sea salt | 2 mL |
| ½ cup | finely chopped green onions | 125 mL |
| 1 tbsp | finely grated lemon zest | 15 mL |
| 1 | large egg, lightly beaten | 1 |
| ¼ cup | milk or plain non-dairy milk (such as soy, almond, rice or hemp) | 60 mL |
| 2 tbsp | unsalted butter, melted | 30 mL |

1. *Soup:* In a large pot, combine carrots, celery, thyme and broth. Bring to a boil over medium-high heat. Reduce heat to low, cover and simmer for 8 to 10 minutes or until vegetables are just tender.

2. Stir in turkey and lemon juice; return to a simmer. Season to taste with salt and pepper.

3. *Dumplings:* Meanwhile, in a medium bowl, whisk together quinoa flour, cornmeal, baking powder and salt. Stir in green onions and lemon zest. Add egg, milk and butter, stirring just until a dough forms.

4. Roll dough into 1-inch (2.5 cm) balls. Add all at once to simmering broth. Cover and simmer, without stirring, for 18 to 20 minutes or until dumplings appear somewhat dry and are cooked through.

# Unstuffed Green Pepper Soup

**Makes
6 servings**

*I've recast the ingredients
from one of my favorite
comfort-food dinners —
stuffed green peppers —
in an extra-easy
weeknight soup. I could
eat this once a week,
every week, during the
chilly winter months.*

## Storage Tip

Store the cooled soup in
an airtight container in
the refrigerator for up to
2 days or in the freezer
for up to 6 months.
Thaw overnight in the
refrigerator or in the
microwave using the
Defrost function. Warm
soup in a medium
saucepan over
medium-low heat.

| | | |
|---|---|---|
| 2 tsp | olive oil | 10 mL |
| 12 oz | Italian turkey sausage (bulk or casings removed) | 375 g |
| 2 | green bell peppers, chopped | 2 |
| 1½ cups | chopped onions | 375 mL |
| 2 | zucchini, diced | 2 |
| ¾ cup | quinoa, rinsed | 175 mL |
| 1 tbsp | dried Italian seasoning | 15 mL |
| 1 | can (14 to 19 oz/398 to 540 mL) white beans, drained and rinsed | 1 |
| 1 | jar (26 oz/700 mL) marinara sauce | 1 |
| 4 cups | ready-to-use reduced-sodium chicken or vegetable broth (GF, if needed) | 1 L |
| | Fine sea salt and freshly ground black pepper | |
| ⅔ cup | crumbled feta cheese | 150 mL |

1. In a large pot, heat oil over medium-high heat. Add sausage and cook, breaking it up with a spoon, for 3 to 5 minutes or until no longer pink. Drain off any excess fat. Add green peppers and onions; cook, stirring, for 6 to 8 minutes or until softened.

2. Stir in zucchini, quinoa, Italian seasoning, beans, marinara sauce and broth; bring to a boil. Reduce heat to low, cover and simmer, stirring occasionally, for 15 to 20 minutes or until quinoa is tender. Season to taste with salt and pepper. Serve sprinkled with cheese.

# Sausage, White Bean and Quinoa Soup

*Tiny curlicues of quinoa hold their own in this sausage, bean and vegetable soup. No need to make any sides: this is a definitive one-bowl meal.*

## Storage Tip

Store the cooled soup in an airtight container in the refrigerator for up to 3 days or in the freezer for up to 6 months. Thaw overnight in the refrigerator or in the microwave using the Defrost function. Warm soup in a medium saucepan over medium-low heat.

| | | |
|---|---|---|
| 2 tsp | olive oil | 10 mL |
| 1 lb | Italian turkey sausage (bulk or casings removed) | 500 g |
| 1½ cups | chopped onions | 375 mL |
| 1½ cups | chopped carrots | 375 mL |
| 3 | cloves garlic, minced | 3 |
| 1 tbsp | dried basil | 15 mL |
| ¼ tsp | freshly ground black pepper | 1 mL |
| 1 cup | quinoa, rinsed | 250 mL |
| 1 | can (14 to 19 oz/398 to 540 mL) white beans, drained and rinsed | 1 |
| 1 | can (28 oz/796 mL) diced tomatoes, with juice | 1 |
| 6 cups | ready-to-use reduced-sodium chicken or vegetable broth (GF, if needed) | 1.5 L |
| 8 cups | packed baby spinach | 2 L |
| | Fine sea salt and freshly ground black pepper | |
| | Freshly grated Parmesan cheese (optional) | |

1. In a large pot, heat oil over medium-high heat. Add sausage and cook, breaking it up with a spoon, for 3 to 5 minutes or until no longer pink. Drain off any excess fat. Add onions and carrots; cook, stirring, for 6 to 8 minutes or until softened. Add garlic and basil; cook, stirring, for 1 minute.

2. Stir in quinoa, beans, tomatoes and broth; bring to a boil. Reduce heat to low, cover and simmer, stirring occasionally, for 15 to 20 minutes or until quinoa is tender. Stir in spinach and simmer, stirring constantly, for 1 to 2 minutes or until wilted. Season to taste with salt and pepper. Serve sprinkled with cheese, if using.

# Ancho Chile Quinoa, Pork and Hominy Soup

*A wonderful assortment of ingredients and flavors — hominy, quinoa, pork, ancho chile and oregano — gives this soup Southwestern style and spice. Each element is terrific, but it's the hominy that steals the show.*

## Tip

Hominy (also called pozole) consists of big, chewy kernels of dried corn that are soaked in slaked lime to remove their hull and germ.

## Storage Tip

Store the cooled soup in an airtight container in the refrigerator for up to 3 days or in the freezer for up to 6 months. Thaw overnight in the refrigerator or in the microwave using the Defrost function. Warm soup in a medium saucepan over medium-low heat.

| | | |
|---|---|---:|
| 2 tbsp | ancho chile powder | 30 mL |
| 2 tsp | dried oregano | 10 mL |
| 2 tsp | ground cumin | 10 mL |
| 1 tsp | fine sea salt | 5 mL |
| ¼ tsp | cayenne pepper | 1 mL |
| 1 lb | pork tenderloin, trimmed and cut into ¼-inch (0.5 cm) cubes | 500 g |
| 4 tsp | olive oil, divided | 20 mL |
| 1½ cups | chopped onions | 375 mL |
| 3 | cloves garlic, minced | 3 |
| 2 cups | frozen corn kernels | 500 mL |
| 1 cup | quinoa, rinsed | 250 mL |
| 1 | can (28 oz/796 mL) diced tomatoes, with juice | 1 |
| 1 | can (15 oz/425 mL) white hominy, drained | 1 |
| 6 cups | ready-to-use reduced-sodium beef or vegetable broth (GF, if needed) | 1.5 L |
| | Fine sea salt and freshly ground black pepper | |

1. In a medium bowl, combine chile powder, oregano, cumin, salt and cayenne. Set aside 1 tbsp (15 mL) of the spice mixture. Add pork to the remaining spice mixture, tossing to coat.
2. In a large pot, heat half the oil over medium-high heat. Add pork and cook, stirring, for 4 to 6 minutes or until browned on all sides. Using a slotted spoon, transfer pork to a plate.
3. Add the remaining oil to the pot. Add onions and cook, stirring, for 3 to 5 minutes or until softened. Add garlic and cook, stirring, for 1 minute.
4. Stir in corn, quinoa, the reserved spice mixture, tomatoes, hominy and broth; bring to a boil. Reduce heat to low, cover and simmer, stirring occasionally, for 15 to 20 minutes or until quinoa is tender. Season to taste with salt and black pepper.

# Puerto Rican Pigeon Pea and Ham Soup

*Peas are staples at the Puerto Rican table, and this soup is at once pull-out-the-stops-special and everyday.*

## Storage Tip

Store the cooled soup in an airtight container in the refrigerator for up to 3 days or in the freezer for up to 6 months. Thaw overnight in the refrigerator or in the microwave using the Defrost function. Warm soup in a medium saucepan over medium-low heat.

| | | |
|---|---|---|
| 1 | sweet potato (about 12 oz/375 g), peeled and cut into 1/4-inch (0.5 cm) cubes | 1 |
| 2/3 cup | quinoa, rinsed | 150 mL |
| 2 tsp | dried oregano | 10 mL |
| 1 tsp | ground cumin | 5 mL |
| 4 cups | ready-to-use reduced-sodium vegetable or chicken broth (GF, if needed) | 1 L |
| 1 cup | diced lean ham | 250 mL |
| 2 | cans (each 14 to 19 oz/398 to 540 mL) black-eyed peas, drained and rinsed | 2 |
| 2 | cans (each 10 oz/284 mL) diced tomatoes with chiles, with juice | 2 |
| 1 tbsp | red wine vinegar | 15 mL |
| | Fine sea salt and freshly ground black pepper | |
| | Fresh cilantro leaves and/or chopped green onions (optional) | |

1. In a large pot, combine sweet potato, quinoa, oregano, cumin and broth. Bring to a boil over medium-high heat. Reduce heat to low, cover and simmer for 15 to 20 minutes or until sweet potato and quinoa are tender.

2. Stir in ham, peas and tomatoes with juice; simmer, uncovered, for 3 to 4 minutes to blend the flavors. Stir in vinegar. Season to taste with salt and pepper. Serve sprinkled with cilantro and/or green onions, if desired.

# Cajun Quinoa Soup

**Makes
6 servings**

*This beautiful soup features a classic combination of Cajun flavors with a modern twist: quinoa in place of traditional long-grain rice. Though lightened to be healthier, it is still rich and zesty.*

## Storage Tip

Store the cooled soup in an airtight container in the refrigerator for up to 3 days or in the freezer for up to 6 months. Thaw overnight in the refrigerator or in the microwave using the Defrost function. Warm soup in a medium saucepan over medium-low heat.

| 2 tsp | olive oil | 10 mL |
|---|---|---|
| 1 | large red bell pepper, chopped | 1 |
| 1 cup | chopped onions | 250 mL |
| 4 | cloves garlic, minced | 4 |
| 2 tsp | dried thyme | 10 mL |
| 2 cups | fresh or frozen sliced okra | 500 mL |
| 1 cup | quinoa, rinsed | 250 mL |
| 2 | cans (each 10 oz/284 mL) diced tomatoes with chiles, with juice | 2 |
| 6 cups | ready-to-use reduced-sodium vegetable or chicken broth (GF, if needed) | 1.5 L |
| 8 oz | reduced-fat smoked sausage, diced | 250 g |
| | Fine sea salt and freshly ground black pepper | |

1. In a large pot, heat oil over medium-high heat. Add red pepper and onions; cook, stirring, for 6 to 8 minutes or until softened. Add garlic and thyme; cook, stirring, for 30 seconds.

2. Stir in okra, quinoa, tomatoes with juice and broth; bring to a boil. Reduce heat to low, cover and simmer, stirring occasionally, for 15 to 20 minutes or until quinoa is tender.

3. Stir in sausage and simmer, uncovered, for 3 to 5 minutes to warm through and blend the flavors. Season to taste with salt and pepper.

# Chinese Seared Beef Soup

**Makes
6 servings**

*This soup will draw
you in every time: the
clean flavors of napa
cabbage, carrots and
bean sprouts accentuate
the seared beef and play
off the earthiness of the
mushrooms and quinoa.*

## Tip

In a pinch, an equal
amount of shredded
coleslaw mix (shredded
cabbage and carrots) can
be used in place of the
napa cabbage.

## Storage Tip

Store the cooled soup
in an airtight container
in the refrigerator for up
to 24 hours. Warm in a
medium saucepan over
medium-low heat.

| | | |
|---|---|---|
| 1 lb | boneless beef sirloin steak, trimmed and patted dry with paper towels | 500 g |
| | Fine sea salt and freshly ground black pepper | |
| 4 tsp | vegetable oil, divided | 20 mL |
| 1 lb | mushrooms, sliced | 500 g |
| 1 cup | quinoa, rinsed | 250 mL |
| 8 cups | ready-to-use reduced-sodium beef or vegetable broth (GF, if needed) | 2 L |
| 3 tbsp | tamari or soy sauce (GF, if needed) | 45 mL |
| 1 tbsp | unseasoned rice vinegar or cider vinegar | 15 mL |
| 2 tsp | Asian chili-garlic sauce | 10 mL |
| 4 cups | thinly sliced napa cabbage (about $1/2$ head) | 1 L |
| 2 cups | pre-cut matchstick-style carrots | 500 mL |
| 1 cup | bean sprouts | 250 mL |
| $1/2$ cup | thinly sliced green onions | 125 mL |

### Suggested Accompaniments

Fresh cilantro leaves

Additional Asian chili-garlic sauce

Toasted sesame oil

1. Generously season beef on both sides with salt and pepper. In a large pot, heat half the oil over medium-high heat. Add beef and cook, without moving, for 3 to 4 minutes or until seared brown. Turn beef and sear for 3 to 4 minutes or until browned. Remove beef to a cutting board and tent with foil.

2. Add the remaining oil to the pot. Add mushrooms and cook, stirring and scraping up any browned bits, for 3 to 5 minutes or until tender.

3. Stir in quinoa, broth, tamari, vinegar and chili-garlic sauce; bring to a boil. Reduce heat and simmer for 15 to 20 minutes or until quinoa is tender. Season to taste with salt and pepper. Remove from heat and stir in cabbage, carrots, bean sprouts and green onions.

4. Cut beef diagonally across the grain into very thin slices. Ladle soup into bowls and top with sliced beef. Garnish with any of the suggested accompaniments, as desired.

# Quinoa Pho

*In Vietnam, people are
fiercely loyal to their
favorite pho bo. After a
taste of this quick quinoa
version (in which quinoa
replaces the traditional
rice noodles), you may
feel that same sense
of loyalty.*

## Tips

For best results, select
a deli roast beef that
does not have additional
flavorings (such as Italian
herbs or barbecue
seasoning).

For a more traditional
noodle pho, replace the
quinoa with 8 oz (250 g)
quinoa spaghetti, broken.
Add where the quinoa was
added in step 1 and boil,
stirring once or twice, for
6 to 8 minutes or until al
dente. Proceed as directed.

## Storage Tip

Store the cooled soup
(without the roast beef
and toppings) in an
airtight container in the
refrigerator for up to
2 days. Warm in a medium
saucepan over medium-
low heat. Serve as directed
in step 2.

| | | |
|---|---|---|
| 2 tbsp | finely grated gingerroot | 30 mL |
| 1 tbsp | natural cane sugar or packed light brown sugar | 15 mL |
| 3 cups | ready-to-use reduced-sodium chicken broth (GF, if needed) | 750 mL |
| 3 cups | water | 750 mL |
| 2 tbsp | Asian fish sauce or soy sauce (GF, if needed) | 30 mL |
| 1 cup | quinoa, rinsed | 250 mL |
| 2 tbsp | freshly squeezed lime juice | 30 mL |
| | Fine sea salt and freshly ground black pepper | |
| 8 oz | sliced deli roast beef, halved crosswise and cut lengthwise into 1-inch (2.5 cm) strips | 250 g |
| 1 cup | bean sprouts | 250 mL |
| 1 cup | packed fresh basil leaves, sliced | 250 mL |
| ½ cup | packed fresh cilantro leaves | 125 mL |
| ½ cup | chopped green onions | 125 mL |

1. In a large pot, combine ginger, sugar, broth, water and fish sauce. Bring to a boil over medium-high heat. Add quinoa, reduce heat to low, cover and simmer, stirring once or twice, for 15 to 20 minutes or until quinoa is tender. Stir in lime juice. Season to taste with salt and pepper.

2. Divide roast beef among four bowls. Ladle hot soup over top. Top with bean sprouts, basil, cilantro and green onions.

### Variation

This soup is easily converted to a vegetarian dish: simply use vegetable broth in place of the chicken broth and replace the roast beef with 8 oz (250 g) firm tofu or tempeh (GF, if needed), diced.

# Quinoa Scotch Broth

*Here, a Scottish classic —
hearty, meaty Scotch
broth — is retrofitted for
light, healthy, anytime
eating. Using ground
lamb instead of lamb stew
meat drastically cuts both
the fat and the overall
cooking time.*

## Storage Tip

Store the cooled soup in
an airtight container in
the refrigerator for up to
2 days or in the freezer
for up to 6 months.
Thaw overnight in the
refrigerator or in the
microwave using the
Defrost function. Warm
soup in a medium
saucepan over
medium-low heat.

| | | |
|---|---|---|
| 12 oz | lean ground lamb | 375 g |
| 2 cups | chopped onions | 500 mL |
| 2 cups | chopped carrots | 500 mL |
| 6 cups | chopped kale or collard greens (tough stems and center ribs removed) | 1.5 L |
| ¾ cup | quinoa, rinsed | 175 mL |
| 1 | bottle (12 oz/341 mL) lager-style beer (GF, if needed) | 1 |
| 4 cups | ready-to-use reduced-sodium beef or vegetable broth (GF, if needed) | 1 L |
| 1 tbsp | malt vinegar or cider vinegar | 15 mL |
| | Fine sea salt and freshly ground black pepper | |

1. In a large pot, cook lamb over medium-high heat, breaking it up with a spoon, for 3 to 5 minutes or until no longer pink. Drain off any excess fat. Add onions and carrots; cook, stirring, for 6 to 8 minutes or until softened.

2. Stir in kale, quinoa, beer and broth; bring to a boil. Reduce heat to low, cover and simmer, stirring occasionally, for 15 to 20 minutes or until quinoa is tender. Stir in vinegar. Season to taste with salt and pepper.

# Sweet Potato, Quinoa and Edamame Zosui

*Zosui is a thick Japanese porridge typically made with leftover rice. Not unlike a risotto, it is often studded with chicken or pork and a smattering of tender, bite-size vegetables — in sum, it's everything a comfort food should be. I've taken the essential idea and run with it, replacing the rice with quinoa and forgoing meat in favor of sweet potatoes and edamame. A quick ginger and green onion relish adds the perfect complementary zing.*

## Storage Tip

Store the cooled soup, without the relish, in an airtight container in the refrigerator for up to 3 days. Warm in a medium saucepan over medium-low heat.

### Zosui

| | | |
|---|---|---|
| 2 tsp | toasted sesame oil | 10 mL |
| 1 | red bell pepper, cut into 1-inch (2.5 cm) pieces | 1 |
| 1½ cups | chopped onions | 375 mL |
| 3 cups | cubed peeled sweet potatoes (½-inch/1 cm cubes) | 750 mL |
| 1 cup | quinoa, rinsed | 250 mL |
| ¼ tsp | freshly cracked black pepper | 1 mL |
| 4 cups | water | 1 L |
| 2 cups | ready-to-use reduced-sodium vegetable or chicken broth (GF, if needed) | 500 mL |
| 1½ cups | frozen shelled edamame | 375 mL |
| 3 tbsp | white or yellow miso | 45 mL |
| | Fine sea salt and freshly ground black pepper | |

### Relish

| | | |
|---|---|---|
| 1 tbsp | vegetable oil | 15 mL |
| 1 cup | minced green onions | 250 mL |
| 3 tbsp | minced fresh gingerroot | 45 mL |
| ⅛ tsp | fine sea salt | 0.5 mL |
| 1 tsp | unseasoned rice vinegar or cider vinegar | 5 mL |

**1.** *Zosui:* In a large pot, heat oil over medium-high heat. Add red pepper and onions; cook, stirring, for 6 to 8 minutes or until softened.

**2.** Stir in sweet potatoes, quinoa, pepper, water and broth; bring to a boil. Reduce heat and simmer for 15 minutes or until sweet potatoes are just tender. Stir in edamame and simmer for 8 to 10 minutes or until sweet potatoes are very tender. Remove from heat and stir in miso. Season to taste with salt and pepper.

**3.** *Relish:* In a small saucepan, heat oil over medium-high heat. Add green onions, ginger and salt; cook, stirring, for about 1 minute or until onions are wilted but still bright green. Stir in vinegar.

**4.** Serve zosui in bowls, dolloped with relish.

# African Quinoa and Groundnut Stew

*This vegetarian showstopper will bowl you over with its layers of flavor — with one bite you'll understand why groundnut stews are heralded in West African cuisine. And while quinoa is a non-traditional addition, it's a sensible one given that seeds in general (especially varieties of millet) are central to West African cooking. The result is a dish with wonderful texture and flavor and a beguiling complexity.*

## Storage Tip

Store the cooled stew in an airtight container in the refrigerator for up to 3 days. Warm in a medium saucepan over medium-low heat.

| | | |
|---|---|---|
| ¼ cup | minced fresh chives or green onions | 60 mL |
| 1 cup | plain Greek yogurt | 250 mL |
| 2 tsp | vegetable oil | 10 mL |
| 1¼ cups | thinly sliced onions | 300 mL |
| ¾ cup | chopped red bell pepper | 175 mL |
| 3 | cloves garlic, minced | 3 |
| 1 cup | chopped unsalted dry-roasted peanuts | 250 mL |
| ½ tsp | hot pepper flakes | 2 mL |
| 4 cups | diced peeled sweet potatoes (about 1½ lbs/750 g) | 1 L |
| 1 | can (28 oz/796 mL) diced tomatoes, with juice | 1 |
| 3 cups | ready-to-use reduced-sodium vegetable broth (GF, if needed) | 750 mL |
| 4 cups | hot cooked quinoa (see page 10) | 1 L |
| | Fine sea salt and freshly ground black pepper | |

1. In a small bowl, combine chives and yogurt; cover and refrigerate until ready to use.
2. In a large pot, heat oil over medium-high heat. Add onions and red pepper; cook, stirring, for 6 to 8 minutes or until softened. And garlic and cook, stirring, for 1 minute. Stir in peanuts and hot pepper flakes.
3. Stir in sweet potatoes, tomatoes with juice and broth; bring to a boil. Reduce heat to low, cover and simmer, stirring occasionally, for 35 to 40 minutes or until sweet potatoes are just tender. Uncover and simmer, stirring occasionally, for 15 to 20 minutes or until thickened and sweet potatoes are very tender. Season to taste with salt and black pepper.
4. Divide quinoa among six bowls and ladle stew over top. Top with dollops of yogurt mixture.

# Winter Quinoa Stew with Swiss Chard

*This is one of my favorite mid-winter stews, a hearty concoction that relies on readily available winter vegetables.*

## Tip

An equal amount of white beans may be used in place of the butter beans.

## Storage Tip

Store the cooled stew in an airtight container in the refrigerator for up to 3 days or in the freezer for up to 6 months. Thaw overnight in the refrigerator or in the microwave using the Defrost function. Warm stew in a medium saucepan over medium-low heat.

| | | |
|---|---|---|
| 1 tbsp | olive oil | 15 mL |
| 1½ cups | chopped onions | 375 mL |
| 1½ cups | chopped fennel bulb (about 1 large bulb), fronds reserved | 375 mL |
| 1 cup | chopped Swiss chard stems | 250 mL |
| 2 | cloves garlic, finely chopped | 2 |
| 3 cups | diced peeled yellow-fleshed potatoes (such as Yukon gold) | 750 mL |
| 1 | can (28 oz/796 mL) diced tomatoes, with juice | 1 |
| 8 cups | ready-to-use reduced-sodium vegetable or chicken broth (GF, if needed) | 2 L |
| 4 cups | packed coarsely chopped Swiss chard leaves | 1 L |
| 2 | cans (each 14 to 19 oz/398 to 540 mL) butter beans, drained and rinsed | 2 |
| 1 tbsp | red wine vinegar | 15 mL |
| | Fine sea salt and freshly ground black pepper | |
| 4 cups | hot cooked quinoa (see page 10) | 1 L |
| ½ cup | crumbled goat cheese | 125 mL |

1. In a large pot, heat oil over medium-high heat. Add onions, chopped fennel bulb and Swiss chard stems; cook, stirring, for 6 to 8 minutes or until vegetables are softened. Add garlic and cook, stirring, for 30 seconds.

2. Stir in potatoes, tomatoes with juice and broth; bring to a boil. Reduce heat to low, cover and simmer, stirring occasionally, for 25 to 30 minutes or until potatoes are tender. Stir in Swiss chard leaves and beans; cover and simmer for 5 minutes or until greens are wilted. Stir in vinegar. Season to taste with salt and pepper.

3. Meanwhile, finely chop the reserved fennel fronds.

4. Divide quinoa among six bowls and ladle stew over top. Sprinkle with goat cheese and fennel fronds.

# Gingered Lentil Stew with Jalapeño Quinoa

*Steeping ginger and curry powder in the broth as the lentils cook is a quick way to achieve depth of flavor. The stew is spooned over spicy, herbed quinoa and enriched with yogurt, cucumbers and a number of optional add-ons. Best of all, this satisfying meal is easy enough to pull together after work.*

## Tip

For a spicier dish, leave in some or all of the jalapeño seeds.

## Storage Tip

Store the cooled stew in an airtight container in the refrigerator for up to 3 days or in the freezer for up to 6 months. Thaw overnight in the refrigerator or in the microwave using the Defrost function. Warm stew in a medium saucepan over medium-low heat.

| | | |
|---|---|---|
| 1 | 2-inch (5 cm) piece gingerroot, minced | 1 |
| 2 cups | dried red lentils, rinsed | 500 mL |
| 1 tbsp | mild yellow curry powder | 15 mL |
| 7½ cups | ready-to-use reduced-sodium vegetable or chicken broth (GF, if needed), divided | 1.875 L |
| | Fine sea salt and freshly ground black pepper | |
| 1¼ cups | quinoa, rinsed | 300 mL |
| 1½ tbsp | minced seeded jalapeño pepper | 22 mL |
| ¾ cup | packed fresh cilantro leaves, chopped | 175 mL |
| 1 cup | plain Greek yogurt | 250 mL |
| 1 cup | diced peeled seedless cucumber | 250 mL |

### Suggested Accompaniments

Mango chutney

Chopped fresh mint

Thinly sliced green onions

Chopped radishes

1. In a large pot, combine ginger, lentils, curry powder and 5 cups (1.25 L) of the broth. Bring to a boil over medium heat. Reduce heat to medium-low, cover, leaving lid ajar, and simmer, stirring occasionally, for 15 to 20 minutes or until lentils are tender. Season to taste with salt and pepper.

2. Meanwhile, in a medium saucepan, combine quinoa, jalapeño and the remaining broth. Bring to a boil over medium-high heat. Reduce heat to low, cover and simmer for 12 to 15 minutes or until liquid is absorbed. Remove from heat and let stand, covered, for 5 minutes. Stir in cilantro, fluffing quinoa with a fork.

3. Divide quinoa among six bowls and ladle stew over top. Garnish with yogurt, cucumber, and any of the suggested accompaniments, as desired.

# Mushroom, Miso and Butternut Squash Stew

*Thanks to a few simple additions — miso, mushrooms and leafy kale — this butternut squash stew has real verve. Served over hot quinoa, it is comfort in a bowl. Best of all, the dish requires little more than a brief sauté and simmer.*

## Storage Tip

Store the cooled stew in an airtight container in the refrigerator for up to 2 days or in the freezer for up to 6 months. Thaw overnight in the refrigerator or in the microwave using the Defrost function. Warm stew in a medium saucepan over medium-low heat.

| | | |
|---|---|---|
| 1 tbsp | extra virgin olive oil | 15 mL |
| 1 | butternut squash (about 2 lbs/1 kg), peeled and cut into 1-inch (2.5 cm) cubes | 1 |
| 1 lb | cremini or button mushrooms, sliced | 500 g |
| 2 cups | chopped onions | 500 mL |
| 4 cups | ready-to-use reduced-sodium vegetable or chicken broth (GF, if needed) | 1 L |
| 3 tbsp | yellow or white miso | 45 mL |
| 1 | large bunch kale, tough stems and center ribs removed, leaves very thinly sliced crosswise (about 6 cups/1.5 L) | 1 |
| 2 | cans (each 14 to 19 oz/398 to 540 mL) white beans, drained and rinsed | 2 |
| | Fine sea salt and freshly ground black pepper | |
| 4 cups | hot cooked quinoa (see page 10) | 1 L |
| | Asian chili-garlic sauce (optional) | |

1. In a large pot, heat oil over medium-high heat. Add squash, mushrooms and onions; cook, stirring, for 12 to 15 minutes or until squash is slightly softened.

2. Stir in broth and miso; bring to a boil. Reduce heat to low, cover and simmer, stirring occasionally, for 15 to 20 minutes or until squash is tender.

3. Stir in kale and beans; cover and simmer, stirring occasionally, for 5 to 6 minutes or until kale is wilted. Season to taste with salt and pepper.

4. Divide quinoa among eight bowls and ladle stew over top. Drizzle with chili-garlic sauce, if desired.

# Lemon Fennel Fish and Quinoa Stew

*This sensational spin on simple fish stew is made even better with a few innovative additions: delicate quinoa, fresh lemon and the subtle licorice flavor of fennel. Frozen fish fillets make it easy enough for a harried weeknight.*

## Tip

For reasons of both convenience and frugality, consider using thawed frozen fish fillets in this recipe.

## Storage Tip

Store the cooled stew in an airtight container in the refrigerator for up to 1 day. Warm in a medium saucepan over medium-low heat.

| | | |
|---|---|---:|
| 2 tsp | extra virgin olive oil | 10 mL |
| 1½ cups | chopped onions | 375 mL |
| 1½ cups | chopped fennel bulb (about 1 large bulb), fronds reserved | 375 mL |
| 3 | cloves garlic, minced | 3 |
| ⅔ cup | quinoa, rinsed | 150 mL |
| 1 | can (28 oz/796 mL) diced tomatoes, with juice | 1 |
| 2 cups | ready-to-use reduced-sodium chicken or vegetable broth (GF, if needed) | 500 mL |
| 1 lb | skinless cod or halibut fillets, cut into 1-inch (2.5 cm) pieces | 500 g |
| 2 tsp | finely grated lemon zest | 10 mL |
| 2 tbsp | freshly squeezed lemon juice | 30 mL |
| | Fine sea salt and freshly ground black pepper | |

1. In a large pot, heat oil over medium-high heat. Add onions and chopped fennel; cook, stirring, for 7 to 8 minutes or until softened. Add garlic and cook, stirring, for 30 seconds.

2. Stir in quinoa, tomatoes with juice and broth; bring to a boil. Reduce heat to low, cover and simmer for 15 minutes.

3. Stir in cod and lemon zest; cover and simmer for about 5 minutes or until quinoa is tender and fish is opaque and flakes easily when tested with a fork.

4. Meanwhile, chop enough of the reserved fennel fronds to measure ¼ cup (60 mL). Stir fennel fronds and lemon juice into stew. Season to taste with salt and pepper.

# Chicken, Quinoa and Green Olive Stew

*Mediterranean flavors shine in this comforting fall stew. Final additions of briny green olives and a flurry of orange zest lend bright bursts of flavor.*

## Storage Tip

Store the cooled stew in an airtight container in the refrigerator for up to 2 days or in the freezer for up to 6 months. Thaw overnight in the refrigerator or in the microwave using the Defrost function. Warm stew in a medium saucepan over medium-low heat.

| | | |
|---|---|---|
| 5 cups | ready-to-use reduced-sodium chicken or vegetable broth (GF, if needed) | 1.25 L |
| 2 lbs | boneless skinless chicken thighs | 1 kg |
| 1 tbsp | olive oil | 15 mL |
| 2 cups | chopped onions | 500 mL |
| 3 | cloves garlic, minced | 3 |
| 2 tsp | chili powder | 10 mL |
| 2 tsp | ground cumin | 10 mL |
| 1 tsp | ground coriander | 5 mL |
| 1 tsp | dried oregano | 5 mL |
| ½ cup | quinoa, rinsed | 125 mL |
| 1 | can (14 to 19 oz/398 to 540 mL) chickpeas, drained and rinsed | 1 |
| 1 | can (14 to 15 oz/398 to 425 mL) diced tomatoes, with juice | 1 |
| 1 cup | small pimento-stuffed green olives | 250 mL |
| 1 tbsp | finely grated orange zest | 15 mL |
| | Fine sea salt and freshly ground black pepper | |

1. In a large pot, bring broth to a boil over medium-high heat. Add chicken, reduce heat to low, cover and simmer for 15 to 20 minutes or until no longer pink inside. Transfer chicken to a plate. Pour broth into a large bowl and set aside. Wipe out pot.

2. In the same pot, heat oil over medium-high heat. Add onions and cook, stirring, for 6 to 8 minutes or until softened. Add garlic, chili powder, cumin, coriander and oregano; cook, stirring, for 1 minute.

3. Add quinoa and the reserved broth; bring to a boil. Reduce heat to low, cover and simmer for 15 minutes.

4. Meanwhile, shred the chicken. Return chicken and any accumulated juices to the pot, along with chickpeas, tomatoes with juice, olives and orange zest. Simmer, uncovered, stirring often, for 5 minutes to heat through and blend the flavors. Season to taste with salt and pepper.

# Portuguese Sausage and Kale Stew

**Makes 8 servings**

*Here's a streamlined version of caldo verde, a Portuguese stew served frequently in Brazil. It's often served over a scoop of hot cooked rice; I contend that nutty quinoa makes it all the better.*

## Tip

For 4 cups (1 L) diced potatoes, you'll need about 2¼ lbs (1.125 kg).

## Storage Tip

Store the cooled stew in an airtight container in the refrigerator for up to 2 days. Warm in a medium saucepan over medium-low heat.

| | | |
|---|---|---|
| 4 tsp | olive oil, divided | 20 mL |
| 12 oz | reduced-fat smoked sausage, halved lengthwise and thinly sliced | 375 g |
| 2 cups | chopped onions | 500 mL |
| 4 | cloves garlic, minced | 4 |
| 1 | sweet potato (about 12 oz/375 g), peeled and cut into ½-inch (1 cm) cubes | 1 |
| 4 cups | diced peeled yellow-fleshed potatoes (such as Yukon gold) | 1 L |
| 6 cups | ready-to-use reduced-sodium vegetable or chicken broth (GF, if needed) | 1.5 L |
| 1 | large bunch kale, tough stems and center ribs removed, leaves very thinly sliced crosswise (about 6 cups/1.5 L) | 1 |
| | Fine sea salt and freshly ground black pepper | |
| 4 cups | hot cooked quinoa (see page 10) | 1 L |

1. In a large pot, heat half the oil over medium-high heat. Add sausage and cook, stirring, for 3 to 5 minutes or until browned. Using a slotted spoon, transfer sausage to a plate lined with paper towels.

2. Add the remaining oil to the pot. Add onions and cook, stirring, for 6 to 8 minutes or until softened. Add garlic and cook, stirring, for 30 seconds.

3. Stir in sweet potato, potatoes and broth; bring to a boil. Reduce heat and simmer for 20 to 25 minutes or until sweet potatoes and potatoes are just tender. Using a potato masher, roughly mash half of the potatoes in the pot.

4. Stir in sausage and kale; simmer, stirring occasionally, for 10 to 15 minutes or until kale is wilted. Season to taste with salt and pepper.

5. Divide quinoa among eight bowls and ladle stew over top.

# Green Chile Quinoa Pozole

*With its notes of garlic, cumin and cilantro playing off the gentle spice of jalapeño, this meatless pozole combines the best parts of a chili and a soup. Its rich body — in large part thanks to the quinoa and hominy — makes it a seriously satisfying dinner any night of the week.*

## Storage Tip

Store the cooled pozole in an airtight container in the refrigerator for up to 3 days or in the freezer for up to 6 months. Thaw overnight in the refrigerator or in the microwave using the Defrost function. Warm pozole in a medium saucepan over medium-low heat.

• **Food processor**

| | | |
|---|---|---|
| 2 | cans (each 12 oz/340 mL) whole tomatillos, with juice | 2 |
| 2 tsp | vegetable oil | 10 mL |
| 2 cups | chopped onions | 500 mL |
| 4 | cloves garlic, minced | 4 |
| 1 tbsp | minced seeded jalapeño pepper | 15 mL |
| 1 tbsp | ground cumin | 15 mL |
| 1 cup | quinoa, rinsed | 250 mL |
| 1 cup | packed fresh cilantro leaves, chopped, divided | 250 mL |
| 2 | cans (each 15 oz/425 mL) yellow hominy, drained | 2 |
| 3 cups | ready-to-use reduced-sodium vegetable or chicken broth (GF, if needed) | 750 mL |
| | Fine sea salt and freshly ground black pepper | |
| | Crumbled queso fresco (optional) | |
| | Lime wedges (optional) | |

1. In food processor, purée tomatillos and their juice. Set aside.
2. In a large pot, heat oil over medium-high heat. Add onions and cook, stirring, for 6 to 8 minutes or until softened. Add garlic, jalapeño and cumin; cook, stirring, for 1 minute.
3. Stir in tomatillo purée, quinoa, half the cilantro, hominy and broth; bring to a boil. Reduce heat to medium-low, cover, leaving lid ajar, and simmer, stirring occasionally, for 15 to 20 minutes or until quinoa is tender. Season to taste with salt and pepper. Serve sprinkled with the remaining cilantro and queso fresco (if using), with lime wedges on the side, if desired.

# Moroccan Squash and Quinoa Chili

*This North African chili includes an easily assembled laundry list of sensational flavors and textures, including tender quinoa and velvety butternut squash, as well as a bevy of spices that have been staples in Morocco for generations. The ensemble is cooked in one pot, then topped with flavorful accompaniments for extra oomph. Sound easy and delicious? That's because it is.*

## Storage Tip

Store the cooled chili in an airtight container in the refrigerator for up to 2 days or in the freezer for up to 6 months. Thaw overnight in the refrigerator or in the microwave using the Defrost function. Warm chili in a medium saucepan over medium-low heat.

| | | |
|---|---|---|
| 2 tsp | extra virgin olive oil | 10 mL |
| 1 | large red bell pepper, finely chopped | 1 |
| 1½ cups | chopped onions | 375 mL |
| 1½ cups | chopped carrots | 375 mL |
| 4 | cloves garlic, minced | 4 |
| 3 cups | diced butternut squash | 750 mL |
| 3 tbsp | chili powder | 45 mL |
| 1 tbsp | ground cumin | 15 mL |
| 1 tbsp | ground coriander | 15 mL |
| 2 tsp | ground cinnamon | 10 mL |
| 1 cup | quinoa, rinsed | 250 mL |
| ½ cup | golden raisins | 125 mL |
| 3 | cans (each 14 to 19 oz/398 to 540 mL) chickpeas, drained and rinsed | 3 |
| 1 | can (28 oz/796 mL) crushed tomatoes | 1 |
| 3 cups | ready-to-use reduced-sodium vegetable or chicken broth (GF, if needed) | 750 mL |
| | Fine sea salt and freshly ground black pepper | |

**Suggested Accompaniments**

Plain Greek yogurt

Chopped kalamata olives

Chopped fresh cilantro or mint

1. In a large pot, heat oil over medium-high heat. Add red pepper, onions and carrots; cook, stirring, for 8 to 10 minutes or until softened. Add garlic, squash, chili powder, cumin, coriander and cinnamon; cook, stirring, for 2 minutes.

2. Stir in quinoa, raisins, chickpeas, tomatoes and broth; bring to a boil. Reduce heat to medium-low, cover, leaving lid ajar, and simmer, stirring occasionally, for 30 minutes. Season to taste with salt and pepper. Serve garnished with any of the suggested accompaniments, as desired.

# Black Bean Quinoa Chipotle Chili

*No one will ask, "Where's the beef?" when sampling this incredibly delicious vegetarian dish. Simmering hearty black beans and quinoa with onions, garlic, herbs and spices creates a wonderfully complex chili that's finished with fresh lime and topped off with tangy yogurt and an assortment of fresh flourishes.*

## Tip

If using the larger 19-oz (540 mL) cans of beans, you may want to add up to ½ cup (125 mL) vegetable broth or water to thin the chili.

## Storage Tip

Store the cooled chili in an airtight container in the refrigerator for up to 2 days or in the freezer for up to 6 months. Thaw overnight in the refrigerator or in the microwave using the Defrost function. Warm chili in a medium saucepan over medium-low heat.

| | | |
|---|---|---:|
| 2 tsp | vegetable oil | 10 mL |
| 2 cups | chopped onions | 500 mL |
| 4 | cloves garlic, minced | 4 |
| 3 tbsp | chili powder | 45 mL |
| 1½ tbsp | ground cumin | 22 mL |
| 2 tsp | dried oregano | 10 mL |
| 1½ tsp | chipotle chile powder | 7 mL |
| 3 | cans (each 14 to 19 oz/398 to 540 mL) black beans, drained and rinsed | 3 |
| 1 cup | quinoa, rinsed | 250 mL |
| 1 | can (28 oz/796 mL) crushed tomatoes | 1 |
| 3 cups | ready-to-use reduced-sodium vegetable or chicken broth (GF, if needed) | 750 mL |
| 1 tbsp | finely grated lime zest | 15 mL |
| ¼ cup | freshly squeezed lime juice | 60 mL |
| | Fine sea salt and freshly ground black pepper | |
| 1 cup | plain Greek yogurt | 250 mL |

### Suggested Accompaniments

Fresh cilantro leaves
Chopped green onions
Chopped radishes
Crumbled queso fresco

1. In a large pot, heat oil over medium-high heat. Add onions and cook, stirring, for 6 to 8 minutes or until softened. Add garlic, chili powder, cumin, oregano and chipotle chile powder; cook, stirring, for 1 minute.

2. In a small bowl, coarsely mash one-third of the beans with a potato masher or fork. Stir mashed beans, whole beans, quinoa, tomatoes and broth into the pot. Bring to a boil. Reduce heat and simmer, stirring often, for about 30 minutes to blend the flavors. Stir in lime zest and lime juice. Season to taste with salt and pepper. Serve topped with yogurt and any of the suggested accompaniments, as desired.

# Hominy Quinoa Red Pork Chili

*An ample amount of chili powder and tomatoes gives the broth a stunning brick-red color, and oregano and cumin contribute authentic Mexican flavor to this streamlined chili. Ground pork, quinoa, hominy and a touch of smoky bacon make the chili hearty without being heavy.*

## Storage Tip

Store the cooled chili in an airtight container in the refrigerator for up to 2 days or in the freezer for up to 6 months. Thaw overnight in the refrigerator or in the microwave using the Defrost function. Warm chili in a medium saucepan over medium-low heat.

| | | |
|---|---|---|
| 2 | slices bacon, chopped | 2 |
| 1½ cups | chopped onions | 375 mL |
| 4 | cloves garlic, minced | 4 |
| ¼ cup | chili powder | 60 mL |
| 1 tbsp | ground cumin | 15 mL |
| 2 tsp | dried oregano | 10 mL |
| 1 lb | extra-lean ground pork | 500 g |
| ¼ cup | tomato paste (GF, if needed) | 60 mL |
| ¾ cup | quinoa, rinsed | 175 mL |
| 1 | can (28 oz/796 mL) crushed tomatoes | 1 |
| 2 | cans (each 15 oz/425 mL) yellow hominy, drained and rinsed | 2 |
| 3 cups | ready-to-use reduced-sodium vegetable or chicken broth (GF, if needed) | 750 mL |
| | Fine sea salt and freshly ground black pepper | |

**Suggested Accompaniments**

Chopped green onions

Plain Greek yogurt

Crumbled queso fresco

1. In a large pot, cook bacon over medium-high heat, stirring, until crisp. Add onions and cook, stirring, for 5 to 6 minutes or until softened. Add garlic, chili powder, cumin and oregano; cook, stirring, for 1 minute. Add pork and tomato paste; cook, breaking pork up with a spoon, for 7 to 10 minutes or until pork is no longer pink.

2. Stir in quinoa, tomatoes, hominy and broth; bring to a boil. Reduce heat to medium-low, cover, leaving lid ajar, and simmer, stirring occasionally, for 15 to 20 minutes or until quinoa is tender and chili is slightly thickened. Season to taste with salt and pepper. Serve with any of the suggested accompaniments, as desired.

# Black-Eyed Pea and Smoked Sausage Chili

*This Louisiana-inspired chili resonates with the deep notes of tomato, garlic and thyme. Black-eyed peas and smoked sausage are natural components, but it's the generous amount of parsley added at the end that's the real revelation, adding a zesty top note. A bed of hot cooked quinoa to soak up all of the flavorful juices completes the picture.*

## Storage Tip

Store the cooled chili in an airtight container in the refrigerator for up to 2 days or in the freezer for up to 6 months. Thaw overnight in the refrigerator or in the microwave using the Defrost function. Warm chili in a medium saucepan over medium-low heat.

| | | |
|---|---|---|
| 2 tsp | vegetable oil | 10 mL |
| 8 oz | reduced-fat smoked sausage, chopped | 250 g |
| 1 | red bell pepper, chopped | 1 |
| 2 cups | chopped onions | 500 mL |
| 4 | cloves garlic, minced | 4 |
| 2 tbsp | chili powder | 30 mL |
| 1 tbsp | ground cumin | 15 mL |
| 2 tsp | dried thyme | 10 mL |
| ¼ tsp | cayenne pepper | 1 mL |
| 3 | cans (each 14 to 19 oz/398 to 540 mL) black-eyed peas, drained and rinsed | 3 |
| 2 | cans (each 10 oz/284 mL) diced tomatoes with chiles, with juice | 2 |
| 1 cup | water | 250 mL |
| ¾ cup | packed fresh flat-leaf (Italian) parsley leaves, chopped | 175 mL |
| 2 tbsp | red wine vinegar | 30 mL |
| | Fine sea salt and freshly ground black pepper | |
| 4 cups | hot cooked quinoa (see page 10) | 1 L |

1. In a large pot, heat oil over medium-high heat. Add sausage, red pepper and onions; cook, stirring, for 7 to 8 minutes or until vegetables are softened. Add garlic, chili powder, cumin, thyme and cayenne; cook, stirring, for 1 minute.

2. In a small bowl, coarsely mash half the peas with a potato masher or fork. Stir mashed peas, whole peas, tomatoes with juice and water into the pot. Bring to a boil. Reduce heat to medium-low, cover, leaving lid ajar, and simmer, stirring occasionally, for 10 to 15 minutes or until slightly thickened. Stir in parsley and vinegar; simmer, uncovered, for 2 minutes. Season to taste with salt and black pepper.

3. Divide quinoa among eight bowls and ladle chili over top.

# Salads and Sides

# Spiced Lentil, Quinoa and Currant Salad

*French green lentils are prized for their meaty texture and deep green color. Here, they work in harmony with quinoa, currants and a spiced vinaigrette to produce a sophisticated salad that is equally at home as a Meatless Monday main dish or as the starring dish at a dinner party.*

## Tip

Regular brown lentils may be used if green lentils are unavailable.

| | | |
|---|---|---|
| 3 cups | water | 750 mL |
| ¾ cup | dried green lentils, rinsed | 175 mL |
| 2 cups | cooked quinoa (see page 10), cooled | 500 mL |
| 4 cups | packed arugula | 1 L |
| ½ cup | dried currants or chopped raisins | 125 mL |
| 2 | cloves garlic, minced | 2 |
| 1 tsp | hot smoked paprika | 5 mL |
| 1 tsp | ground coriander | 5 mL |
| ½ tsp | ground cumin | 2 mL |
| ½ tsp | ground cinnamon | 2 mL |
| 3 tbsp | extra virgin olive oil | 45 mL |
| 2 tbsp | sherry vinegar or white wine vinegar | 30 mL |
| 1 tbsp | liquid honey or agave nectar | 15 mL |
| | Fine sea salt and freshly cracked black pepper | |

1. In a medium saucepan, bring water to a boil over high heat. Add lentils, reduce heat and simmer for about 30 minutes or until tender but not mushy. Drain and let cool completely.

2. In a large bowl, combine lentils, quinoa, arugula and currants.

3. In a small bowl, whisk together garlic, paprika, coriander, cumin, cinnamon, oil, vinegar and honey. Add to lentil mixture and gently toss to coat. Season to taste with salt and pepper.

# Warm Red Lentil, Quinoa and Eggplant Salad

*Here, red lentils —
which cook in about
half the time of brown
lentils — combine with
meaty eggplant and nutty
quinoa for a hearty main
dish that is guaranteed
to enhance your salad
repertoire.*

## Tip

Lentils are members of the
protein-rich legume family.
They are high in fiber and
complex carbohydrates
and relatively low in fat.
They offer a substantial
amount of vitamins A
and B, as well as calcium,
and are a particularly
good source of iron and
phosphorous.

| | | |
|---|---|---|
| 1 cup | dried red lentils, rinsed | 250 mL |
| 5 cups | ready-to-use reduced-sodium vegetable or chicken broth (GF, if needed), divided | 1.25 L |
| 1 cup | quinoa, rinsed | 250 mL |
| 2 tbsp | extra virgin olive oil | 30 mL |
| 1½ cups | chopped onions | 375 mL |
| 1 | large eggplant, trimmed and diced (about 3 cups/750 mL) | 1 |
| 1 tsp | ground cumin | 5 mL |
| ¼ cup | tomato paste (GF, if needed) | 60 mL |
| 2 tbsp | freshly squeezed lemon juice | 30 mL |
| | Fine sea salt and freshly cracked black pepper | |
| ½ cup | plain Greek yogurt | 125 mL |
| 1 | cucumber, peeled, seeded and diced | 1 |
| 1 cup | chopped tomato | 250 mL |
| ½ cup | packed fresh mint leaves, chopped | 125 mL |

1. In a medium saucepan, combine lentils and 3½ cups (875 mL) of the broth. Bring to a boil over medium-high heat. Reduce heat and simmer for 10 minutes. Stir in quinoa, cover and cook over low heat for 12 to 15 minutes or until liquid is absorbed. Remove from heat and let stand, covered, for 5 minutes. Fluff with a fork and transfer to a large bowl. Let cool.

2. Meanwhile, in a large nonstick skillet, heat oil over medium-high heat. Add onions and cook, stirring, for 5 to 6 minutes or until softened. Add eggplant and cook, stirring, for 2 minutes.

3. Stir in cumin, tomato paste and the remaining broth; bring to a boil. Reduce heat and simmer, stirring occasionally, for 15 to 20 minutes or until eggplant is very soft. Remove from heat and stir into lentil mixture. Let cool slightly, then stir in lemon juice. Season to taste with salt and pepper.

4. Divide lentil mixture among shallow bowls. Dollop with yogurt and sprinkle with cucumber, tomato and mint.

# Greek Quinoa Salad

*This hearty quinoa salad features a medley of classic Greek flavors, including cucumber, tomato, feta, brine-cured olives and fresh dill. To make the salad even more main-dish-worthy, I've added a can of chickpeas.*

## Tip

If you don't have fresh dill on hand, you can substitute 2 tsp (10 mL) dried dillweed.

| | | |
|---|---|---|
| 3 cups | cooked black or white quinoa (see page 10), cooled | 750 mL |
| 1 | cucumber, peeled, seeded and cubed | 1 |
| 1 | red bell pepper, chopped | 1 |
| 1 cup | halved grape or cherry tomatoes | 250 mL |
| ⅔ cup | finely chopped red onion | 150 mL |
| ⅔ cup | coarsely crumbled feta cheese | 150 mL |
| ½ cup | pitted brine-cured black olives (such as kalamata), roughly chopped | 125 mL |
| 1 | can (14 to 19 oz/398 to 540 mL) chickpeas, drained and rinsed | 1 |
| 2 tbsp | chopped fresh dill | 30 mL |
| 3 tbsp | red wine vinegar | 45 mL |
| 3 tbsp | extra virgin olive oil | 45 mL |
| 1 tsp | Dijon mustard | 5 mL |
| | Fine sea salt and freshly cracked black pepper | |

1. In a large bowl, combine quinoa, cucumber, red pepper, tomatoes, red onion, cheese, olives and chickpeas.

2. In a small bowl, whisk together dill, vinegar, oil and mustard. Add to quinoa mixture and gently toss to coat. Season to taste with salt and pepper. Cover and refrigerate for at least 30 minutes, until chilled, or for up to 2 hours.

# Green Pea and Quinoa Salad

*This elegant quinoa salad, with pungent radishes, sweet-tender peas and nutty chickpeas, is the perfect option for hot summer nights: cool, yet eminently satisfying.*

**Tip**

One 15-oz (425 mL) can of chickpeas or beans, drained and rinsed, yields about 1⅔ cups (400 mL).

| | | |
|---|---|---|
| 3 cups | cooked quinoa (see page 10), cooled | 750 mL |
| 2 cups | frozen petite peas, thawed | 500 mL |
| 1 cup | chopped red radishes | 250 mL |
| 1⅔ cups | rinsed drained canned chickpeas | 400 mL |
| ⅓ cup | buttermilk | 75 mL |
| 1 tbsp | extra virgin olive oil | 15 mL |
| 1 tbsp | white wine vinegar | 15 mL |
| ½ cup | crumbled feta cheese | 125 mL |
| ¼ cup | chopped fresh dill | 60 mL |
| | Fine sea salt and freshly cracked black pepper | |

1. In a large bowl, combine quinoa, peas, radishes and chickpeas.
2. In a small bowl, whisk together buttermilk, oil and vinegar. Stir in cheese and dill. Add to quinoa mixture and gently toss to coat. Season to taste with salt and pepper. Cover and refrigerate for at least 30 minutes, until chilled, or for up to 2 hours.

# Quinoa and Black Bean Salad

*With black beans, tomatoes, cumin and cilantro, this quick quinoa salad takes a delectable Tex-Mex detour.*

**Tip**

This salad is especially attractive made with red quinoa, but any variety will do.

| | | |
|---|---|---|
| 3 cups | cooked quinoa (see page 10), cooled | 750 mL |
| 2 cups | chopped tomatoes | 500 mL |
| ½ cup | thinly sliced green onions | 125 mL |
| ½ cup | packed fresh cilantro leaves, chopped | 125 mL |
| 1⅔ cups | rinsed drained canned black beans | 400 mL |
| 2 tsp | ground cumin | 10 mL |
| 3 tbsp | extra virgin olive oil | 45 mL |
| 2 tsp | finely grated lime zest | 10 mL |
| 2 tbsp | freshly squeezed lime juice | 30 mL |
| 1 tsp | agave nectar or liquid honey | 5 mL |
| | Fine sea salt and freshly cracked black pepper | |

1. In a large bowl, combine quinoa, tomatoes, green onions, cilantro and beans.
2. In a small bowl, whisk together cumin, oil, lime zest, lime juice and agave nectar. Add to quinoa mixture and gently toss to coat. Season to taste with salt and pepper. Cover and refrigerate for at least 30 minutes, until chilled, or for up to 4 hours.

# Sweet Potato, Quinoa and Black Bean Salad

**Makes 4 main-dish servings**

*These sweet potatoes caramelize slightly in the oven, which gives them a sweet crunch even as their flesh remains creamy. Quinoa and black beans balance their sweetness while making this dish supper-worthy, and a lime dressing lends addictive acid and tart notes.*

- **Preheat oven to 400°F (200°C)**
- **Large rimmed baking sheet, lined with foil and sprayed with nonstick cooking spray**

| | | |
|---|---|---|
| 1 lb | sweet potatoes, peeled and cut into ½-inch (1 cm) cubes | 500 g |
| 3 tbsp | extra virgin olive oil, divided | 45 mL |
| 1 tbsp | chili powder | 15 mL |
| | Fine sea salt and freshly cracked black pepper | |
| 1½ cups | cooked quinoa (see page 10), cooled slightly | 375 mL |
| 1 | large red bell pepper, chopped | 1 |
| ½ cup | thinly sliced green onions | 125 mL |
| 1 | can (14 to 19 oz/398 to 540 mL) black beans, drained and rinsed | 1 |
| 1 tbsp | ground cumin | 15 mL |
| 3 tbsp | freshly squeezed lime juice | 45 mL |
| 1 tbsp | liquid honey or agave nectar | 15 mL |

1. Place sweet potatoes on prepared baking sheet. Drizzle with 1 tbsp (15 mL) of the oil and sprinkle with chili powder. Season with salt and pepper. Gently toss to coat. Spread in a single layer. Roast in preheated oven for 20 to 25 minutes or until golden brown and tender. Let cool completely in pan.

2. In a large bowl, combine sweet potatoes, quinoa, red pepper, green onions and beans.

3. In a small bowl, whisk together cumin, lime juice, honey and the remaining oil. Add to sweet potato mixture and gently toss to coat. Season to taste with salt and pepper.

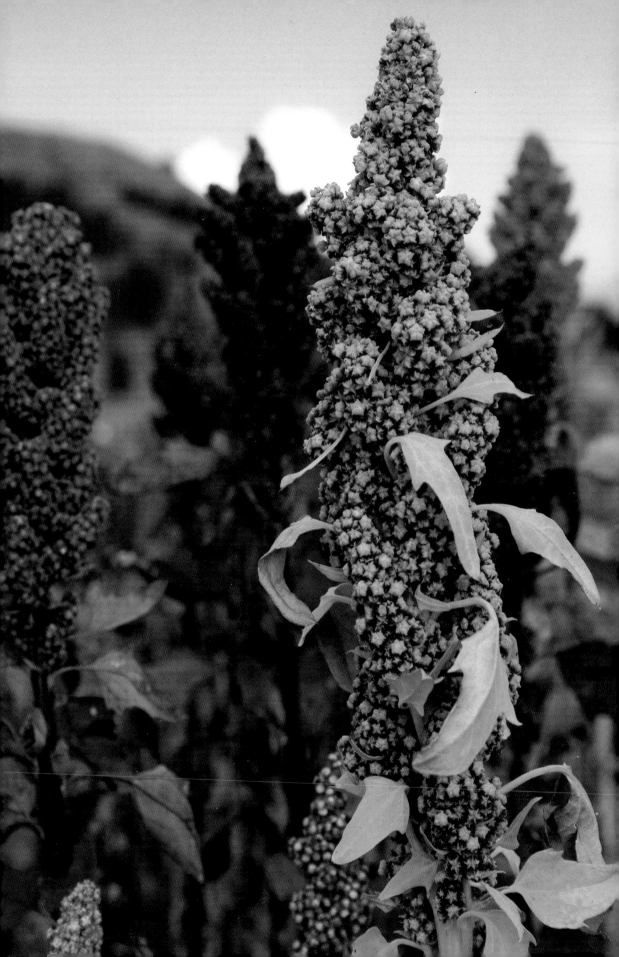

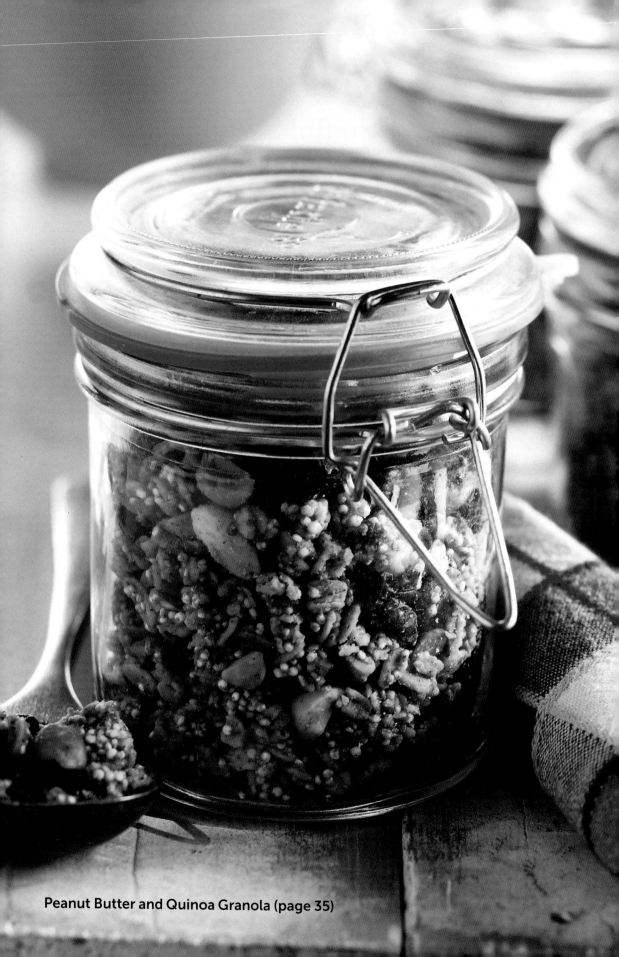

Peanut Butter and Quinoa Granola (page 35)

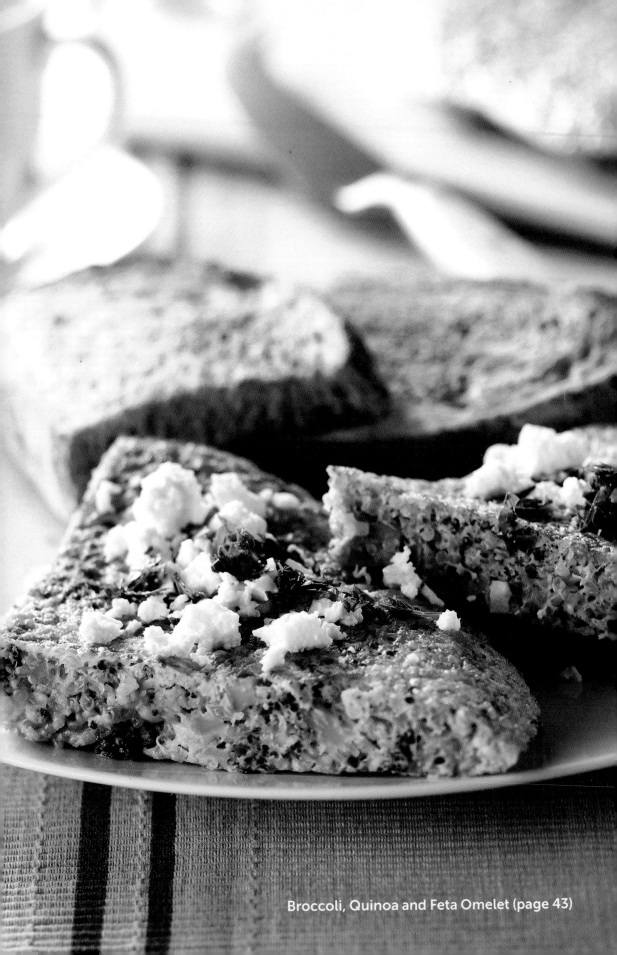

Broccoli, Quinoa and Feta Omelet (page 43)

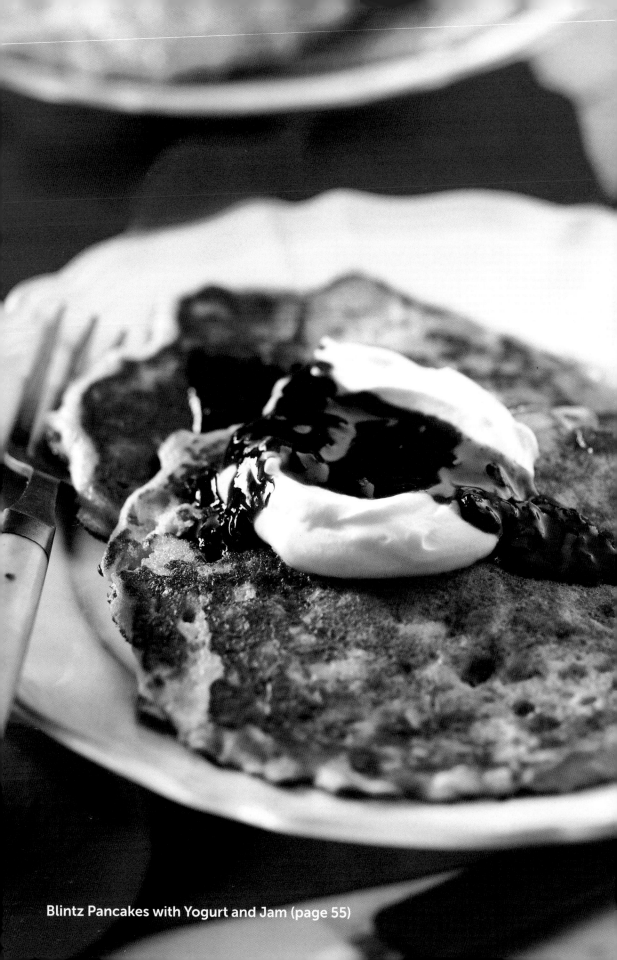

Blintz Pancakes with Yogurt and Jam (page 55)

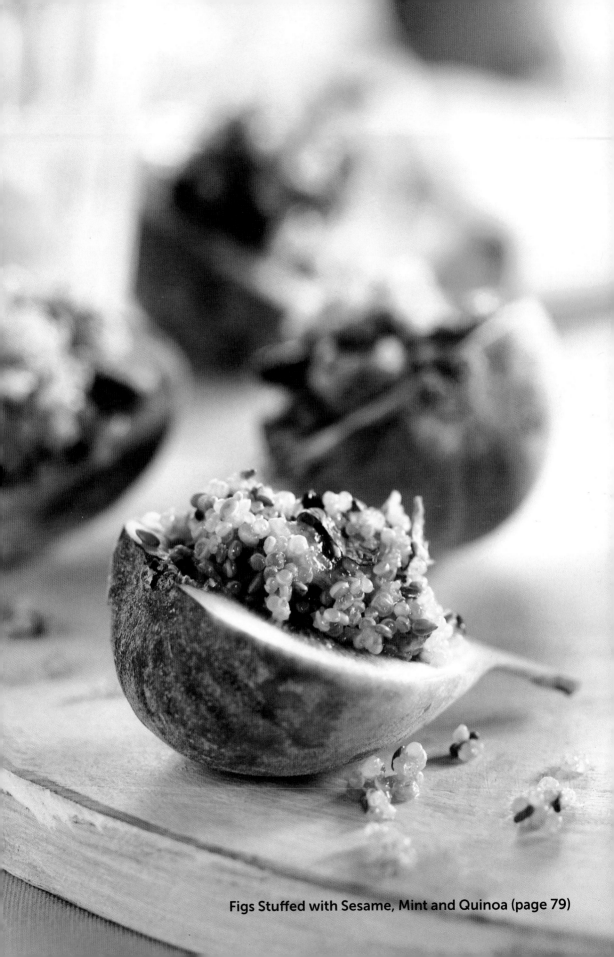

Figs Stuffed with Sesame, Mint and Quinoa (page 79)

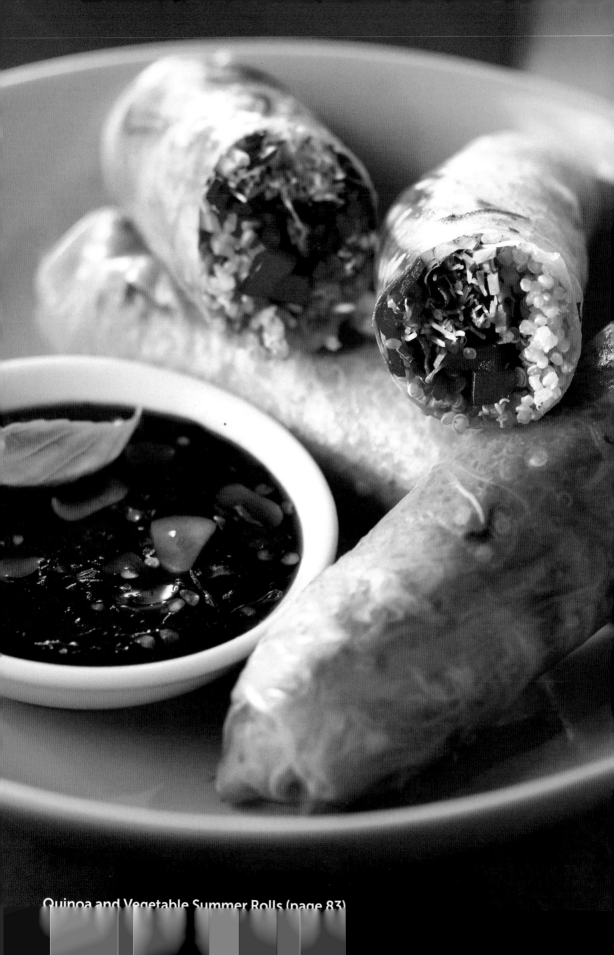

Quinoa and Vegetable Summer Rolls (page 83)

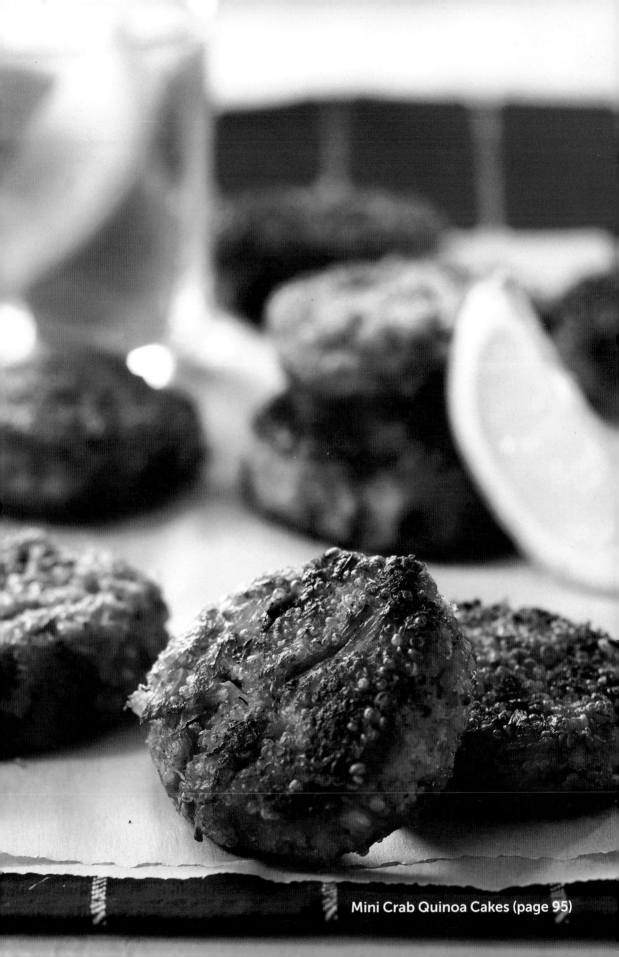

Mini Crab Quinoa Cakes (page 95)

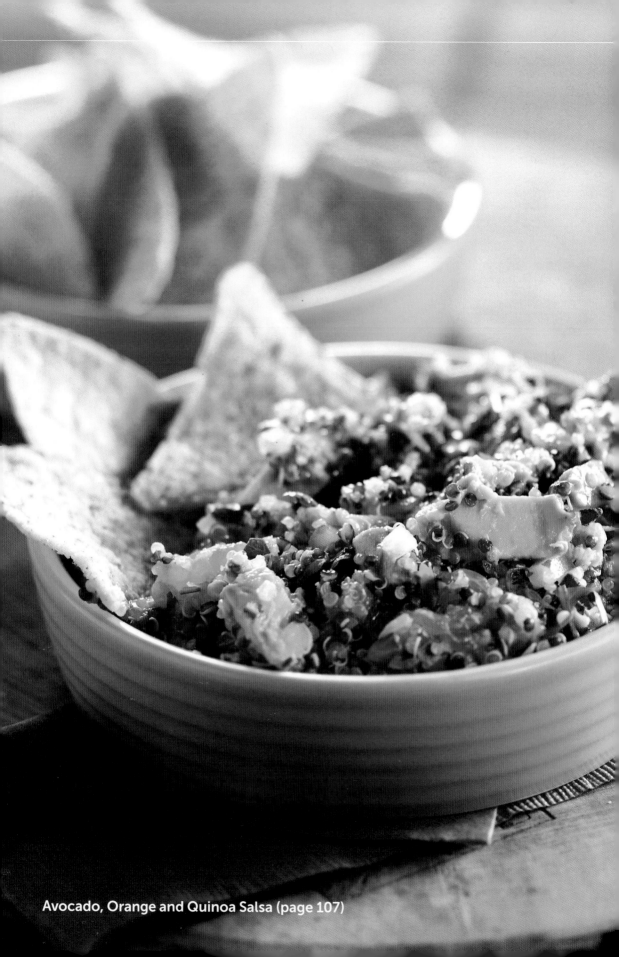

Avocado, Orange and Quinoa Salsa (page 107)

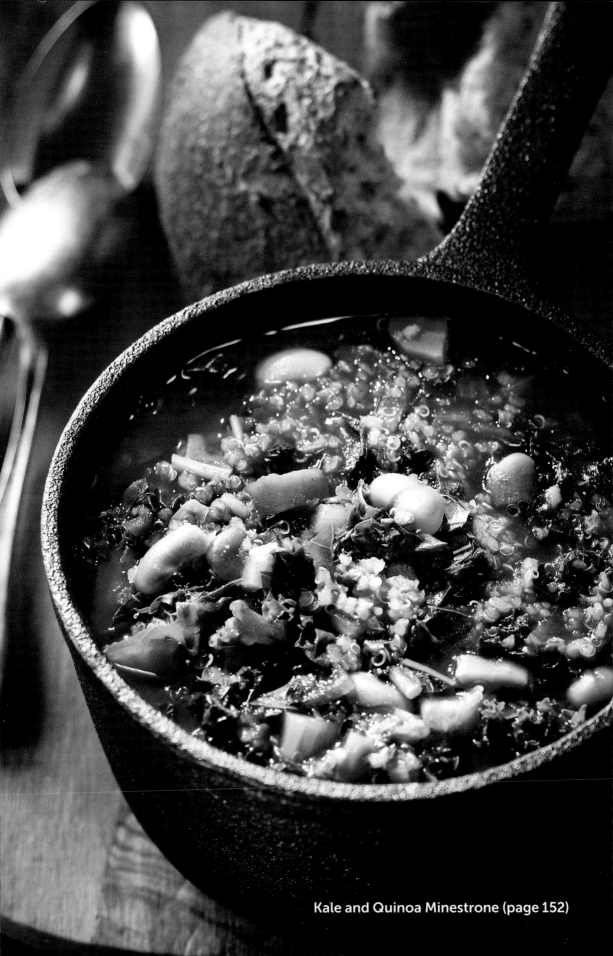

Kale and Quinoa Minestrone (page 152)

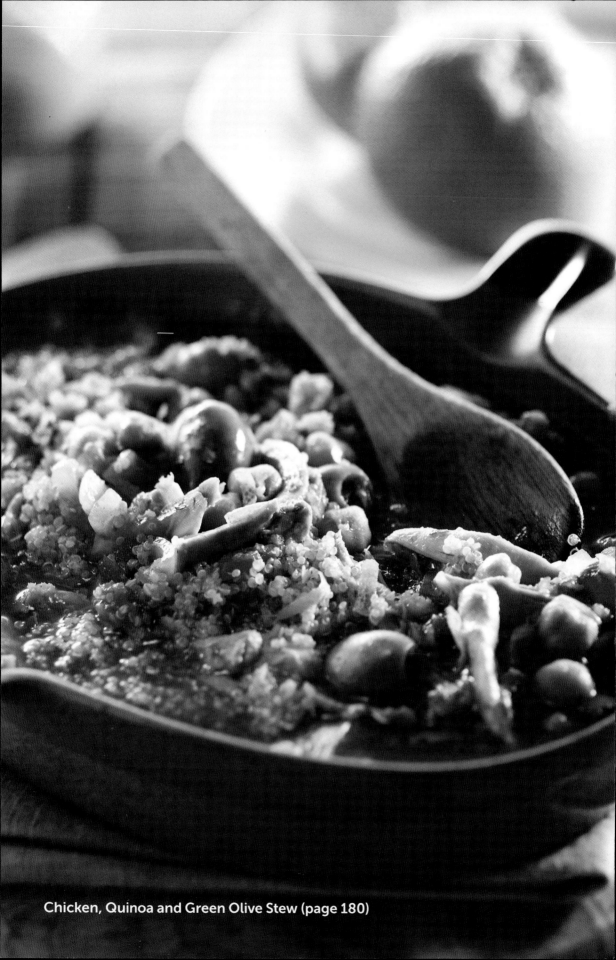

Chicken, Quinoa and Green Olive Stew (page 180)

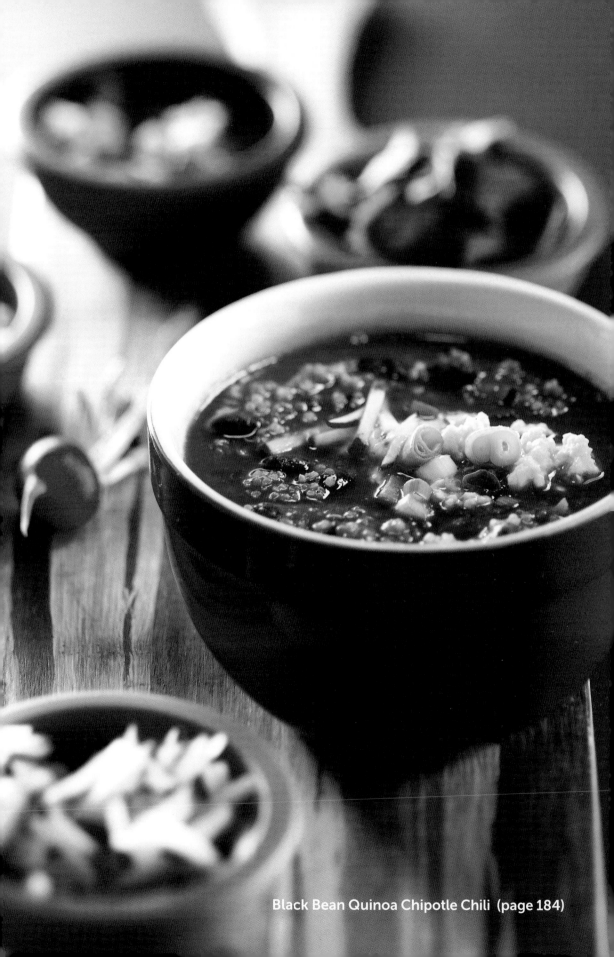

Black Bean Quinoa Chipotle Chili  (page 184)

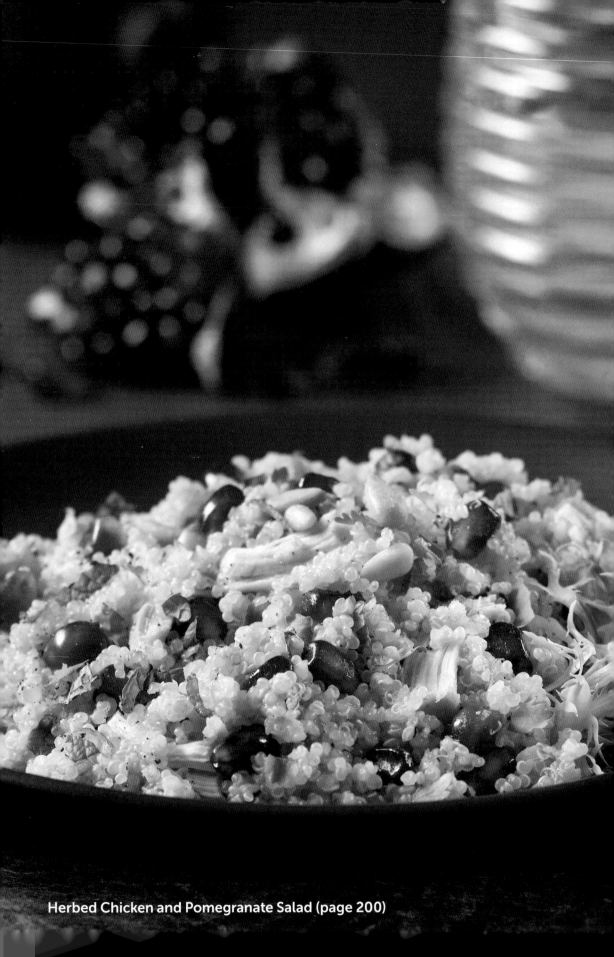

Herbed Chicken and Pomegranate Salad (page 200)

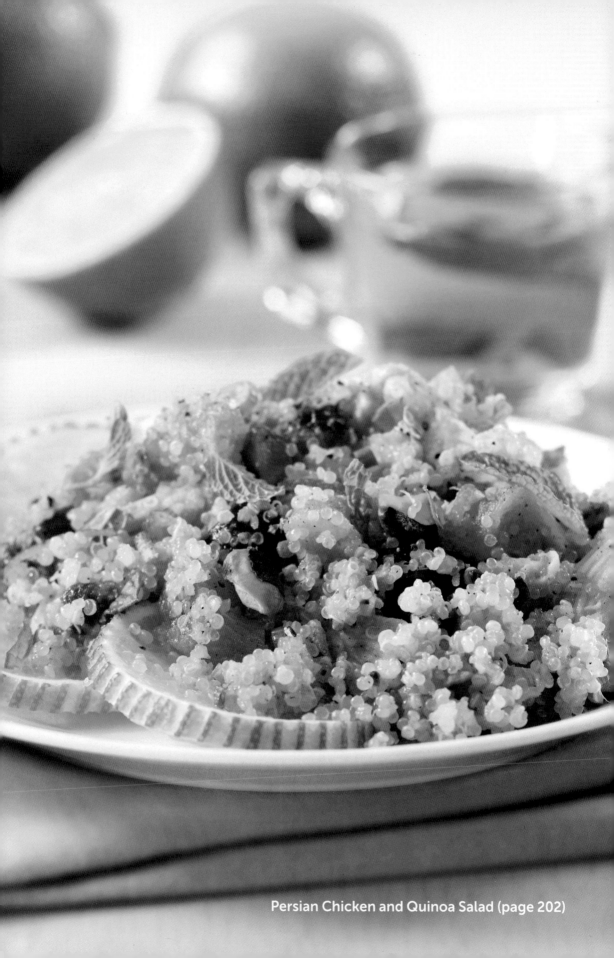

Persian Chicken and Quinoa Salad (page 202)

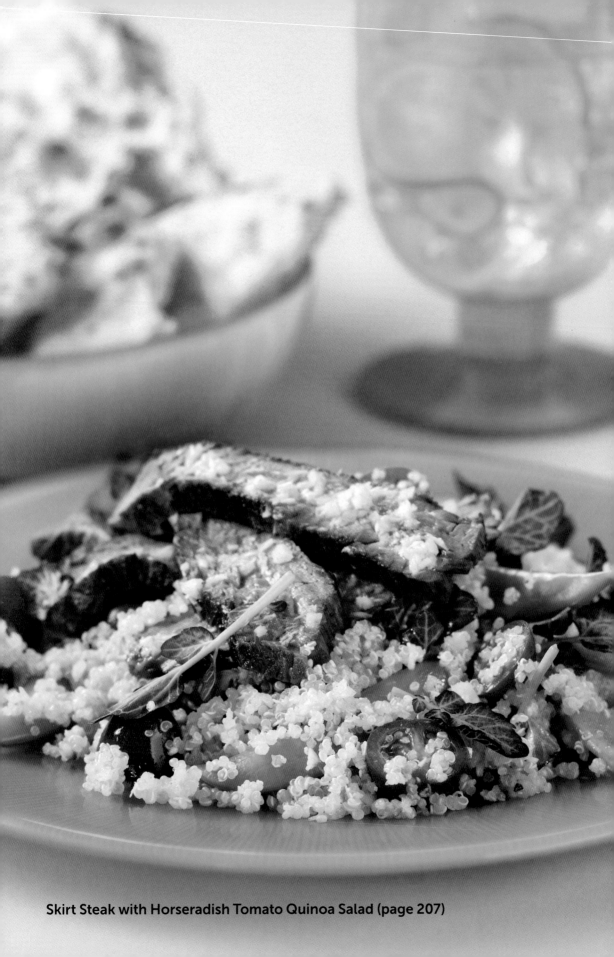

Skirt Steak with Horseradish Tomato Quinoa Salad (page 207)

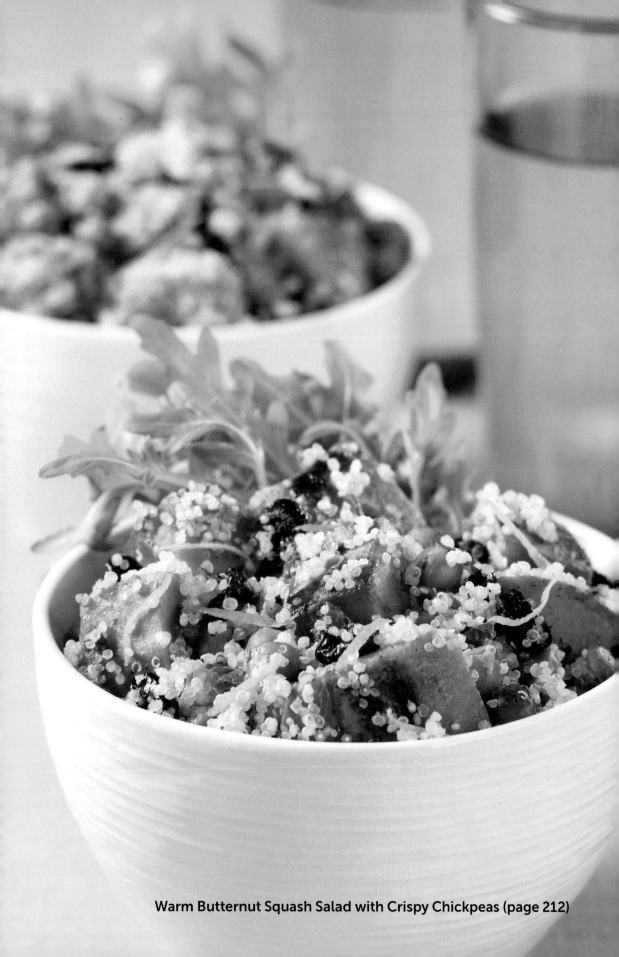

Warm Butternut Squash Salad with Crispy Chickpeas (page 212)

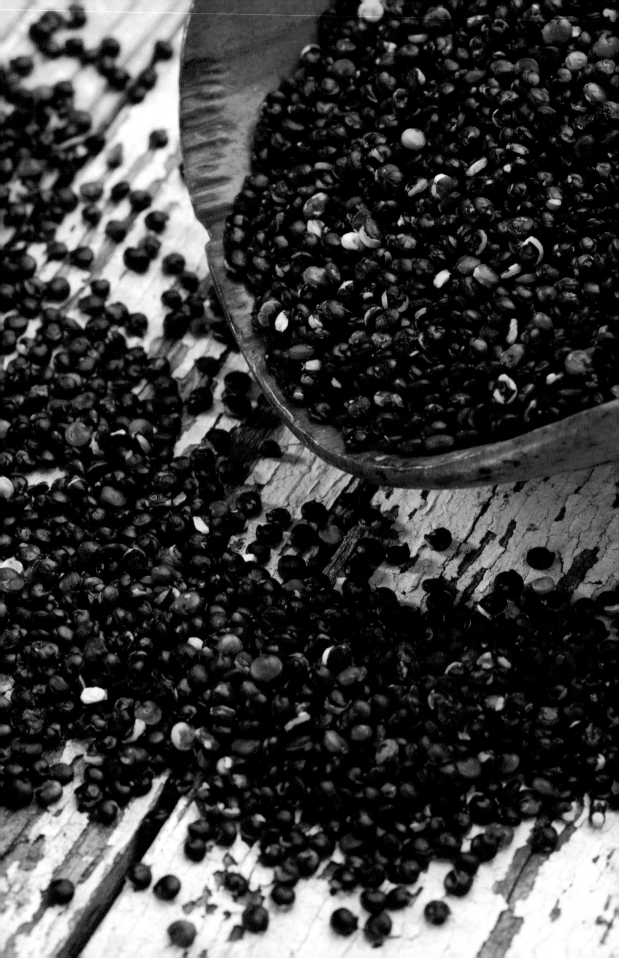

# Tofu, Quinoa and Miso Salad

*Here, the crisp-creamy taste and texture of pan-fried tofu escapes the 1970s health food cliché to find new expression in a sophisticated Asian-inspired quinoa salad. Miso in the dressing adds instant depth, accentuating both the fresh (broccoli, carrots, snap peas) and earthy (quinoa, tofu) elements simultaneously.*

## Tip

If the package of tofu you buy is slightly larger or smaller than 14 oz (400 g), just use the entire package (there is no need to add or subtract tofu to equal 14 oz/400 g).

| | | |
|---|---|---|
| 1 cup | black, red or white quinoa, rinsed | 250 mL |
| 12 oz | sugar snap peas, strings removed | 375 g |
| 2 cups | broccoli florets | 500 mL |
| 3 tbsp | vegetable oil, divided | 45 mL |
| 14 oz | extra-firm tofu, drained, patted dry and cut into 1/2-inch (1 cm) cubes | 400 g |
| 1 | red bell pepper, chopped | 1 |
| 1 1/2 cups | shredded carrots | 375 mL |
| 3 tbsp | unseasoned rice vinegar | 45 mL |
| 2 tbsp | white or yellow miso (GF, if needed) | 30 mL |
| 1 tsp | Asian chili-garlic sauce | 5 mL |
| | Fine sea salt and freshly cracked black pepper | |

1. In a large saucepan of boiling salted water, cook quinoa for 11 minutes. Add peas and broccoli; boil for 1 minute. Drain and rinse under cold water until cool. Transfer to a large bowl.

2. In a large skillet, heat 1 tbsp (15 mL) of the oil over medium-high heat. Add tofu and cook, stirring, for 3 to 4 minutes or until golden. Add to quinoa mixture, along with red pepper and carrots.

3. In a small bowl, whisk together vinegar, miso, chili-garlic sauce and the remaining oil. Add to quinoa mixture and gently toss to coat. Season to taste with salt and pepper. Let cool to room temperature, then cover and refrigerate for at least 1 hour, until chilled, or for up to 2 hours.

# Tuna, Quinoa and White Bean Salad

**Makes 4 main-dish servings**

*Even those who prefer their tuna salad dressed with mayonnaise and a bit of pickle relish will be won over by this preparation. Combined with quinoa for texture, the tuna flavor is deepened by using the packing oil in an easy, lemony dressing. The bold flavors continue with the colorful additions of celery, red onion, white beans and fresh herbs.*

## Tip

For the white beans, you could use Great Northern beans, cannellini (white kidney) beans or white pea (navy) beans.

| | | |
|---|---|---|
| 2 | cans (each 6 oz/170 g) tuna packed in olive oil, with oil | 2 |
| 2 tbsp | red wine vinegar | 30 mL |
| 1 tsp | Dijon mustard | 5 mL |
| 3 cups | cooked red, black or white quinoa (see page 10), cooled | 750 mL |
| 1 cup | finely chopped celery | 250 mL |
| 1/2 cup | finely chopped red onion | 125 mL |
| 3/4 cup | packed fresh flat-leaf (Italian) parsley leaves, chopped | 175 mL |
| 1 1/2 tsp | minced fresh rosemary | 7 mL |
| 1 | can (14 to 19 oz/398 to 540 mL) white beans, drained and rinsed | 1 |
| | Fine sea salt and freshly cracked black pepper | |

1. Drain tuna, reserving 3 tbsp (15 mL) oil. In a small bowl, whisk together the reserved oil, vinegar and mustard.

2. In a large bowl, combine tuna, quinoa, celery, red onion, parsley, rosemary and beans. Add dressing and gently toss to coat. Season to taste with salt and pepper.

## Variation

Use chickpeas in place of the white beans and replace the celery with 1 cup (250 mL) halved cherry or grape tomatoes.

# Sicilian Tuna and Quinoa Salad

**Makes 4 main-dish servings**

*Quinoa replaces the rice in this riff on a popular Sicilian tuna and egg salad. Capers and olives, common cooking ingredients in Sicily, give the salad a tangy, briny flavor.*

## Tip

To hard-cook eggs, place eggs in a saucepan large enough to hold them in a single layer. Add enough cold water to cover eggs by 1 inch (2.5 cm). Heat over high heat until water is just boiling. Remove from heat and cover pan. Let stand for about 12 minutes for large eggs (9 minutes for medium eggs; 15 minutes for extra-large eggs). Drain eggs and cool completely under cold running water or in a bowl of ice water. Refrigerate until ready to eat.

| | | |
|---|---|---:|
| 2 | cans (each 6 oz/170 g) tuna packed in olive oil, with oil | 2 |
| 2 tsp | finely grated lemon zest | 10 mL |
| 1/4 cup | freshly squeezed lemon juice | 60 mL |
| 3 cups | cooked quinoa (see page 10), cooled | 750 mL |
| 1 | large red bell pepper, chopped | 1 |
| 1 cup | thinly sliced green onions | 250 mL |
| 1 cup | chopped celery | 250 mL |
| 1/2 cup | pitted kalamata or other brine-cured black olives, chopped | 125 mL |
| 3 tbsp | drained capers | 45 mL |
| | Fine sea salt and freshly cracked black pepper | |
| 2 | hard-cooked large eggs, peeled and chopped | 2 |
| 1 cup | packed fresh flat-leaf (Italian) parsley leaves, chopped | 250 mL |

1. Drain tuna, reserving 3 tbsp (45 mL) oil. In a small bowl, whisk together the reserved oil, lemon zest and lemon juice.
2. In a large bowl, combine tuna, quinoa, red pepper, green onions, celery, olives and capers. Add dressing and gently toss to coat. Season to taste with salt and pepper. Cover and refrigerate for at least 1 hour, until chilled, or for up to 6 hours.
3. Just before serving, add eggs and parsley, gently tossing to combine.

# Tuna, Quinoa and Spinach Salad

*A flavorful tarragon vinaigrette makes this newfangled tuna salad as sophisticated as it is easy.*

| 2 | cans (each 6 oz/170 g) tuna packed in olive oil, with oil | 2 |
|---|---|---|
| 3 tbsp | white wine vinegar | 45 mL |
| 1 tsp | Dijon mustard | 5 mL |
| 2 tsp | dried tarragon | 10 mL |
| 3 cups | cooked quinoa (see page 10), cooled | 750 mL |
| | Fine sea salt and freshly cracked black pepper | |
| 6 cups | packed baby spinach | 1.5 L |

1. Drain tuna, reserving 3 tbsp (45 mL) oil. In a small bowl, whisk together the reserved oil, vinegar, mustard and tarragon.
2. In a medium bowl, combine tuna and quinoa, gently tossing to combine. Add two-thirds of the dressing and gently toss to coat. Season to taste with salt and pepper.
3. In a large bowl, toss spinach with the remaining dressing until coated. Season to taste with salt and pepper.
4. Divide spinach among four dinner plates and top with quinoa mixture.

# Shrimp, Mango and Quinoa Salad

*Hello, summer. The secret to this otherwise simple shrimp and quinoa salad's decadent taste is creamy avocado, which is rich in heart-healthy unsaturated fat. Chunks of tart-sweet mango, a shot of fresh lime juice and a kick of chile-garlic sauce brighten the flavor.*

| 1 lb | medium shrimp, peeled, deveined and cooked | 500 g |
|---|---|---|
| 3 cups | cooked black or white quinoa (see page 10), cooled | 750 mL |
| 2 | large firm-ripe mangos, diced | 2 |
| 2 | small firm-ripe Hass avocados, diced | 2 |
| 3 tbsp | extra virgin olive oil | 45 mL |
| 3 tbsp | freshly squeezed lime juice | 45 mL |
| 1 tbsp | agave nectar or liquid honey | 15 mL |
| 1½ tsp | Asian chili-garlic sauce | 7 mL |
| | Fine sea salt and freshly cracked black pepper | |

1. In a large bowl, combine shrimp, quinoa, mangos and avocados.
2. In a small bowl, whisk together oil, lime juice, honey and chili-garlic sauce. Add to shrimp mixture and gently toss to coat. Season to taste with salt and pepper. Cover and refrigerate for at least 30 minutes, until chilled, or for up to 2 hours.

# Crab and Quinoa Salad with Basil Vinaigrette

*The delicate sweetness of crab is front and center in this easy summer salad. To make the dish sing, use the freshest corn and best-quality crab you can find.*

## Tips

Jumbo lump crabmeat is typically larger chunks of crabmeat from larger crabs. It works well in salads and crab cakes.

Three 6-oz (175 g) cans of lump crabmeat, drained, may be used in place of the fresh crabmeat.

| | | |
|---|---|---|
| 12 oz | cooked jumbo lump crabmeat, picked over | 375 g |
| 3 cups | cooked quinoa (see page 10), cooled | 750 mL |
| 1½ cups | halved cherry or grape tomatoes | 375 mL |
| 1½ cups | cooked fresh corn kernels | 375 mL |
| 3 tbsp | extra virgin olive oil | 45 mL |
| 2 tbsp | white wine vinegar | 30 mL |
| 1 tbsp | prepared horseradish | 15 mL |
| 2 tsp | liquid honey | 10 mL |
| ½ cup | packed fresh basil leaves, chopped | 125 mL |
| | Fine sea salt and freshly cracked black pepper | |

1. In a large bowl, combine crab, quinoa, tomatoes and corn.

2. In a small bowl, whisk together oil, vinegar, horseradish and honey. Stir in basil. Add to crab mixture and gently toss to coat. Season to taste with salt and pepper. Cover and refrigerate for at least 30 minutes, until chilled, or for up to 2 hours.

# Provençal Chicken and Quinoa Salad

*Chicken, artichoke hearts, currants, olives and tomato come together in this main-dish quinoa salad, a nod to the warm and sunny flavors of Provence. A bright tarragon dressing unites all of the elements in harmony.*

## Tip

The remaining artichoke marinade may be stored in the refrigerator (in the original jar) and used in salad dressings.

| | | |
|---|---|---|
| 1 | jar (6 oz/170 mL) marinated artichoke hearts, with marinade | 1 |
| 3 cups | cooked quinoa (see page 10), cooled | 750 mL |
| 2 cups | diced roasted or poached chicken breast | 500 mL |
| 1½ cups | halved cherry or grape tomatoes | 375 mL |
| ½ cup | pitted brine-cured black olives (such as kalamata), coarsely chopped | 125 mL |
| ¼ cup | dried currants or chopped raisins | 60 mL |
| 1 tbsp | chopped fresh tarragon | 15 mL |
| 2 tbsp | white wine vinegar | 30 mL |
| 2 tsp | Dijon mustard | 10 mL |
| | Fine sea salt and freshly cracked black pepper | |

1. Drain artichoke hearts, reserving 3 tbsp (45 mL) marinade. Roughly chop artichoke hearts.
2. In a large bowl, combine artichoke hearts, quinoa, chicken, tomatoes, olives and currants.
3. In a small bowl, whisk together tarragon, vinegar, mustard and the reserved marinade. Add to artichoke mixture and gently toss to coat. Season to taste with salt and pepper. Cover and refrigerate for at least 30 minutes, until chilled, or for up to 4 hours.

## Variation

Replace the chicken with 12 oz (375 g) tempeh (GF, if needed), diced.

# Nectarine, Chicken and Quinoa Salad

*Nectarines are a subspecies of peaches and generally have a more pronounced, intense flavor. This newfangled chicken-quinoa salad is studded with chunks of nectarines, their summery, sunshiny essence enhanced by goat cheese and an equally summery fresh basil dressing.*

## Tip

Two large peeled peaches can be used in place of the nectarines.

| | | |
|---|---|---|
| 3 cups | cooked black or white quinoa (see page 10), cooled | 750 mL |
| 2 cups | diced roasted or poached chicken breast | 500 mL |
| 2 | large firm-ripe nectarines, diced | 2 |
| 3 tbsp | walnut or extra virgin olive oil | 45 mL |
| 3 tbsp | white wine vinegar | 45 mL |
| 1 tsp | Dijon mustard | 5 mL |
| | Fine sea salt and freshly cracked black pepper | |
| ¾ cup | crumbled goat cheese | 175 mL |
| ⅔ cup | packed fresh basil leaves, chopped | 150 mL |
| ½ cup | chopped toasted pecans | 125 mL |

1. In a large bowl, combine quinoa, chicken and nectarines.
2. In a small bowl, whisk together oil, vinegar and mustard. Add to quinoa mixture and gently toss to coat. Season to taste with salt and pepper. Cover and refrigerate for at least 30 minutes, until chilled, or for up to 24 hours.
3. Just before serving, add cheese, basil and pecans, gently tossing to combine.

## Variation

Replace the chicken with 12 oz (375 g) tempeh (GF, if needed), diced.

# Herbed Chicken and Pomegranate Salad

*This stellar salad relies on varied tastes and textures — nutty quinoa, succulent roast chicken, aromatic fresh herbs, tart, crunchy pomegranate seeds and rich, slightly sweet pine nuts — to impress one and all.*

## Tip

To remove pomegranate seeds from the fruit, score the pomegranate around the circumference and place it in a large bowl of water. Break the pomegranate open underwater to free the white seed sacs. The seeds will sink to the bottom of the bowl, and the membrane will float to the top. Strain out the seeds and put them in a separate bowl. You can refrigerate or freeze any remaining seeds for another use.

| | | |
|---|---|---|
| 3 cups | cooked quinoa (see page 10), cooled | 750 mL |
| 2 cups | shredded rotisserie, grilled or poached chicken breast | 500 mL |
| 1 cup | pomegranate seeds | 250 mL |
| 2 tsp | finely grated lime zest | 10 mL |
| 2 tbsp | freshly squeezed lime juice | 30 mL |
| 2 tbsp | extra virgin olive oil | 30 mL |
| 1 tbsp | liquid honey | 15 mL |
| | Fine sea salt and freshly cracked black pepper | |
| ¼ cup | packed fresh mint leaves, chopped | 60 mL |
| ¼ cup | packed fresh cilantro leaves, chopped | 60 mL |
| ⅓ cup | toasted pine nuts or sliced almonds | 75 mL |

1. In a large bowl, combine quinoa, chicken and pomegranate seeds.
2. In a small bowl, whisk together lime zest, lime juice, oil and honey. Add to quinoa mixture and gently toss to coat. Season to taste with salt and pepper. Cover and refrigerate for at least 30 minutes, until chilled, or for up to 4 hours.
3. Just before serving, add mint and cilantro, gently tossing to combine. Sprinkle with pine nuts.

## Variation

An equal amount of dried cranberries or chopped dried cherries may be used in place of the pomegranate seeds.

# Snap Pea and Chicken Salad with Tahini Dressing

### Makes 4 main-dish servings

*The many components of this big, beautiful salad — definitely filling enough for a main dish — all have quite different flavors and textures, but once mixed, they go together brilliantly.*

## Tip

To toast sesame seeds, place up to 3 tbsp (45 mL) seeds in a medium skillet set over medium heat. Cook, shaking the skillet, for 3 to 5 minutes or until seeds are golden brown and fragrant. Let cool completely before use.

| | | |
|---|---|---|
| 1 cup | black or white quinoa, rinsed | 250 mL |
| 8 oz | sugar snap peas, strings removed | 250 g |
| 1 | red bell pepper, chopped | 1 |
| 2 cups | diced roasted or poached chicken breast | 500 mL |
| 2 | cloves garlic, minced | 2 |
| 1/3 cup | well-stirred tahini | 75 mL |
| 3 tbsp | freshly squeezed lemon juice | 45 mL |
| 2 tbsp | water | 30 mL |
| 2 tsp | liquid honey | 10 mL |
| | Fine sea salt and freshly cracked black pepper | |
| 2 tbsp | toasted sesame seeds (see tip, at left) | 30 mL |

1. In a large saucepan of boiling salted water, cook quinoa for 11 minutes. Add peas and boil for 1 minute. Drain and rinse under cold water until cool.
2. In a large bowl, combine quinoa mixture, red pepper and chicken.
3. In a small bowl, whisk together garlic, tahini, lemon juice, water and honey. Add to quinoa mixture and gently toss to coat. Season to taste with salt and pepper. Cover and refrigerate for at least 30 minutes, until chilled, or for up to 2 hours.
4. Just before serving, sprinkle with sesame seeds.

## Variation

Replace the chicken with 12 oz (375 g) tempeh (GF, if needed), diced.

# Persian Chicken and Quinoa Salad

*Tired of the typical chicken salad with mayonnaise and celery? Prepare to have your affection rekindled by this lively quinoa-enhanced version, studded with crunchy pistachios, plump dates and dried apricots, and emerald herbs.*

| | | |
|---|---|---|
| 3 cups | cooked black, red or white quinoa (see page 10), cooled | 750 mL |
| 2 cups | shredded rotisserie or poached chicken breast | 500 mL |
| ½ cup | chopped dried apricots | 125 mL |
| ½ cup | chopped pitted dates | 125 mL |
| 1 tsp | ground cardamom | 5 mL |
| 1 tsp | finely grated lime zest | 5 mL |
| 3 tbsp | freshly squeezed lime juice | 45 mL |
| 3 tbsp | extra virgin olive oil | 45 mL |
| 1 tbsp | liquid honey | 15 mL |
| | Fine sea salt and freshly cracked black pepper | |
| ¾ cup | thinly sliced green onions | 175 mL |
| ¾ cup | packed fresh mint leaves, chopped | 175 mL |
| ½ cup | lightly salted roasted pistachios, coarsely chopped | 125 mL |

1. In a large bowl, combine quinoa, chicken, apricots and dates.
2. In a small bowl, whisk together cardamom, lime zest, lime juice, oil and honey. Add to quinoa mixture and gently toss to coat. Season to taste with salt and pepper. Cover and refrigerate for at least 30 minutes, until chilled, or for up to 24 hours.
3. Just before serving, add green onions, mint and pistachios, gently tossing to combine.

# Thai Chicken Quinoa Salad

*You may be wondering why a Thai-inspired salad needs to include so many ingredients. Why not just drizzle store-bought Thai peanut sauce over bagged salad greens and call it a day? One forkful reveals the answer: this salad has many layers of complexity, and the overall effect is well worth every moment of chopping and whisking. Adding generous amounts of chicken and quinoa might not be strictly traditional, but it transforms the salad into a hearty meal.*

| | | |
|---|---|---|
| 3 cups | cooked red, black or white quinoa (see page 10), cooled | 750 mL |
| 2 cups | diced roasted or poached chicken breast | 500 mL |
| 1 | cucumber, seeded and diced | 1 |
| 3 cups | chopped purple cabbage | 750 mL |
| 1 cup | shredded carrots | 250 mL |
| ½ cup | chopped green onions | 125 mL |
| ½ cup | packed fresh mint or cilantro leaves, chopped | 125 mL |
| ⅓ cup | freshly squeezed lime juice | 75 mL |
| ¼ cup | tamari or soy sauce (GF, if needed) | 60 mL |
| 3 tbsp | unsweetened natural peanut butter | 45 mL |
| 2 tbsp | vegetable oil | 30 mL |
| 2 tbsp | liquid honey | 30 mL |
| 2 tsp | Asian chili-garlic sauce | 10 mL |
| | Fine sea salt and freshly ground black pepper | |
| ⅓ cup | coarsely chopped lightly salted roasted peanuts | 75 mL |

1. In a large bowl, combine quinoa, chicken, cucumber, cabbage, carrots, green onions and mint.

2. In a small bowl, whisk together lime juice, tamari, peanut butter, oil, honey and chili-garlic sauce. Add to quinoa mixture and gently toss to coat. Season to taste with salt and pepper. Cover and refrigerate for at least 30 minutes, until chilled, or for up to 24 hours.

3. Just before serving, sprinkle with peanuts.

## Variations

Any variety of unsweetened natural nut or seed butter (such as cashew, almond or sunflower) may be used in place of the peanut butter.

Any other roasted or toasted chopped nuts or seeds (such as cashews, almonds, sunflower seeds or pepitas) may be used in place of the peanuts.

Replace the chicken with 12 oz (375 g) tempeh (GF, if needed), diced.

# Ham, Apple and Quinoa Salad

*Apples and sharp mustard are time-honored accompaniments to ham at any time of the year. Add in the nuttiness of quinoa and the crisp mineral quality of celery, plus a handful of toasted pecans, and the dish tastes modern and sassy. It's also very pretty, with the pale green celery, golden apple and pink ham nestled in the ivory quinoa.*

| | | |
|---|---|---|
| 3 cups | cooked quinoa (see page 10), cooled | 750 mL |
| 1½ cups | diced lean ham | 375 mL |
| 1 | large Granny Smith or other tart apple, peeled and diced | 1 |
| 1 cup | thinly sliced celery | 250 mL |
| ½ cup | packed celery leaves, chopped | 125 mL |
| 3 tbsp | extra virgin olive oil | 45 mL |
| 2 tbsp | white wine vinegar | 30 mL |
| 1½ tbsp | Dijon mustard | 22 mL |
| 2 tsp | liquid honey | 10 mL |
| | Fine sea salt and freshly cracked black pepper | |
| ¾ cup | chopped toasted pecans | 175 mL |

**1.** In a large bowl, combine quinoa, ham, apple, celery and celery leaves.

**2.** In a small bowl, whisk together oil, vinegar, mustard and honey. Add to quinoa mixture and gently toss to coat. Season to taste with salt and pepper. Cover and refrigerate for at least 30 minutes, until chilled, or for up to 4 hours.

**3.** Just before serving, sprinkle with pecans.

# Warm Quinoa Kielbasa Salad

*Fresh herbs and delicate quinoa are a perfect balancing act, especially when combined with rich smoked sausage and a sweet-and-sour vinaigrette.*

| | | |
|---|---|---|
| 3 tbsp | extra virgin olive oil, divided | 45 mL |
| 1 lb | reduced-fat kielbasa or other smoked sausage, diced | 500 g |
| 3 cups | cooked quinoa (see page 10), cooled | 750 mL |
| 1 cup | packed fresh flat-leaf (Italian) parsley leaves, chopped | 250 mL |
| 3 tbsp | chopped fresh dill | 45 mL |
| 2 tbsp | cider vinegar | 30 mL |
| 1 tbsp | whole-grain Dijon mustard | 15 mL |
| 1 tsp | liquid honey or agave nectar | 5 mL |
| | Fine sea salt and freshly cracked black pepper | |

1. In a large skillet, heat 1 tbsp (15 mL) of the oil over medium-high heat. Add kielbasa and cook, stirring, for 5 to 6 minutes or until browned and crispy.
2. In a large bowl, combine kielbasa, quinoa, parsley and dill.
3. In a small bowl, whisk together vinegar, mustard, honey and the remaining oil. Add to kielbasa mixture and gently toss to coat. Season to taste with salt and pepper.

# Steak and Quinoa Salad with Chimichurri

*The vibrant flavors of fresh parsley and garlic make chimichurri a favorite accompaniment to Argentine beef. Here, it works its magic both as a sauce for thinly sliced grilled steak and as the dressing for the accompanying quinoa-tomato salad.*

● **Blender**

| | | |
|---|---|---|
| 3 cups | cooked quinoa (see page 10), cooled | 750 mL |
| 1½ cups | halved cherry or grape tomatoes | 375 mL |
| 2 | cloves garlic | 2 |
| 1 cup | packed fresh flat-leaf (Italian) parsley leaves | 250 mL |
| ¾ tsp | chipotle chile powder or hot smoked paprika | 3 mL |
| ¼ cup | extra virgin olive oil | 60 mL |
| 2 tbsp | red wine vinegar | 30 mL |
| | Fine sea salt and freshly ground black pepper | |
| 1 lb | beef flank steak, trimmed | 500 g |

1. In a large bowl, combine quinoa and tomatoes.
2. In blender, combine garlic, parsley, chipotle chile powder, oil and vinegar; purée until smooth.
3. Pour two-thirds of the dressing over quinoa mixture and gently toss to coat. Season to taste with salt and pepper. Separately cover and refrigerate quinoa mixture and the remaining dressing for at least 30 minutes, until chilled, or for up to 2 hours.
4. Preheat barbecue grill to medium-high heat. Season both sides of steak with salt and pepper. Grill steak, turning once, for about 5 minutes per side for medium-rare, or to desired doneness. Transfer steak to a cutting board and let rest for 5 minutes. Thinly slice across the grain on a slight diagonal.
5. Divide quinoa mixture among four plates. Arrange steak on top. Drizzle with the remaining dressing.

# Skirt Steak with Horseradish Tomato Quinoa Salad

**Makes 4 main-dish servings**

*The sweetness of tomatoes is a wonderful foil to the distinctive bite of horseradish and watercress. Thin slices of skirt steak, quickly seared in a skillet, round out this inventive salad.*

## Tip

To mash garlic, working with one clove at a time, place the side of a chef's knife flat against the clove. Place the heel of your hand on the side of the knife and apply pressure so that the clove flattens slightly (this will loosen the peel). Remove and discard the peel, then roughly chop the garlic. Sprinkle a pinch of coarse salt over the garlic. Use the flat part of the knife as before to press the garlic against the cutting board. Repeat until the garlic turns into a fine paste. The mashed garlic is now ready for use in your favorite recipe.

| | | |
|---|---|---|
| 1 cup | quinoa, rinsed | 250 mL |
| 8 oz | sugar snap peas, strings removed | 250 g |
| 3 | cloves garlic, mashed (see tip, at left) | 3 |
| 4 tbsp | extra virgin olive oil, divided | 60 mL |
| 2 tbsp | prepared horseradish | 30 mL |
| 1½ tbsp | white wine vinegar | 22 mL |
| 2 cups | halved grape or cherry tomatoes | 500 mL |
| | Fine sea salt and freshly cracked black pepper | |
| 1 lb | beef skirt steak, cut into 4 pieces | 500 g |
| 4 cups | packed tender watercress sprigs | 1 L |

1. In a large saucepan of boiling salted water, cook quinoa for 11 minutes. Add peas and boil for 1 minute. Drain and rinse under cold water until cool.

2. In a small bowl, whisk together garlic, 3 tbsp (45 mL) of the oil, horseradish and vinegar.

3. In a large bowl, combine quinoa mixture, tomatoes and 2 tbsp (30 mL) of the dressing, gently tossing to combine. Season to taste with salt and pepper. Separately cover and refrigerate salad and the remaining dressing while preparing steak.

4. Generously season steak with salt and pepper. In a large, heavy skillet, heat the remaining oil over high heat. Add steak and cook, turning once, for 3 to 4 minutes per side or until crusty and medium-rare, or to desired doneness. Transfer steak to a cutting board and let rest for 5 minutes. Thinly slice across the grain on a slight diagonal.

5. Add watercress to the quinoa mixture, gently tossing to combine. Divide salad among four plates. Arrange steak on top. Drizzle with the remaining dressing.

# Red Quinoa, Roasted Beet and Orange Salad

*Roasted beets, sweet oranges and crimson quinoa team up in a sophisticated salad that makes a terrific side or main dish for any number of special-occasion meals.*

## Tips

Any type of beet (red, golden or red-and-white-striped Chioggia) will be great in this salad. To avoid stained hands, wear plastic gloves when peeling dark-colored beets.

If you can only find 10-oz (287 mL) cans of mandarin oranges, use 1½ cans.

If you prefer, you can use coarsely chopped fresh navel oranges, but you cannot beat the convenience of ready-to-use mandarin orange segments.

- **Preheat oven to 400°F (200°C)**
- **Large rimmed baking sheet**

| | | |
|---|---|---|
| 4 | beets, with greens attached (about 1½ lbs/750 g) | 4 |
| 2 | cloves garlic, minced | 2 |
| 1 tsp | finely grated orange zest | 5 mL |
| 3 tbsp | freshly squeezed orange juice | 45 mL |
| 2 tbsp | extra virgin olive oil | 30 mL |
| 1 tbsp | coarse-grain mustard | 15 mL |
| 3 cups | cooked red or white quinoa (see page 10), cooled | 750 mL |
| 1 | can (15 oz/425 mL) mandarin oranges, drained and coarsely chopped | 1 |
| | Fine sea salt and freshly cracked black pepper | |

1. Trim greens from beets. Cut off and discard stems, then coarsely chop leaves. Set beet greens aside.
2. Tightly wrap each beet in foil and place on baking sheet. Roast in preheated oven for about 90 minutes or until tender when pierced with a fork. Let cool completely in foil on pan. Peel beets and cut into ¼-inch (0.5 cm) dice.
3. Meanwhile, in a large saucepan of boiling water, cook beet greens for 2 to 3 minutes or until tender. Drain and let cool completely. Squeeze to remove any excess water, then chop.
4. In a small bowl, whisk together garlic, orange zest, orange juice, oil and mustard.
5. In a large bowl, combine beets, beet greens, quinoa and oranges. Add dressing and gently toss to coat. Season to taste with salt and pepper. Cover and refrigerate for at least 30 minutes, until chilled, or overnight.

# Mediterranean Lentil and Quinoa Salad

**Makes 8 side-dish or 4 main-dish servings**

*Here's a sensational spin on lentil salad. Quinoa and lentils get a Mediterranean accent with the addition of sun-dried tomatoes, feta cheese and herbs.*

## Tip

You can use 2 tbsp (30 mL) of the oil the sun-dried tomatoes were packed in instead of the olive oil.

| | | |
|---|---|---:|
| 4 cups | water | 1 L |
| 1 cup | dried green lentils, rinsed | 250 mL |
| 3 cups | cooked black, red or white quinoa (see page 10), cooled | 750 mL |
| ½ cup | chopped drained oil-packed sun-dried tomatoes | 125 mL |
| 2 tbsp | white wine vinegar | 30 mL |
| 2 tbsp | extra virgin olive oil | 30 mL |
| 1 tsp | Dijon mustard | 5 mL |
| | Fine sea salt and freshly cracked black pepper | |
| 4 cups | packed arugula, chopped | 1 L |
| 1 cup | packed fresh mint leaves, chopped | 250 mL |
| 1 cup | crumbled feta cheese | 250 mL |

1. In a medium saucepan, bring water to a boil over high heat. Add lentils, reduce heat and simmer for about 30 minutes or until tender but not mushy. Drain and let cool completely.

2. In a large bowl, combine lentils, quinoa and sun-dried tomatoes.

3. In a small bowl, whisk together vinegar, oil and mustard. Add to lentil mixture and gently toss to coat. Season to taste with salt and pepper. Cover and refrigerate for at least 1 hour, until chilled, or for up to 4 hours.

4. Just before serving, add arugula, mint and cheese, gently tossing to combine.

# Zucchini, Quinoa and Chickpea Salad

*With chunks of delicate zucchini, peppery radishes, meaty chickpeas, lots of fresh chives and mellow coriander and cumin, this appealing salad is a meal unto itself. But you will also adore it in the company of your favorite summer grilled chicken, burgers (beef or veggie) or sausages.*

## Tip

For the best flavor, use small to medium zucchini in this recipe, as they are sweeter when raw than larger ones.

| | | |
|---|---|---|
| 3 cups | cooked black or white quinoa (see page 10), cooled | 750 mL |
| 3 | small zucchini, quartered lengthwise and diced | 3 |
| 1 cup | chopped radishes | 250 mL |
| 1 | can (14 to 19 oz/398 to 540 mL) chickpeas, drained and rinsed | 1 |
| 1 tsp | ground coriander | 5 mL |
| 3/4 tsp | ground cumin | 3 mL |
| 1/4 cup | buttermilk | 60 mL |
| 1 tbsp | white wine vinegar | 15 mL |
| 1 tbsp | extra virgin olive oil | 15 mL |
| 1/3 cup | chopped fresh chives | 75 mL |
| | Fine sea salt and freshly cracked black pepper | |

1. In a large bowl, combine quinoa, zucchini, radishes and chickpeas.
2. In a small bowl, whisk together coriander, cumin, buttermilk, vinegar and oil. Stir in chives. Add to quinoa mixture and gently toss to coat. Season to taste with salt and pepper. Cover and refrigerate for at least 30 minutes, until chilled, or for up to 2 hours.

# Indian-Spiced Chickpea Quinoa Salad

*No-nonsense canned chickpeas are quick-roasted with garam masala and cayenne pepper for an aromatic makeover. Mellow quinoa and cool mint balance the spice, while plump golden raisins offer a sweet counterpoint.*

- **Preheat oven to 450°F (230°C)**
- **Large rimmed baking sheet, lined with foil and sprayed with nonstick cooking spray**

| | | |
|---|---|---|
| 1 | can (14 to 19 oz/398 to 540 mL) chickpeas, drained, rinsed and patted dry | 1 |
| 2 tsp | garam masala, divided | 10 mL |
| ¼ tsp | cayenne pepper | 1 mL |
| 2 tbsp | extra virgin olive oil, divided | 30 mL |
| 2 tsp | finely grated lime zest | 10 mL |
| 3 tbsp | freshly squeezed lime juice | 45 mL |
| 3 cups | cooked black, red or white quinoa (see page 10), cooled | 750 mL |
| ⅔ cup | golden raisins | 150 mL |
| | Fine sea salt and freshly cracked black pepper | |
| ½ cup | packed fresh mint leaves, chopped | 125 mL |
| | Plain yogurt (optional) | |

1. In a medium bowl, combine chickpeas, $1\frac{1}{2}$ tsp (7 mL) of the garam masala, cayenne and half the oil. Spread in a single layer on prepared baking sheet. Roast in preheated oven for 10 to 15 minutes or until golden brown and crisp. Let cool completely in pan.

2. In a small bowl, whisk together the remaining garam masala, lime zest, lime juice and the remaining oil.

3. In a large bowl, combine roasted chickpeas, quinoa and raisins. Add dressing and gently toss to coat. Season to taste with salt and black pepper. Cover and refrigerate for at least 30 minutes, until chilled, or for up to 4 hours.

4. Just before serving, add mint, gently tossing to combine. If desired, dollop with yogurt.

# Warm Butternut Squash Salad with Crispy Chickpeas

*This warm salad combines several of fall's best flavors and textures, with complementary exotic nuances. Sweet roasted squash, tart cranberries and earthy quinoa are irresistible partners for crispy, Indian-spiced chickpeas and citrus yogurt.*

- **Preheat oven to 400°F (200°C)**
- **Large rimmed baking sheet, lined with foil and sprayed with nonstick cooking spray**

| | | |
|---|---|---|
| 1 | large butternut squash, cut into 1-inch (2.5 cm) cubes | 1 |
| 1 | can (14 to 19 oz/398 to 540 mL) chickpeas, drained, rinsed and patted dry | 1 |
| 2 tsp | mild curry powder | 10 mL |
| 1½ tsp | garam masala | 7 mL |
| 3 tbsp | extra virgin olive oil, divided | 45 mL |
| | Fine sea salt and freshly cracked black pepper | |
| 1 cup | plain yogurt | 250 mL |
| 2 tbsp | freshly squeezed lemon juice, divided | 30 mL |
| 3 cups | cooked red or white quinoa (see page 10), cooled | 750 mL |
| ⅔ cup | dried cranberries | 150 mL |
| ½ cup | packed fresh mint leaves, chopped | 125 mL |
| 1 tbsp | finely grated orange zest | 15 mL |
| ¼ cup | freshly squeezed orange juice | 60 mL |
| 6 cups | packed baby arugula leaves | 1.5 L |

1. In a large bowl, combine butternut squash, chickpeas, curry powder, garam masala and 2 tbsp (30 mL) of the oil. Season with salt and pepper. Spread in a single layer on prepared baking sheet. Roast in preheated oven for 35 to 40 minutes, stirring occasionally, until squash is tender and chickpeas are crispy. Let cool in pan for 10 minutes.

2. In a small bowl, combine yogurt and 1 tbsp (15 mL) of the lemon juice.

3. In a large bowl, combine squash mixture and quinoa. Add cranberries, mint, orange zest, orange juice, the remaining oil and the remaining lemon juice, gently tossing to combine. Season to taste with salt and pepper.

4. Arrange arugula on a large rimmed platter or in bowls. Spoon quinoa mixture on top. Drizzle with some of the yogurt mixture and serve the rest on the side.

# Winter White Quinoa Salad

*A play of white winter vegetables, this beautiful salad is worthy of both comfort-food and spa cuisine status. Humble cauliflower takes on a whole new appeal when tossed with earthy quinoa; lots of slightly bitter endive plus fresh lemon makes it bright and refreshing.*

| | | |
|---|---|---|
| 3 tbsp | extra virgin olive oil, divided | 45 mL |
| 4 cups | small cauliflower florets (about 1 medium head) | 1 L |
| 3 | cloves garlic, minced | 3 |
| 1 tsp | minced fresh rosemary | 5 mL |
| | Fine sea salt and fresh cracked black pepper | |
| 3 cups | cooked quinoa (see page 10), cooled | 750 mL |
| 1 | can (14 to 19 oz/398 to 540 mL) white beans, drained and rinsed | 1 |
| 1 tbsp | finely grated lemon zest | 15 mL |
| 3 tbsp | freshly squeezed lemon juice | 45 mL |
| 1 | head Belgian endive | 1 |
| ½ cup | crumbled feta cheese | 125 mL |

1. In a large skillet, heat 2 tbsp (30 mL) of the oil over medium-high heat. Add cauliflower, stirring until florets are coated. Cook for 3 to 4 minutes, without stirring, to brown the cauliflower. Cook, stirring, for 2 to 3 minutes to further brown the cauliflower, adding garlic and rosemary for the last 30 seconds. Season to taste with salt and pepper.

2. In a large bowl, combine cauliflower, quinoa, beans, lemon zest, lemon juice and the remaining oil. Season to taste with salt and pepper. Cover and refrigerate for at least 30 minutes, until chilled, or for up to 4 hours.

3. Just before serving, trim endive, cut in half lengthwise, then thinly slice crosswise. Add endive and cheese to salad, gently tossing to combine.

# Edamame, Black Quinoa and Cashew Salad

**Makes 8 side-dish or 4 main-dish servings**

*Black quinoa provides a healthy whole-grain base to this colorful, hearty salad. The ginger-lime dressing and the play of complementary textures will draw you in, and the triple dose of healthy protein — quinoa, edamame and cashews — will fill you up for hours.*

| | | |
|---|---|---|
| 3 cups | frozen shelled edamame | 750 mL |
| 2 | cloves garlic, minced | 2 |
| 2 tsp | ground ginger | 10 mL |
| 2 tsp | finely grated lime zest | 10 mL |
| 3 tbsp | freshly squeezed lime juice | 45 mL |
| 3 tbsp | extra virgin olive oil | 45 mL |
| 1 tbsp | liquid honey or agave nectar | 15 mL |
| 3 cups | cooked black or white quinoa (see page 10), cooled | 750 mL |
| 1 cup | packed fresh cilantro leaves, chopped | 250 mL |
| 1/2 cup | chopped green onions | 125 mL |
| | Fine sea salt and freshly cracked black pepper | |
| 1/2 cup | lightly salted cashews or peanuts, chopped | 125 mL |

1. In a medium saucepan of boiling water, cook edamame for 4 to 6 minutes or until bright green and tender. Drain and rinse under cold water until cool.

2. In a small bowl, whisk together garlic, ginger, lime zest, lime juice, oil and honey.

3. In a large bowl, combine edamame, quinoa, cilantro and green onions. Add dressing and gently toss to coat. Season to taste with salt and pepper. Cover and refrigerate for at least 30 minutes, until chilled, or for up to 4 hours.

4. Just before serving, sprinkle with cashews.

# Supergreen Quinoa Salad

*Forking up this mélange of über-healthy emerald ingredients is an exercise in both great taste and great health. This innovative salad can stand alone as a main dish, but it would also be a terrific side to grilled fish, chicken or tofu.*

## Tip

Avocados come in several varieties, but Hass are the most widely available. A Hass avocado — notable for its dark, bumpy skin and rich, buttery flesh — is ideal in this simple salad, but any other variety may be used in its place.

| | | |
|---|---|---:|
| 1 cup | black or white quinoa, rinsed | 250 mL |
| 1 cup | frozen shelled edamame | 250 mL |
| 1 | small firm-ripe Hass avocado, diced | 1 |
| 1 cup | thinly sliced celery | 250 mL |
| 1 cup | frozen petite peas, thawed | 250 mL |
| ½ cup | thinly sliced green onions | 125 mL |
| ½ cup | packed fresh flat-leaf (Italian) parsley leaves, chopped | 125 mL |
| ¼ cup | packed fresh mint leaves, chopped | 60 mL |
| 2 tsp | ground cumin | 10 mL |
| 3 tbsp | freshly squeezed lime juice | 45 mL |
| 2 tbsp | extra virgin olive oil | 30 mL |
| | Fine sea salt and freshly cracked black pepper | |

1. In a large saucepan of boiling salted water, cook quinoa for 8 minutes. Add edamame and cook for 4 to 6 minutes or until edamame are bright green and tender. Drain and rinse under cold water until cool.

2. In a large bowl, combine quinoa mixture, avocado, celery, peas, green onions, parsley and mint.

3. In a small bowl, whisk together cumin, lime juice and oil. Add to quinoa mixture and gently toss to coat. Season to taste with salt and pepper. Cover and refrigerate for at least 1 hour, until chilled, or for up to 2 hours.

# Springtime Asparagus, Pea and Quinoa Salad

*This colorful mix of tender quinoa, petite peas, asparagus and hard-cooked eggs, tossed with a garlicky lemon dressing, is the quintessential spring salad — cool, colorful and very fresh.*

## Tip

To hard-cook eggs, place eggs in a saucepan large enough to hold them in a single layer. Add enough cold water to cover eggs by 1 inch (2.5 cm). Heat over high heat until water is just boiling. Remove from heat and cover pan. Let stand for about 12 minutes for large eggs (9 minutes for medium eggs; 15 minutes for extra-large eggs). Drain eggs and cool completely under cold running water or in a bowl of ice water. Refrigerate until ready to eat.

| | | |
|---|---|---:|
| 1 cup | quinoa, rinsed | 250 mL |
| 1 lb | asparagus, trimmed and cut into ¼-inch (0.5 cm) pieces, tips left intact | 500 g |
| 1 cup | frozen petite peas | 250 mL |
| ¼ cup | chopped fresh chives | 60 mL |
| 2 | cloves garlic, minced | 2 |
| 3 tbsp | freshly squeezed lemon juice | 45 mL |
| 3 tbsp | extra virgin olive oil | 45 mL |
| 1 tsp | Dijon mustard | 5 mL |
| | Fine sea salt and freshly cracked black pepper | |
| 2 | hard-cooked large eggs (see tip, at left), peeled and chopped | 2 |
| ⅔ cup | chopped toasted walnuts | 150 mL |

1. In a large saucepan of boiling salted water, cook quinoa for 12 minutes. Add asparagus and peas; cook for 30 seconds. Drain and rinse under cold water until cool.

2. In a large bowl, combine quinoa and chives.

3. In a small bowl, whisk together garlic, lemon juice, oil and mustard. Add to quinoa mixture and gently toss to coat. Season to taste with salt and pepper. Cover and refrigerate for at least 30 minutes, until chilled, or for up to 2 hours.

4. Just before serving, add eggs and walnuts, gently tossing to combine.

# Spicy Quinoa and Three-Bean Salad

*When the weather is sweltering, you can practically live on this salad. It tastes bright and fresh, and is satisfying without being heavy.*

## Tip

For a spicier salad, leave in the jalapeño seeds.

| | | |
|---|---|---|
| 3 cups | cooked red, black or white quinoa (see page 10), cooled | 750 mL |
| 1 | red bell pepper, chopped | 1 |
| 2 cups | chopped celery | 500 mL |
| 1 | can (14 to 19 oz/398 to 540 mL) chickpeas, drained and rinsed | 1 |
| 1 | can (14 to 19 oz/398 to 540 mL) black beans, drained and rinsed | 1 |
| 1 | can (14 to 19 oz/398 to 540 mL) dark red kidney beans, drained and rinsed | 1 |
| 1 tbsp | minced seeded jalapeño pepper | 15 mL |
| 1 tbsp | ground cumin | 15 mL |
| 3 tbsp | extra virgin olive oil | 45 mL |
| 2 tbsp | balsamic vinegar | 30 mL |
| 1½ tbsp | liquid honey, agave nectar or brown rice syrup | 22 mL |
| | Fine sea salt and freshly cracked black pepper | |

1. In a large bowl, combine quinoa, red pepper, celery, chickpeas, black beans and kidney beans.

2. In a small bowl, whisk together jalapeño, cumin, oil, vinegar and honey. Add to quinoa mixture and gently toss to coat. Season to taste with salt and pepper. Cover and refrigerate for at least 1 hour, until chilled, or for up to 24 hours.

# Shredded Beet, Parsley and Quinoa Salad

*It's rare that Italian parsley is treated as a salad green unto itself. But when it's tempered by earthy quinoa, juicy raw beets and an orange vinaigrette, the mineral-tinged flat leaves will surprise and delight.*

## Tip

Use the coarse side of a box grater to shred the beets. Or, to make quick work of the task, use the shredding disk on a food processor.

| | | |
|---|---|---:|
| 2 cups | cooked quinoa (see page 10), cooled | 500 mL |
| 4 | orange, yellow or red beets, peeled and coarsely shredded | 4 |
| 1 tsp | finely grated orange zest | 5 mL |
| 2 tbsp | freshly squeezed orange juice | 30 mL |
| 2 tbsp | extra virgin olive oil | 30 mL |
| 1 tbsp | sherry vinegar or white wine vinegar | 15 mL |
| | Fine sea salt and freshly cracked black pepper | |
| 1½ cups | packed fresh flat-leaf (Italian) parsley leaves, chopped | 375 mL |
| ½ cup | crumbled soft goat cheese | 125 mL |
| ⅓ cup | chopped lightly salted roasted pistachios | 75 mL |

1. In a large bowl, combine quinoa and beets.
2. In a small bowl, whisk together orange zest, orange juice, oil and vinegar. Add to quinoa mixture and gently toss to coat. Season to taste with salt and pepper. Cover and refrigerate for at least 1 hour, until chilled, or for up to 4 hours.
3. Just before serving, add parsley and cheese, gently tossing to combine. Sprinkle with pistachios.

# Broccoli Quinoa Salad

| **Makes 8 side-dish servings** | |
|---|---|

*Broccoli seems like something new in this so-flavorful, satisfyingly eclectic quinoa salad, dolled up with blue cheese and tart cherries.*

● **Steamer basket**

| 3 cups | chopped broccoli florets (about 1 large bunch) | 750 mL |
|---|---|---|
| | Ice water | |
| 2 tbsp | extra virgin olive oil | 30 mL |
| 1 tbsp | white wine vinegar | 15 mL |
| 1 tsp | Dijon mustard | 5 mL |
| 3 cups | cooked quinoa (see page 10), cooled | 750 mL |
| ½ cup | crumbled blue cheese | 125 mL |
| ⅓ cup | dried tart cherries or cranberries, chopped | 75 mL |
| ¼ cup | chopped green onions | 60 mL |
| | Fine sea salt and freshly cracked black pepper | |
| ½ cup | chopped toasted walnuts | 125 mL |

1. Place broccoli in a steamer basket set over a large saucepan of boiling water. Cover and steam for 1 to 2 minutes or until tender-crisp but still bright green. Transfer to a large bowl of ice water to stop the cooking. Drain and pat dry with paper towels.

2. In a small bowl, whisk together oil, vinegar and mustard.

3. In a large bowl, combine broccoli, quinoa, cheese, cherries and green onions. Add dressing and gently toss to coat. Season to taste with salt and pepper. Cover and refrigerate for at least 30 minutes, until chilled, or for up to 2 hours.

4. Just before serving, sprinkle with walnuts.

# Lemony Brussels Sprouts Quinoa Salad

*When Brussels sprouts are lightly cooked — as they are in this simple yet vibrant salad — and then complemented with assertive flavors, such as tart lemon and nutty quinoa, their intense flavor is beautifully balanced.*

## Tip

Trim the root end from Brussels sprouts and cut off any loose, thick outer leaves, then rinse well to remove any grit that may have gathered under loose leaves.

### • Steamer basket

| | | |
|---|---|---|
| 1 lb | Brussels sprouts, trimmed | 500 g |
| | Ice water | |
| 1 tsp | finely grated lemon zest | 5 mL |
| 2 tbsp | freshly squeezed lemon juice | 30 mL |
| 2 tbsp | extra virgin olive oil | 30 mL |
| 2 tbsp | liquid honey | 30 mL |
| 1 tbsp | whole-grain Dijon mustard | 15 mL |
| 2 cups | cooked red, black or white quinoa (see page 10), cooled | 500 mL |
| | Fine sea salt and freshly cracked black pepper | |
| ½ cup | chopped toasted walnuts | 125 mL |

1. Place Brussels sprouts in a steamer basket set over a large saucepan of boiling water. Cover and steam for 5 to 6 minutes or until tender-crisp but still bright green. Transfer to a large bowl of ice water to stop the cooking. Drain and pat dry with paper towels. Using a very sharp knife or a mandolin, thinly slice Brussels sprouts lengthwise.

2. In a small bowl, whisk together lemon zest, lemon juice, oil, honey and mustard.

3. In a large bowl, combine Brussels sprouts and quinoa. Add dressing and gently toss to coat. Season to taste with salt and pepper. Cover and refrigerate for at least 30 minutes, until chilled, or for up to 2 hours.

4. Just before serving, sprinkle with walnuts.

# Warm Cauliflower, Quinoa and Raisin Salad

*Cauliflower boasts plenty of antioxidant, cancer-fighting and heart-healthy properties. But what makes this salad exceptional is the deep, caramelized flavor cauliflower delivers when roasted until golden. Teamed with versatile quinoa, piquant capers and sweet plump golden raisins, it makes a sensational salad.*

## Tip

To mash garlic, working with one clove at a time, place the side of a chef's knife flat against the clove. Place the heel of your hand on the side of the knife and apply pressure so that the clove flattens slightly (this will loosen the peel). Remove and discard the peel, then roughly chop the garlic. Sprinkle a pinch of coarse salt over the garlic. Use the flat part of the knife as before to press the garlic against the cutting board. Repeat until the garlic turns into a fine paste. The mashed garlic is now ready for use in your favorite recipe.

- **Preheat oven to 400°F (200°C)**
- **Large rimmed baking sheet, lined with foil and sprayed with nonstick cooking spray**

| | | |
|---|---|---|
| 4 cups | small cauliflower florets (about 1 medium head) | 1 L |
| 1½ tsp | ground coriander | 7 mL |
| 3 tbsp | extra virgin olive oil, divided | 45 mL |
| | Fine sea salt and freshly cracked black pepper | |
| 2 | cloves garlic, mashed (see tip, at left) | 2 |
| 2 tbsp | drained capers, minced | 30 mL |
| 2 tbsp | sherry vinegar or white wine vinegar | 30 mL |
| 1 tsp | Dijon mustard | 5 mL |
| 3 cups | cooked quinoa (see page 10), cooled | 750 mL |
| ½ cup | golden raisins | 125 mL |
| 1 cup | firmly packed fresh flat-leaf (Italian) parsley leaves, roughly chopped | 250 mL |

1. In a large bowl, toss cauliflower with coriander and half the oil. Sprinkle with salt and pepper. Spread in a single layer on prepared baking sheet. Roast in preheated oven for 35 to 40 minutes, stirring once or twice, until tender and golden brown. Let cool slightly in pan on a wire rack.

2. In a small bowl, whisk together garlic, capers, vinegar and mustard.

3. In a large bowl, combine roasted cauliflower, quinoa and raisins. Add dressing and parsley, gently tossing to coat. Season to taste with salt and pepper. Serve immediately.

# North African Carrot Quinoa Salad

*A Moroccan-inspired carrot and quinoa salad is versatile enough to accompany almost any meal. Although it's wonderful made with regular orange carrots, you could also showcase the rainbow of offerings (shades of scarlet, burgundy and yellow) that beckon at farmers' markets.*

| | | |
|---|---|---|
| 2 cups | cooked black or white quinoa (see page 10), cooled | 500 mL |
| 3 cups | coarsely shredded carrots (about 12 oz/375 g) | 750 mL |
| ¾ cup | packed fresh cilantro or flat-leaf (Italian) parsley leaves, chopped | 175 mL |
| ⅓ cup | golden raisins | 75 mL |
| 3 | cloves garlic, mashed (see tip, page 221) or minced | 3 |
| 1½ tsp | ground cumin | 7 mL |
| ¾ tsp | hot smoked paprika | 3 mL |
| ½ tsp | ground cinnamon | 2 mL |
| 2 tbsp | extra virgin olive oil | 30 mL |
| 2 tbsp | freshly squeezed lemon juice | 30 mL |
| | Fine sea salt and freshly cracked black pepper | |

1. In a large bowl, combine quinoa, carrots, cilantro and raisins.
2. In a small bowl, whisk together garlic, cumin, paprika, cinnamon, oil and lemon juice. Add to quinoa mixture and gently toss to coat. Season to taste with salt and pepper. Cover and refrigerate for at least 1 hour, until chilled, or for up to 4 hours.

# Gingered Carrot and Quinoa Salad

*Carrots and quinoa take on an exotic twist with the flavors of ginger and chile pepper in this easy-to-prepare salad. Quinoa has a subtle sesame flavor already; adding toasted sesame seeds to the salad enhances it.*

**Tip**

For a spicier salad, leave in some or all of the serrano seeds.

| | | |
|---|---|---|
| 2 cups | cooked quinoa (see page 10), cooled | 500 mL |
| 2 cups | coarsely shredded carrots | 500 mL |
| 1 cup | thinly sliced green onions | 250 mL |
| 1 tbsp | grated gingerroot | 15 mL |
| 1 tsp | minced seeded serrano or jalapeño pepper | 5 mL |
| 3 tbsp | unseasoned rice vinegar | 45 mL |
| 1½ tbsp | vegetable oil | 22 mL |
| 2 tsp | liquid honey | 10 mL |
| | Fine sea salt and freshly cracked black pepper | |
| 2 tbsp | toasted sesame seeds (optional) | 30 mL |

1. In a large bowl, combine quinoa, carrots and green onions.
2. In a small bowl, whisk together ginger, serrano pepper, vinegar, oil and honey. Add to quinoa mixture and gently toss to coat. Season to taste with salt and pepper. Cover and refrigerate for at least 30 minutes, until chilled, or for up to 2 hours.
3. Just before serving, sprinkle with sesame seeds, if desired.

# Quinoa Tabbouleh

*Removing the typical bulgur wheat from tabbouleh leaves ample room for nutty, protein-packed quinoa in this modern departure.*

| | | |
|---|---|---|
| 4 cups | cooked quinoa (see page 10), cooled | 1 L |
| 1 | large cucumber, peeled, seeded and diced | 1 |
| 2 cups | chopped tomatoes | 500 mL |
| 1 cup | packed fresh flat-leaf (Italian) parsley leaves, chopped | 250 mL |
| ¾ cup | packed fresh mint leaves, chopped | 175 mL |
| ¾ cup | chopped green onions | 175 mL |
| 2 tsp | ground cumin | 10 mL |
| ¼ cup | freshly squeezed lemon juice | 60 mL |
| 3 tbsp | extra virgin olive oil | 45 mL |
| | Fine sea salt and freshly cracked black pepper | |

1. In a large bowl, combine quinoa, cucumber, tomatoes, parsley, mint, green onions, cumin, lemon juice and oil. Season to taste with salt and pepper. Cover and refrigerate for at least 30 minutes, until chilled, or for up to 4 hours.

# Indian Cucumber Quinoa Salad

*Granted, this East Indian–inspired salad features a less-than-usual combination of flavors, but the sum is far greater than the parts. The toasted cumin seeds in the piquant dressing underscore the earthy flavor of the quinoa while complementing the cool flavor of the cucumbers and mint.*

## Tip

To toast coconut, preheat oven to 300°F (150°C). Spread coconut in a thin, even layer on an ungreased baking sheet. Bake for 15 to 20 minutes, stirring every 5 minutes, until golden brown and fragrant. Transfer to a plate and let cool completely.

| | | |
|---|---|---|
| 3 cups | cooked black, red or white quinoa (see page 10), cooled | 750 mL |
| 2 | cucumbers, peeled, seeded and cubed | 2 |
| ⅔ cup | unsweetened flaked coconut, toasted (see tip, at left) | 150 mL |
| 2 tbsp | unsalted butter or coconut oil, melted | 30 mL |
| 1½ tsp | cumin seeds, toasted | 7 mL |
| 1 tsp | finely grated lime zest | 5 mL |
| 2 tbsp | freshly squeezed lime juice | 30 mL |
| 2 tsp | liquid honey | 10 mL |
| | Fine sea salt and freshly cracked black pepper | |
| ⅓ cup | packed fresh mint or cilantro leaves, chopped | 75 mL |
| ⅔ cup | lightly salted roasted cashews, chopped | 150 mL |

1. In a large bowl, combine quinoa, cucumbers, coconut and butter.
2. In a small bowl, whisk together cumin seeds, lime zest, lime juice and honey. Add to quinoa mixture and gently toss to coat. Season to taste with salt and pepper. Cover and refrigerate for at least 30 minutes, until chilled, or for up to 2 hours.
3. Just before serving, add mint, gently tossing to combine. Sprinkle with cashews.

# Fennel, Quinoa and Radish Salad

*My mother is a wonderful cook and inventive salads are a regular part of her supper repertoire. This recipe is a tribute to her. The fennel has nuanced notes of licorice, the radishes contribute a peppery crisp coolness, and the quinoa and goat cheese provide earthiness. The simple dressing ties the salad together.*

## Tips

Look for fennel bulbs with delicate green fronds still attached to the ends of the stalks.

To prepare the fennel bulb, trim off the tough stalks from the top and the root end before cutting the bulb in half. Chop any feathery fronds from the stalks and add them to the salad, if desired. If the outer layers of the bulb are tough and stringy, you can peel them off with a sharp vegetable peeler.

Fennel tastes best when very thinly sliced and has the best crunch when very cold, so be sure to take your time (and use your sharpest knife) when slicing it for this salad, and chill well before serving.

| | | |
|---|---|---|
| 3 cups | cooked quinoa (see page 10), cooled | 750 mL |
| 1 | large fennel bulb (see tips, at left), halved lengthwise, cored and very thinly sliced crosswise | 1 |
| 1 cup | chopped radishes | 250 mL |
| 1 cup | packed fresh flat-leaf (Italian) parsley leaves, chopped | 250 mL |
| 2 tbsp | extra virgin olive oil | 30 mL |
| 1 tbsp | liquid honey | 15 mL |
| 1 tbsp | white wine vinegar | 15 mL |
| | Fine sea salt and freshly cracked black pepper | |
| ½ cup | crumbled soft goat cheese | 125 mL |

1. In a large bowl, combine quinoa, fennel, radishes and parsley.
2. In a small bowl, whisk together oil, honey and vinegar. Add to quinoa mixture and gently toss to coat. Season to taste with salt and pepper. Cover and refrigerate for at least 1 hour, until chilled, or for up to 4 hours.
3. Just before serving, sprinkle with cheese.

# Summer Green Bean and Quinoa Salad

*The satisfying crunch of almonds gives a helping of quinoa, tomatoes and tender green beans added dimension. Further, the nuts have a natural affinity for the mustardy dressing and the hint of licorice from the tarragon.*

• **Steamer basket**

| | | |
|---|---|---|
| 12 oz | green beans, trimmed and halved crosswise | 375 g |
| | Ice water | |
| 1 tbsp | minced fresh tarragon | 15 mL |
| 3 tbsp | extra virgin olive oil | 45 mL |
| 2 tbsp | freshly squeezed lemon juice | 30 mL |
| 2 tsp | Dijon mustard | 10 mL |
| 3 cups | cooked quinoa (see page 10), cooled | 750 mL |
| 2 cups | halved yellow and red cherry or grape tomatoes | 500 mL |
| | Fine sea salt and freshly cracked black pepper | |
| ½ cup | lightly salted roasted almonds, chopped | 125 mL |

1. Place green beans in a steamer basket set over a large saucepan of boiling water. Cover and steam for 4 to 6 minutes or until tender-crisp. Transfer to a large bowl of ice water to stop the cooking. Drain and pat dry with paper towels.
2. In a small bowl, whisk together tarragon, oil, lemon juice and mustard.
3. In a large bowl, combine green beans, quinoa and tomatoes. Add dressing and gently toss to coat. Season to taste with salt and pepper. Cover and refrigerate for at least 30 minutes, until chilled, or for up to 2 hours.
4. Just before serving, sprinkle with almonds.

# French Green Bean, Walnut and Quinoa Salad

*This is an excellent picnic salad because it can be served cold or at room temperature. Just pack the quinoa mixture and dressing separately, then toss and sprinkle with walnuts before serving.*

## Tip

If you have fresh tarragon on hand, you can substitute 1 tbsp (15 mL) chopped fresh tarragon for the dried.

• **Steamer basket**

| | | |
|---|---|---|
| 1 lb | green beans, trimmed and cut into 2-inch (5 cm) pieces | 500 g |
| | Ice water | |
| 1 tsp | dried tarragon | 5 mL |
| 2 tbsp | white wine vinegar | 30 mL |
| 2 tbsp | walnut oil or extra virgin olive oil | 30 mL |
| 1 tsp | Dijon mustard | 5 mL |
| 3 cups | cooked quinoa (see page 10), cooled | 750 mL |
| 2 cups | halved grape or cherry tomatoes | 500 mL |
| ¾ cup | packed fresh flat-leaf (Italian) parsley leaves, chopped | 175 mL |
| ½ cup | thinly sliced red onion | 125 mL |
| | Fine sea salt and freshly cracked black pepper | |
| ¾ cup | chopped toasted walnuts | 175 mL |

1. Place green beans in a steamer basket set over a large saucepan of boiling water. Cover and steam for 4 to 6 minutes or until tender-crisp. Transfer to a large bowl of ice water to stop the cooking. Drain and pat dry with paper towels.

2. In a small bowl, whisk together tarragon, vinegar, oil and mustard.

3. In a large bowl, combine green beans, quinoa, tomatoes, parsley and red onion. Add dressing and gently toss to coat. Season to taste with salt and pepper. Serve immediately or cover and refrigerate for at least 1 hour, until chilled, or for up to 4 hours.

4. Just before serving, sprinkle with walnuts.

# Quinoa Sushi Salad

There's certainly nothing traditional about using quinoa in a "sushi salad," but once you see how wonderful it tastes in tandem with a familiar lineup of California roll ingredients — cucumber, carrot, pickled ginger, nori and wasabi — you'll be a convert.

## Tips

To toast sesame seeds, place up to 3 tbsp (45 mL) seeds in a medium skillet set over medium heat. Cook, shaking the skillet, for 3 to 5 minutes or until seeds are golden brown and fragrant. Let cool completely before use.

Use a very sharp knife or kitchen shears to cut the nori into strips (its dryness can make it somewhat tough to cut).

| | | |
|---|---|---|
| 3 cups | cooked quinoa (see page 10), cooled | 750 mL |
| 1/4 cup | unseasoned rice vinegar | 60 mL |
| 2 tbsp | agave nectar | 30 mL |
| 1 tsp | fine sea salt | 5 mL |
| 1 1/2 tbsp | vegetable oil | 22 mL |
| 1 1/2 tbsp | water | 22 mL |
| 1 1/4 tsp | wasabi paste | 6 mL |
| 2 cups | diced seeded peeled cucumber | 500 mL |
| 1 cup | coarsely shredded carrots | 250 mL |
| 1 cup | thinly sliced green onions | 250 mL |
| 3 tbsp | chopped drained pickled ginger | 45 mL |
| 1 tbsp | toasted sesame seeds (see tip, at left) | 15 mL |
| | Fine sea salt and freshly cracked black pepper | |
| 1 | firm-ripe Hass avocado | 1 |
| 1 | 6-inch (15 cm) square toasted nori, cut into very thin strips | 1 |

1. Place quinoa in a large bowl.
2. In a small saucepan, combine vinegar, agave nectar and salt. Bring just to a boil over medium heat. Pour over quinoa and gently stir to combine. Let cool completely.
3. In a small cup, whisk together oil, water and wasabi paste.
4. To the quinoa, add cucumber, carrots, green onions, ginger and sesame seeds. Drizzle with wasabi mixture and gently toss to coat. Season to taste with salt and pepper. Cover and refrigerate for at least 1 hour, until chilled, or for up to 2 hours.
5. Just before serving, dice avocado and sprinkle over salad, along with nori strips.

# Mixed Herb Quinoa Salad with Fresh Mozzarella

*So simple to prepare, this salad showcases red quinoa and a bright trio of fresh herbs that's pleasing to the eye and the palate. Fresh mozzarella adds mellow creaminess to each bite.*

| | | |
|---|---|---|
| 3 cups | cooked red or white quinoa (see page 10), cooled | 750 mL |
| ¾ cup | packed fresh flat-leaf (Italian) parsley leaves, chopped | 175 mL |
| ½ cup | chopped fresh chives | 125 mL |
| 3 tbsp | chopped fresh dill | 45 mL |
| 2 tbsp | extra virgin olive oil | 30 mL |
| 1 tbsp | white wine vinegar or sherry vinegar | 15 mL |
| | Fine sea salt and freshly cracked black pepper | |
| 6 oz | water-packed mozzarella, drained and diced | 175 g |

1. In a large bowl, combine quinoa, parsley, chives and dill. Drizzle with oil and vinegar, gently tossing to coat. Season to taste with salt and pepper. Cover and refrigerate for at least 30 minutes, until chilled, or for up to 2 hours.

2. Just before serving, add cheese, gently tossing to combine.

# Bok Choy Quinoa Salad with Miso Dressing

*Asian accents can be found in the dressing's miso, ginger and toasted sesame oil, as well as the salad's crisp bok choy. Add quinoa, and this salad makes a good partner for grilled fish or tofu.*

| | | |
|---|---|---|
| 2 cups | cooked quinoa (see page 10), cooled | 500 mL |
| 8 cups | chopped bok choy (about 1 large head) | 2 L |
| 1 tbsp | minced gingerroot | 15 mL |
| 2 tbsp | unseasoned rice vinegar | 30 mL |
| 1½ tbsp | white or yellow miso (GF, if needed) | 22 mL |
| 1 tbsp | toasted sesame oil | 15 mL |
| 1 tbsp | agave nectar or liquid honey | 15 mL |
| | Fine sea salt and freshly ground black pepper | |

1. In a large bowl, combine quinoa and bok choy.

2. In a small bowl, whisk together ginger, vinegar, miso, oil and agave nectar. Add to quinoa mixture and gently toss to coat. Let stand for 10 minutes to blend the flavors.

# Red Cabbage and Quinoa Salad

*Welcome, fall! Crisp, sweet red cabbage, apples and toasted walnuts add depth of flavor and significant crunch to quinoa infused with a mustardy maple dressing.*

## Tip

Make measuring and cleanup easy by measuring the oil in the tablespoon (15 mL) measure before measuring the maple syrup, so the oil coats the spoon and the sticky maple syrup slides out easily.

| | | |
|---|---|---|
| 2 cups | cooked quinoa (see page 10), cooled | 500 mL |
| 2 | tart-sweet apples (such as Braeburn or Gala), peeled and coarsely chopped | 2 |
| 6 cups | chopped red cabbage | 1.5 L |
| 1/2 cup | chopped green onions | 125 mL |
| 1/2 cup | dried cherries or cranberries, chopped | 125 mL |
| 3 tbsp | cider vinegar | 45 mL |
| 2 tbsp | extra virgin olive oil | 30 mL |
| 3 tbsp | pure maple syrup | 45 mL |
| 2 tsp | Dijon mustard | 10 mL |
| | Fine sea salt and freshly cracked black pepper | |
| 3/4 cup | chopped toasted walnuts | 175 mL |

1. In a large bowl, combine quinoa, apples, cabbage, green onions and cherries.
2. In a small bowl, whisk together vinegar, oil, maple syrup and mustard. Add to quinoa mixture and gently toss to coat. Season to taste with salt and pepper. Cover and refrigerate for at least 1 hour, until chilled, or for up to 4 hours.
3. Just before serving, sprinkle with walnuts.

# Wilted Kale, Quinoa and Chorizo Salad

*A bit of Spanish chorizo goes a long way, lending another dimension to an Andalusian-inspired quinoa salad full of wilted greens, tangy olives and a lively orange dressing.*

## Tip

Unlike other greens, kale stems are so tough they are virtually inedible. Hence, they, along with the tougher part of the center rib, must be removed before cooking. To do so, lay a leaf upside down on a cutting board and use a paring knife to cut a V shape along both sides of the rib, cutting it and the stem free from the leaf.

| | | |
|---|---|---|
| 1 cup | quinoa, rinsed | 250 mL |
| 2 cups | ready-to-use reduced-sodium chicken or vegetable broth (GF, if needed) | 500 mL |
| 1 | large bunch kale, tough stems and center ribs removed, leaves very thinly sliced crosswise (about 6 cups/1.5 L) | 1 |
| 1 tsp | finely grated orange zest | 5 mL |
| 2 tbsp | freshly squeezed orange juice | 30 mL |
| 2 tbsp | extra virgin olive oil | 30 mL |
| 2 tsp | sherry vinegar or white wine vinegar | 10 mL |
| 1 tsp | Dijon mustard | 5 mL |
| 4 oz | cured spicy Spanish chorizo, chopped | 125 g |
| 1/3 cup | pitted green olives, chopped | 75 mL |
| | Fine sea salt and freshly cracked black pepper | |

1. In a large pot, combine quinoa and broth. Bring to a boil over medium-high heat. Reduce heat to low, cover and simmer for 12 to 15 minutes or until liquid is absorbed. Remove from heat. Place kale on top of quinoa, cover and let stand for 15 minutes. Fluff with a fork and transfer to a large bowl. Let cool completely.

2. In a small bowl, whisk together orange zest, orange juice, oil, vinegar and mustard.

3. To the quinoa mixture, add chorizo and olives. Add dressing and gently toss to coat. Season to taste with salt and pepper.

# Quinoa Salad with Dates, Radicchio and Goat Cheese

*Slightly bitter, softly crunchy radicchio matches deliciously with slightly sweet, nutty quinoa, and its deep reddish purple color is a gorgeous contrast to the off-white quinoa seeds. Sweet dates, crunchy hazelnuts and creamy goat cheese seal the deal, making this a star salad by any measure.*

## Tip

Plump, tender Medjool dates are the most commonly available soft dates in the U.S. and Canada, but any other variety of soft, fresh dates may be used in their place.

| | | |
|---|---|---|
| 3 cups | cooked quinoa (see page 10), cooled | 750 mL |
| ½ cup | pitted Medjool dates, quartered lengthwise | 125 mL |
| 2 tbsp | extra virgin olive oil | 30 mL |
| 1 tbsp | sherry vinegar or white wine vinegar | 15 mL |
| 1 tsp | Dijon mustard | 5 mL |
| | Fine sea salt and freshly cracked black pepper | |
| 1 | small head radicchio, leaves separated and torn | 1 |
| ½ cup | chopped toasted hazelnuts or almonds | 125 mL |
| ½ cup | crumbled soft goat cheese | 125 mL |

1. In a large bowl, combine quinoa and dates.
2. In a small bowl, whisk together oil, vinegar and mustard. Add to quinoa mixture and gently toss to coat. Season to taste with salt and pepper. Cover and refrigerate for at least 30 minutes, until chilled, or for up to 2 hours.
3. Just before serving, add radicchio and hazelnuts, gently tossing to combine. Sprinkle with cheese.

# Wilted Swiss Chard Quinoa Salad

**Makes 6 side-dish servings**

*A classic combination — sweet raisins and briny olives — team up with Swiss chard and quinoa in a terrific salad that will sway anyone who typically shies away from greens and grains.*

## Tip

Dark raisins may be used in place of the golden raisins.

| | | |
|---|---|---|
| 1 | large bunch Swiss chard, tough stems and center ribs removed, leaves thinly sliced crosswise (about 5 cups/1.25 L) | 1 |
| 3 cups | cooked quinoa (see page 10), cooled | 750 mL |
| ½ cup | pitted green olives, coarsely chopped | 125 mL |
| ¼ cup | golden raisins, chopped | 60 mL |
| ¼ tsp | fine sea salt | 1 mL |
| 2 tbsp | extra virgin olive oil | 30 mL |
| 1 tbsp | liquid honey | 15 mL |
| 1 tbsp | sherry vinegar or white wine vinegar | 15 mL |
| ⅓ cup | chopped toasted walnuts or pecans (optional) | 75 mL |

1. In a large saucepan of boiling salted water, cook Swiss chard for 1 to 2 minutes or until wilted. Drain and rinse under cold water until cool. Thoroughly squeeze chard to remove excess liquid, then chop.

2. In a large bowl, combine Swiss chard, quinoa, olives and raisins.

3. In a small bowl, whisk together salt, oil, honey and vinegar. Add to quinoa mixture and gently toss to coat. Let stand for 10 minutes to blend the flavors. If desired, sprinkle with walnuts.

# Apricot Quinoa Salad with Watercress

*Apricots and almonds have an affinity for each other, as you'll discover in this happy marriage of the plump dried fruit and toasted sliced nuts. Quinoa underscores the flavor of the almonds, while watercress balances the sweetness of the apricots with peppery depth.*

## Tip

To toast sliced almonds, place up to ½ cup (125 mL) almonds in a medium skillet set over medium heat. Cook, shaking the skillet, for 2 to 3 minutes or until almonds are golden brown and fragrant. Let cool completely before use.

| | | |
|---|---|---|
| 2 cups | cooked black or white quinoa (see page 10), cooled | 500 mL |
| 1 cup | chopped dried apricots | 250 mL |
| 1 tsp | dried thyme | 5 mL |
| 3 tbsp | extra virgin olive oil | 45 mL |
| 2½ tbsp | white balsamic or white wine vinegar | 37 mL |
| | Fine sea salt and freshly cracked black pepper | |
| 6 cups | packed tender watercress sprigs or arugula leaves | 1.5 L |
| ½ cup | sliced almonds, toasted (see tip, at left) | 125 mL |

1. In a large bowl, combine quinoa and apricots.
2. In a small bowl, whisk together thyme, oil and vinegar. Add to quinoa mixture and gently toss to coat. Season to taste with salt and pepper. Cover and refrigerate for at least 30 minutes, until chilled, or for up to 4 hours.
3. Just before serving, add watercress, gently tossing to combine. Sprinkle with almonds.

# Cherry, Quinoa and Pepita Salad

*Quinoa and pepitas give this salad a heartiness that leaves you feeling satisfied, not stuffed. Meanwhile, dried cherries and a maple-cider vinaigrette play against delicate onion flavor from the chives.*

| | | |
|---|---|---|
| 3 cups | cooked black or white quinoa (see page 10), cooled | 750 mL |
| 1/2 cup | dried cherries, chopped | 125 mL |
| 3/4 tsp | dried rubbed sage | 3 mL |
| 2 tbsp | extra virgin olive oil | 30 mL |
| 2 tbsp | cider vinegar | 30 mL |
| 1 tbsp | pure maple syrup or brown rice syrup | 15 mL |
| | Fine sea salt and freshly cracked black pepper | |
| 1/2 cup | lightly salted roasted green pumpkin seeds (pepitas) | 125 mL |
| 1/4 cup | chopped fresh chives | 60 mL |

1. In a large bowl, combine quinoa and cherries.
2. In a small bowl, whisk together sage, oil, vinegar and maple syrup. Add to quinoa mixture and gently toss to coat. Season to taste with salt and pepper. Cover and refrigerate for at least 1 hour, until chilled, or for up to 24 hours.
3. Just before serving, add pumpkin seeds and chives, gently tossing to combine.

# Avocado, Grapefruit and Quinoa Salad

*Pretty in shades of pink and green, plus the polka-dot accents of poppy seeds, this easy salad is refreshing and satisfying at the same time. The quinoa and avocados give the salad real substance, and the grapefruit, mustard and red onion provide zest.*

## Tip

Avocados come in several varieties, but Hass are the most widely available. A Hass avocado — notable for its dark, bumpy skin and rich, buttery flesh — is ideal in this simple salad, but any other variety may be used in its place.

| | | |
|---|---|---|
| 2 | large ruby red grapefruits | 2 |
| 1 tsp | ground cumin | 5 mL |
| 3 tbsp | extra virgin olive oil | 45 mL |
| 1 tbsp | agave nectar or liquid honey | 15 mL |
| 2 tsp | Dijon mustard | 10 mL |
| 3 cups | cooked quinoa (see page 10), cooled | 750 mL |
| 2 | small firm-ripe Hass avocados, diced | 2 |
| 1/3 cup | finely chopped red onion | 75 mL |
| 2 tbsp | chopped fresh mint | 30 mL |
| | Fine sea salt and freshly cracked black pepper | |
| 1 tbsp | poppy seeds | 15 mL |

1. Using a sharp knife, cut peel and pith from grapefruits. Working over a small bowl, cut between membranes to release segments. Squeeze the membranes to release any remaining juice into the bowl. Remove segments and coarsely chop.

2. To the grapefruit juice, whisk in cumin, oil, agave nectar and mustard.

3. In a large bowl, combine grapefruit segments, quinoa, avocados, red onion and mint. Add dressing and gently toss to coat. Season to taste with salt and pepper. Cover and refrigerate for at least 30 minutes, until chilled, or for up to 2 hours.

4. Just before serving, sprinkle with poppy seeds.

# Orange and Jicama Quinoa Salad

*This Central American–influenced salad is drenched in bright, fresh flavors: tart-sweet mandarin oranges, crisp jicama, aromatic cilantro and a tart and spicy dressing to coat mildly nutty quinoa. It's super-easy to make, too.*

## Tip

For a spicier salad, add some or all of the jalapeño seeds.

| | | |
|---|---|---|
| 3 cups | cooked black or white quinoa (see page 10), cooled | 750 mL |
| 1½ cups | diced peeled jicama | 375 mL |
| ½ cup | packed fresh cilantro leaves, chopped | 125 mL |
| ⅓ cup | chopped red onion | 75 mL |
| 1 | can (15 oz/425 mL) mandarin oranges, drained and coarsely chopped | 1 |
| 1 tbsp | minced seeded jalapeño pepper | 15 mL |
| 3 tbsp | freshly squeezed lime juice | 45 mL |
| 2 tbsp | extra virgin olive oil | 30 mL |
| 1 tbsp | agave nectar or liquid honey | 15 mL |
| | Fine sea salt and freshly cracked black pepper | |

1. In a large bowl, combine quinoa, jicama, cilantro, red onion and oranges.
2. In a small bowl, whisk together jalapeño, lime juice, oil and agave nectar. Add to quinoa mixture and gently toss to coat. Season to taste with salt and pepper. Cover and refrigerate for at least 30 minutes, until chilled, or for up to 4 hours.

# Asian Pear, Quinoa and Feta Salad

*Sweet Asian pears and tangy feta cheese play off each other deliciously in this early autumn salad.*

## Tip

Asian pears are round like apples, with a crisp texture and a flavor similar to regular pears. If you cannot find them, use Bosc pears in their place.

| | | |
|---|---|---|
| 3 cups | cooked quinoa (see page 10), cooled | 750 mL |
| 2 | Asian pears, peeled and diced | 2 |
| 3 tbsp | extra virgin olive oil | 45 mL |
| 3 tbsp | freshly squeezed lemon juice | 45 mL |
| 1 tbsp | liquid honey | 15 mL |
| | Fine sea salt and freshly cracked black pepper | |
| 4 cups | packed baby spinach | 1 L |
| ¾ cup | crumbled feta cheese | 175 mL |
| ½ cup | chopped toasted walnuts | 125 mL |

1. In a large bowl, combine quinoa and pears.
2. In a small bowl, whisk together oil, lemon juice and honey. Add to quinoa mixture and gently toss to coat. Season to taste with salt and pepper. Cover and refrigerate for at least 30 minutes, until chilled, or for up to 2 hours.
3. Just before serving, add spinach, cheese and walnuts, gently tossing to combine.

# Waldorf Quinoa Salad

**Makes 6 side-dish servings**

*The rich, nutty taste of quinoa brings out the sweet-tart flavors of the apples and red grapes. Bittersweet radicchio, toasted walnuts and a crumble of blue cheese further enhance this reinvention of a New York City original.*

| | | |
|---|---|---|
| 3 cups | cooked quinoa (see page 10), cooled | 750 mL |
| 2 | large Granny Smith or other tart apples, peeled and diced | 2 |
| 1½ cups | thinly sliced celery | 375 mL |
| 1½ cups | red seedless grapes, halved | 375 mL |
| 3 tbsp | extra virgin olive oil | 45 mL |
| 2 tbsp | sherry vinegar or cider vinegar | 30 mL |
| 2 tsp | Dijon mustard | 10 mL |
| 2 tsp | liquid honey | 10 mL |
| | Fine sea salt and freshly cracked black pepper | |
| 1½ cups | torn radicchio | 375 mL |
| ½ cup | chopped toasted walnuts | 125 mL |
| ½ cup | crumbled blue cheese | 125 mL |

1. In a large bowl, combine quinoa, apples, celery and grapes.
2. In a small bowl, whisk together oil, vinegar, mustard and honey. Add to quinoa mixture and gently toss to coat. Season to taste with salt and pepper. Cover and refrigerate for at least 30 minutes, until chilled, or for up to 2 hours.
3. Just before serving, add radicchio and walnuts, gently tossing to combine. Sprinkle with cheese.

# Mango Coconut Quinoa Salad

*If quinoa took a trip to Thailand, it might come back looking a lot like this. With sunshiny mangos, a trinity of Thai herbs (basil, cilantro and mint) and a toasty duo of coconut and peanuts adding rich depth, this quinoa salad is packed with flavor.*

## Tip

To toast coconut, preheat oven to 300°F (150°C). Spread coconut in a thin, even layer on an ungreased baking sheet. Bake for 15 to 20 minutes, stirring every 5 minutes, until golden brown and fragrant. Transfer to a plate and let cool completely.

| | | |
|---|---|---|
| 3 cups | cooked black or white quinoa (see page 10), cooled | 750 mL |
| 2 | large firm-ripe mangos, diced | 2 |
| 1 | red bell pepper, chopped | 1 |
| ¼ tsp | cayenne pepper | 1 mL |
| 3 tbsp | freshly squeezed lime juice | 45 mL |
| 1 tbsp | vegetable oil | 15 mL |
| 1 tbsp | liquid honey | 15 mL |
| | Fine sea salt and freshly cracked black pepper | |
| 1 cup | packed fresh basil leaves, chopped | 250 mL |
| ½ cup | packed fresh cilantro leaves, chopped | 125 mL |
| ¼ cup | packed fresh mint leaves, chopped | 60 mL |
| ⅔ cup | unsweetened flaked coconut, toasted (see tip, at left) | 150 mL |
| ½ cup | lightly salted roasted peanuts or cashews, chopped | 125 mL |

1. In a large bowl, combine quinoa, mangos and red pepper.
2. In a small bowl, whisk together cayenne, lime juice, oil and honey. Add to quinoa mixture and gently toss to coat. Season to taste with salt and black pepper. Cover and refrigerate for at least 1 hour, until chilled, or for up to 4 hours.
3. Just before serving, add basil, cilantro, mint and coconut, gently tossing to combine. Sprinkle with peanuts.

# Watermelon, Quinoa and Feta Salad

*Watermelon provides bursts of sweetness and gorgeous color in this summery salad; feta cheese provides pungent contrast. This dish is particularly striking made with black quinoa.*

## Tip

If you prefer, you can substitute 4 tsp (20 mL) chopped fresh tarragon for the dried.

| | | |
|---|---|---|
| 2 cups | cooked black or white quinoa (see page 10), cooled | 500 mL |
| 4 cups | cubed seedless watermelon ($^3/_4$-inch/2 cm cubes) | 1 L |
| 1 cup | packed fresh flat-leaf (Italian) parsley leaves, chopped | 250 mL |
| 1½ tsp | dried tarragon | 7 mL |
| 2 tbsp | freshly squeezed lime juice | 30 mL |
| 1 tbsp | extra virgin olive oil | 15 mL |
| 1 tbsp | liquid honey | 15 mL |
| | Fine sea salt and freshly cracked black pepper | |
| ½ cup | crumbled feta or goat cheese | 125 mL |

1. In a large bowl, combine quinoa, watermelon and parsley.
2. In a small bowl, whisk together tarragon, lime juice, oil and honey. Add to quinoa mixture and gently toss to coat. Season to taste with salt and pepper. Cover and refrigerate for at least 30 minutes, until chilled, or for up to 2 hours.
3. Just before serving, sprinkle with cheese.

# Piperade Quinoa Salad

**Makes 8 side-dish servings**

*A modern spin on the classic Basque dish, this gorgeous quinoa salad takes additional Spanish cues from sherry vinegar, smoked paprika and brine-cured olives.*

| | | |
|---|---|---|
| ¼ cup | extra virgin olive oil | 60 mL |
| 1 | large red bell pepper, thinly sliced | 1 |
| 1 | large yellow bell pepper, thinly sliced | 1 |
| 1 | large red onion, halved and thinly sliced | 1 |
| 2 | cloves garlic, thinly sliced | 2 |
| ¾ tsp | hot smoked paprika | 3 mL |
| 2 tbsp | sherry vinegar or white wine vinegar | 30 mL |
| 3 cups | cooked quinoa (see page 10), cooled | 750 mL |
| ⅓ cup | pitted brine-cured black olives (such as kalamata), coarsely chopped | 75 mL |
| | Fine sea salt and freshly cracked black pepper | |
| ½ cup | packed fresh flat-leaf (Italian) parsley leaves, roughly chopped | 125 mL |

1. In a large skillet, heat oil over medium-high heat. Add red pepper, yellow pepper and red onion; cook, stirring, for 7 to 10 minutes or until tender. Add garlic and paprika; cook, stirring, for 1 minute. Remove from heat and stir in vinegar.

2. In a large bowl, combine red pepper mixture, quinoa and olives, gently tossing to combine. Season to taste with salt and pepper. Let cool completely, then add parsley, gently tossing to combine.

# Quinoa Pilaf

*Meet your new go-to side dish. This easy dish is endlessly versatile: vary the nuts and herbs, stir in leftover roasted or grilled vegetables, or add a touch of sweetness with dried fruit. You can even transform it into a main dish simply by adding your favorite protein, from cooked beans to grilled meat to canned tuna.*

| | | |
|---|---|---|
| 1 cup | white, red or black quinoa, rinsed | 250 mL |
| 2 cups | ready-to-use reduced-sodium chicken or vegetable broth (GF, if needed) | 500 mL |
| 1 tbsp | extra virgin olive oil | 15 mL |
| 1¼ cups | chopped onions | 300 mL |
| 1 | clove garlic, minced | 1 |
| ½ cup | packed fresh flat-leaf (Italian) parsley leaves, chopped | 125 mL |
| ⅓ cup | lightly salted roasted almonds, chopped | 75 mL |
| | Fine sea salt and freshly cracked black pepper | |

1. In a medium saucepan, combine quinoa and broth. Bring to a boil over medium-high heat. Reduce heat to low, cover and simmer for 12 to 15 minutes or until liquid is absorbed. Remove from heat and let stand, covered, for 5 minutes. Fluff with a fork.

2. Meanwhile, in a large nonstick skillet, heat oil over medium-high heat. Add onions and cook, stirring, for 6 to 8 minutes or until softened. Add garlic and cook, stirring, for 1 minute. Add quinoa and cook, stirring, for 2 minutes. Remove from heat and stir in parsley and almonds. Season to taste with salt and pepper.

# Cilantro-Ginger Quinoa

*A stir-in of cilantro, sesame, ginger and lime transforms plain quinoa into a lively side that's an ideal accompaniment for Asian main dishes.*

● **Blender**

| | | |
|---|---|---|
| 1 cup | black or white quinoa, rinsed | 250 mL |
| 2 cups | ready-to-use reduced-sodium chicken or vegetable broth (GF, if needed) | 500 mL |
| 1 | clove garlic, minced | 1 |
| 1 | 1-inch (2.5 cm) piece gingerroot, roughly chopped | 1 |
| 1 cup | packed fresh cilantro leaves | 250 mL |
| 2 tbsp | freshly squeezed lime juice | 30 mL |
| 1 tbsp | toasted sesame oil | 15 mL |
| | Fine sea salt and freshly ground black pepper | |

1. In a medium saucepan, combine quinoa and broth. Bring to a boil over medium-high heat. Reduce heat to low, cover and simmer for 12 to 15 minutes or until liquid is absorbed. Remove from heat and let stand, covered, for 5 minutes. Fluff with a fork. Transfer to a medium bowl.

2. Meanwhile, in blender, combine garlic, ginger, cilantro, lime juice and oil; pulse until smooth. Add to quinoa, tossing with a fork to combine. Season to taste with salt and pepper.

## Variation

*Cilantro-Jalapeño Quinoa:* Replace the sesame oil with vegetable oil and add 1 tbsp (15 mL) minced jalapeño pepper to the blender in step 2. Depending on the level of heat you like, you can omit or include some or all of the jalapeño seeds.

# Quinoa and Greens Gratin

*In this newfangled rendition of a classic gratin, quinoa and greens soak up all the goodness of a an easy egg and Gruyère mixture scented with garlic and thyme.*

## Tip

Other finely chopped greens, such as kale, collard greens or spinach, may be used in place of the chard.

- **Preheat oven to 375°F (190°C)**
- **8-cup (2 L) baking dish, sprayed with nonstick cooking spray**

| | | |
|---|---|---|
| ⅔ cup | quinoa, rinsed | 150 mL |
| 1⅓ cups | ready-to-use reduced-sodium vegetable or chicken broth (GF, if needed) | 325 mL |
| 1 tbsp | extra virgin olive oil | 15 mL |
| 1½ cups | chopped onions | 375 mL |
| 2 to 3 | cloves garlic, minced | 2 to 3 |
| 1 | large bunch Swiss chard, tough stems and center ribs removed, leaves finely chopped (about 2 cups/500 mL) | 1 |
| 2 tsp | dried thyme | 10 mL |
| | Fine sea salt and freshly cracked black pepper | |
| 4 | large eggs | 4 |
| ¾ cup | shredded Gruyère or white Cheddar cheese | 175 mL |

1. In a medium saucepan, combine quinoa and broth. Bring to a boil over medium-high heat. Reduce heat to low, cover and simmer for 12 to 15 minutes or until liquid is absorbed. Remove from heat and let stand, covered, for 5 minutes. Fluff with a fork.

2. In a large skillet, heat oil over medium-high heat. Add onions and cook, stirring, for 5 to 6 minutes or until softened. Add garlic to taste, Swiss chard and thyme; cook, stirring, for 2 minutes or until chard is slightly wilted. Let cool slightly. Season to taste with salt and pepper.

3. In a large bowl, whisk eggs. Stir in quinoa, chard mixture and cheese. Spread evenly in prepared baking dish.

4. Bake in preheated oven for 25 to 30 minutes or until browned on top and just set. Let cool on a wire rack for at least 10 minutes before cutting. Serve warm or let cool completely.

# Corn and Quinoa Polenta

*Consider this recipe a template, much as you would a basic recipe for corn polenta. Add cheese, herbs, vegetables — whatever inspires you and suits your taste.*

| | | |
|---|---|---|
| 1 cup | polenta or other coarse cornmeal (not instant) | 250 mL |
| 1 cup | water | 250 mL |
| 3 cups | milk or plain non-dairy milk (such as soy, almond, rice or hemp) | 750 mL |
| 1 tsp | fine sea salt | 5 mL |
| 1 cup | hot cooked black, red or white quinoa (see page 10) | 250 mL |
| | Freshly cracked or ground black pepper | |

1. In a medium bowl, whisk together polenta and water.
2. In a medium saucepan, bring milk and salt to a simmer over medium-high heat. Gradually add polenta mixture, whisking constantly until it comes to boil. Reduce heat and simmer, stirring occasionally, for 10 to 12 minutes or until very thick. Stir in quinoa. Season to taste with pepper.

## Variations

*Cheese and Chives Polenta:* Add ¾ cup (175 mL) grated or shredded cheese (such as Parmesan, Romano, sharp Cheddar or Gruyère, or crumbled goat or blue cheese) and 3 tbsp (45 mL) minced fresh chives with the quinoa.

*Broiled Parmesan Quinoa Polenta Sticks:* Prepare quinoa polenta and immediately pour into a 13- by 9-inch (33 by 23 cm) baking pan sprayed with nonstick cooking spray, spreading polenta evenly with a spatula. Let cool completely. (The polenta can be covered and refrigerated for up to 3 days at this point.) Invert onto a baking sheet sprayed with nonstick cooking spray. Preheat broiler, with rack set 4 inches (10 cm) from the heat source. Brush polenta with 1 tbsp (15 mL) extra virgin olive oil and sprinkle with ½ cup (125 mL) freshly grated Parmesan cheese. Broil for 5 to 7 minutes or until golden. Let cool for 5 minutes, then cut into 3- by 1½-inch (7.5 by 4 cm) sticks.

# Caribbean Peas and Quinoa

*Peas and rice is a staple dish throughout the Caribbean, and despite its name is as often made with red kidney beans as with pigeon peas. Here, it is reimagined with quinoa in place of the rice. Coconut milk, allspice and thyme give this so-easy side dish its island flavor.*

| | | |
|---|---|---|
| 1 cup | quinoa, rinsed | 250 mL |
| 1 | clove garlic, minced | 1 |
| 1 tsp | dried thyme | 5 mL |
| ½ tsp | ground allspice | 2 mL |
| 1 cup | light coconut milk | 250 mL |
| 1 cup | ready-to-use reduced-sodium chicken or vegetable broth (GF, if needed) | 250 mL |
| ¼ tsp | hot pepper sauce | 1 mL |
| 1 | can (14 to 19 oz/398 to 540 mL) dark red kidney beans, drained and rinsed | 1 |
| | Fine sea salt and freshly cracked black pepper | |

1. In a medium saucepan, combine quinoa, garlic, thyme, allspice, coconut milk, broth and hot pepper sauce. Bring to a boil over medium-high heat. Reduce heat to low, cover and simmer for 12 to 15 minutes or until liquid is absorbed. Remove from heat and let stand, covered, for 5 minutes. Fluff with a fork.

2. Gently stir in beans. Season to taste with salt and pepper. Cover and let stand for 5 minutes to warm the beans.

# Parmesan Lemon Chickpeas and Quinoa

*This protein-rich dish is wonderful plain, but can be elevated further with a small dollop of prepared basil pesto or chopped fresh tomatoes on top.*

## Tip

This dish also works well as a main dish, in which case it serves four.

| | | |
|---|---|---|
| 2 tsp | vegetable oil | 10 mL |
| ¾ cup | quinoa, rinsed | 175 mL |
| 1½ tsp | ground coriander | 7 mL |
| 1½ cups | water | 375 mL |
| 1 | can (14 to 19 oz/398 to 540 mL) chickpeas, drained and rinsed | 1 |
| | Fine sea salt and freshly cracked black pepper | |
| ½ cup | packed fresh flat-leaf (Italian) parsley leaves, chopped | 125 mL |
| 1 tsp | finely grated lemon zest | 5 mL |
| 1 tbsp | freshly squeezed lemon juice | 15 mL |
| ¼ cup | freshly grated Parmesan cheese | 60 mL |

1. In a medium saucepan, heat oil over medium-high heat. Add quinoa, coriander and water; bring to a boil. Reduce heat to low, cover and simmer for 10 to 11 minutes or until liquid is almost absorbed.

2. Stir in chickpeas and simmer, uncovered, for 2 to 3 minutes or until liquid is absorbed. Remove from heat and let stand, covered, for 5 minutes. Fluff with a fork. Season to taste with salt and pepper. Stir in parsley, lemon zest and lemon juice. Serve sprinkled with Parmesan.

# Black and White Quinoa Dressing

*This riff on holiday dressing will surprise you with its depth of flavor and its incredible ease of preparation. Using a combination of quinoa (black and white) heightens the beauty of the dish, but you can certainly keep the quinoa monochromatic.*

| | | |
|---|---|---|
| ¾ cup | white quinoa, rinsed | 175 mL |
| ¾ cup | black quinoa, rinsed | 175 mL |
| 3 cups | ready-to-use reduced-sodium chicken or vegetable broth (GF, if needed) | 750 mL |
| ½ cup | chopped dried apricots | 125 mL |
| ½ cup | dried cherries | 125 mL |
| 1 tbsp | extra virgin olive oil | 15 mL |
| 1¼ cups | chopped onions | 300 mL |
| 1 | clove garlic, minced | 1 |
| 1½ tsp | minced fresh rosemary | 7 mL |
| 1 cup | chopped toasted pecans | 250 mL |
| ½ cup | packed fresh flat-leaf (Italian) parsley leaves, chopped | 125 mL |
| | Fine sea salt and freshly cracked black pepper | |

1. In a medium saucepan, combine white quinoa, black quinoa and broth. Bring to a boil over medium-high heat. Reduce heat to low, cover and simmer for 12 to 15 minutes or until liquid is absorbed. Remove from heat and sprinkle with apricots and cherries. Cover and let stand for 5 minutes. Fluff with a fork.

2. Meanwhile, in a large nonstick skillet, heat oil over medium-high heat. Add onions and cook, stirring, for 6 to 8 minutes or until golden. Add garlic and rosemary; cook, stirring, for 1 minute. Add quinoa mixture and cook, stirring, for 2 minutes. Remove from heat and stir in pecans and parsley. Season to taste with salt and pepper.

# Vegetarian Main Dishes

# Roasted Grape and Walnut Quinoa

**Makes 4 servings**

*Grapes for dinner? Believe it. In this surprising entrée, plump grapes are roasted to near bursting with an intoxicating flavor combination of balsamic vinegar, honey, black pepper and rosemary. Toss with quinoa and fresh parsley, sprinkle with a bit of cheese and toasted walnuts, and ordinary ingredients are transformed into an extraordinary dinner.*

- Preheat oven to 400°F (200°C)
- Rimmed baking sheet, lined with foil and sprayed with nonstick cooking spray

| | | |
|---|---|---|
| 2 cups | red seedless grapes | 500 mL |
| 1½ tsp | chopped fresh rosemary | 7 mL |
| 1 tbsp | balsamic vinegar | 15 mL |
| 1 tsp | olive oil | 5 mL |
| 1 tsp | liquid honey | 5 mL |
| | Fine sea salt and freshly ground black pepper | |
| 1 cup | quinoa, rinsed | 250 mL |
| 2 cups | ready-to-use reduced-sodium vegetable broth (GF, if needed) | 500 mL |
| ¾ cup | packed fresh flat-leaf (Italian) parsley leaves, chopped | 175 mL |
| ¾ cup | chopped toasted walnuts | 175 mL |
| ½ cup | crumbled blue cheese or goat cheese | 125 mL |

1. In a medium bowl, combine grapes, rosemary, vinegar, oil and honey. Season to taste with salt and pepper. Spread in a single layer on prepared baking sheet. Roast in preheated oven for 18 to 21 minutes, stirring occasionally, until grape skins begin to burst.

2. In a medium saucepan, combine quinoa and broth. Bring to a boil over medium-high heat. Reduce heat to low, cover and simmer for 12 to 15 minutes or until liquid is absorbed. Remove from heat and let stand, covered, for 5 minutes. Fluff with a fork.

3. To the quinoa, add roasted grapes and parsley, tossing to combine. Serve sprinkled with walnuts and cheese.

# Quinoa Risotto with Asparagus and Lemon

*In this innovative "quinotto," the bright flavors of lemon, peas and asparagus play against the rustic flavor of quinoa. Quinoa does not release starch to create the signature, creamy consistency of risotto, but the dilemma is solved by the addition of soft garlic- and herb-flavored cheese, which imparts both creaminess and flavor.*

| | | |
|---|---|---|
| 2 tsp | olive oil | 10 mL |
| 1 cup | finely chopped onion | 250 mL |
| 1 cup | quinoa, rinsed | 250 mL |
| 1 tsp | dried thyme | 5 mL |
| ½ cup | dry white wine | 125 mL |
| 2 cups | ready-to-use reduced-sodium vegetable broth (GF, if needed) | 500 mL |
| 1 lb | asparagus, trimmed and cut into 1-inch (2.5 cm) pieces | 500 g |
| 1 cup | frozen petite peas, thawed | 250 mL |
| ½ cup | soft garlic- and herb-flavored cheese (such as Boursin) | 125 mL |
| 1 tsp | finely grated lemon zest | 5 mL |
| 2 tbsp | freshly squeezed lemon juice | 30 mL |
| | Fine sea salt and freshly cracked black pepper | |
| ¼ cup | freshly grated Parmesan cheese | 60 mL |

1. In a large saucepan, heat oil over medium-high heat. Add onion and quinoa; cook, stirring, for 5 to 6 minutes or until onion is softened. Add thyme and wine; cook, stirring, for 3 to 5 minutes or until liquid is evaporated.

2. Stir in broth and bring to a boil, stirring often. Reduce heat and simmer, stirring occasionally, for 8 minutes. Stir in asparagus and simmer, stirring occasionally, for 4 to 5 minutes or until tender. Stir in peas, garlic- and herb-flavored cheese, lemon zest and lemon juice; simmer for 1 minute or until heated through. Season to taste with salt and pepper. Serve sprinkled with Parmesan.

# Roasted Asparagus, Tomato and Olive Quinoa

**Makes 4 servings**

*Delivering a lot of punch for very little effort, this dish balances the toasty flavor of quinoa with the grassy, fresh flavor of asparagus and the acidity of roasted tomatoes.*

- **Preheat oven to 400°F (200°C)**
- **Rimmed baking sheet, lined with foil and sprayed with nonstick cooking spray**

| | | |
|---|---|---|
| 12 oz | asparagus, trimmed and cut into 1-inch (2.5 cm) pieces | 375 g |
| 1½ cups | cherry or grape tomatoes | 375 mL |
| ½ tsp | fine sea salt | 2 mL |
| ½ tsp | hot pepper flakes | 2 mL |
| 1 tbsp | olive oil | 15 mL |
| 1 cup | quinoa, rinsed | 250 mL |
| 2 cups | ready-to-use reduced-sodium vegetable broth (GF, if needed) | 500 mL |
| ¼ cup | pitted brine-cured black olives (such as kalamata), chopped | 60 mL |
| ½ cup | crumbled soft mild goat cheese | 125 mL |

1. In a medium bowl, combine asparagus, tomatoes, salt, hot pepper flakes and oil. Spread in a single layer on prepared baking sheet. Roast in preheated oven for 13 to 16 minutes, stirring occasionally, until vegetables begin to brown.

2. In a medium saucepan, combine quinoa and broth. Bring to a boil over medium-high heat. Reduce heat to low, cover and simmer for 12 to 15 minutes or until liquid is absorbed. Remove from heat and let stand, covered, for 5 minutes. Fluff with a fork.

3. To the quinoa, add roasted asparagus mixture and olives, tossing to combine. Serve sprinkled with cheese.

# Crimson Quinoa with Beets and Goat Cheese

*I love the contrasts at play in this dish — from the deep, sweet flavors of the beets and beet greens to the tender bite of the nutty quinoa to the crumbly finish of tangy goat cheese.*

## Tip

An equal amount of chopped raisins or dried cranberries may be used in place of the currants.

| | | |
|---|---|---|
| 1 tbsp | olive oil | 15 mL |
| 4 cups | thinly sliced onions | 1 L |
| 6 | beets (about 2 inches/5 cm in diameter), with green tops attached | 6 |
| 3 | cloves garlic, minced | 3 |
| | Fine sea salt and freshly cracked black pepper | |
| 1 cup | red or white quinoa, rinsed | 250 mL |
| 2 cups | ready-to-use reduced-sodium vegetable broth (GF, if needed) | 500 mL |
| ¼ cup | dried currants | 60 mL |
| 2 tsp | balsamic vinegar | 10 mL |
| ½ cup | crumbled feta or goat cheese | 125 mL |

1. In a large skillet, heat oil over medium-low heat. Add onions and cook, stirring occasionally, for about 25 minutes or until dark golden brown.

2. Meanwhile, trim leaves and stems from beets, reserving leaves and tender stems. Scrub beets. Rinse and spin-dry beet greens and tender stems, then coarsely chop. Peel beets and cut each into 8 wedges.

3. In a large pot of boiling salted water, cook beets for about 10 minutes or until tender. Drain beets and transfer to a medium bowl.

4. Add garlic to the onions and season with salt and pepper. Cook, stirring, for 2 minutes. Stir in beet greens, cover and cook for about 5 minutes or until tender. Remove from heat.

5. In a large saucepan, combine quinoa and broth. Bring to a boil over medium-high heat. Reduce heat to low, cover and simmer for 12 to 15 minutes or until liquid is absorbed. Remove from heat and let stand, covered, for 5 minutes. Fluff with a fork.

6. To the quinoa, add beets, onion mixture, currants and vinegar. Cook over medium-low heat, tossing to combine, for 1 minute. Serve sprinkled with cheese.

# Broccoli with Sesame Quinoa and Tahini Miso Dressing

*This easy supper is packed with both nutrition and flavor. The broccoli is chock full of beta carotene — a powerful antioxidant that the body converts to vitamin A — the miso is a very good source of vitamin $B_{12}$, and quinoa is rich in protein.*

## Tip

To toast sesame seeds, place up to 3 tbsp (45 mL) seeds in a medium skillet set over medium heat. Cook, shaking the skillet, for 3 to 5 minutes or until seeds are golden brown and fragrant. Let cool completely before use.

- **Steamer basket**

| | | |
|---|---|---|
| 1½ lbs | broccoli (about 1 large bunch), tough stems trimmed off | 750 g |
| 1 | clove garlic, minced | 1 |
| ¼ cup | tahini | 60 mL |
| 2 tbsp | water | 30 mL |
| 1½ tbsp | yellow or white miso | 22 mL |
| 2 tsp | freshly squeezed lemon juice | 10 mL |
| 3 tbsp | toasted sesame seeds (see tip, at left) | 45 mL |
| 3 cups | hot cooked quinoa (see page 10) | 750 mL |
| | Fine sea salt and freshly cracked black pepper | |

1. Cut broccoli into small florets. Use a vegetable peeler to peel the stem, then cut the stem crosswise into ¼-inch (0.5 cm) thick slices. Place in a steamer basket set over a large pot of boiling water. Cover and steam for 5 to 7 minutes or until tender.
2. Meanwhile, in a small bowl, whisk together garlic, tahini, water, miso and lemon juice.
3. Stir sesame seeds into hot quinoa. Season to taste with salt and pepper. Divide among four bowls and top with broccoli. Drizzle with dressing.

# Roasted Cauliflower Quinoa

*Try this modern spin on roasted cauliflower. Green olives and golden raisins are the wild cards here, contributing unexpected depth of flavor.*

## Tip

Chopped pitted brine-cured black olives (such as kalamata) may be used in place of the green olives.

- **Preheat oven to 450°F (230°C)**
- **Large rimmed baking sheet, lined with foil and sprayed with nonstick cooking spray (preferably olive oil)**

| | | |
|---|---|---|
| 4 cups | roughly chopped cauliflower florets (about 1 medium head) | 1 L |
| 1 tbsp | olive oil | 15 mL |
| | Fine sea salt and freshly cracked black pepper | |
| 1 cup | quinoa, rinsed | 250 mL |
| 2 cups | ready-to-use reduced-sodium vegetable broth (GF, if needed) | 500 mL |
| ½ cup | packed fresh flat-leaf (Italian) parsley leaves, chopped | 125 mL |
| ½ cup | chopped toasted walnuts | 125 mL |
| ¼ cup | chopped pitted green olives | 60 mL |
| ¼ cup | golden raisins | 60 mL |

1. In a large bowl, combine cauliflower and oil. Season to taste with salt and pepper. Spread in a single layer on prepared baking sheet. Roast in preheated oven for 20 to 25 minutes, stirring once or twice, until golden brown and tender.

2. Meanwhile, in a medium saucepan, combine quinoa and broth. Bring to a boil over medium-high heat. Reduce heat to low, cover and simmer for 12 to 15 minutes or until liquid is absorbed. Remove from heat and let stand, covered, for 5 minutes. Fluff with a fork.

3. To the quinoa, add roasted cauliflower, parsley, walnuts, olives and raisins, tossing to combine. Season to taste with salt and pepper.

# Quinoa al Norma

*Fresh basil and Romano cheese form a flawless Italian duo that boldly punctuates this quinoa riff on pasta al Norma.*

## Tip

When selecting an eggplant, choose one with firm, shiny, blemish-free skin and a mostly green (not brown) stem top. The eggplant should feel heavier than it looks; the greater the moisture, the fresher the eggplant.

- **Preheat oven to 500°F (260°C)**
- **Large rimmed baking sheet, lined with foil and sprayed with nonstick cooking spray (preferably olive oil)**

| | | |
|---|---|---|
| 1 | large eggplant, trimmed and cut into 1-inch (2.5 cm) cubes | 1 |
| 2 tsp | olive oil | 10 mL |
| | Fine sea salt and freshly cracked black pepper | |
| 1 cup | quinoa, rinsed | 250 mL |
| 2 cups | ready-to-use reduced-sodium vegetable broth (GF, if needed) | 500 mL |
| ⅓ cup | chopped drained oil-packed sun-dried tomatoes | 75 mL |
| ¼ tsp | hot pepper flakes | 1 mL |
| ¼ cup | dry white wine | 60 mL |
| ⅓ cup | freshly grated Romano cheese | 75 mL |
| ⅓ cup | packed fresh basil leaves, torn | 75 mL |

1. In a large bowl, combine eggplant and oil. Season to taste with salt and pepper. Spread in a single layer on prepared baking sheet. Roast in preheated oven for 15 to 20 minutes or until tender and golden brown.

2. Meanwhile, in a large, deep skillet, combine quinoa and broth. Bring to a boil over medium-high heat. Reduce heat to low, cover and simmer for 12 to 15 minutes or until liquid is absorbed. Remove from heat and let stand, covered, for 5 minutes. Fluff with a fork.

3. To the quinoa, add roasted eggplant, sun-dried tomatoes, hot pepper flakes and wine, tossing to combine. Cook over medium-low heat, stirring constantly, for 2 to 3 minutes or until liquid is evaporated. Serve sprinkled with cheese and basil.

# Spiced Eggplant Ragù over Quinoa

**Makes 4 servings**

*This wonderfully rich ragù layers the flavors of eggplant, mushrooms and exotic spices with nutty quinoa and a tangy yogurt-walnut sauce.*

## Tip

To mash garlic, working with one clove at a time, place the side of a chef's knife flat against the clove. Place the heel of your hand on the side of the knife and apply pressure so that the clove flattens slightly (this will loosen the peel). Remove and discard the peel, then roughly chop the garlic. Sprinkle a pinch of coarse salt over the garlic. Use the flat part of the knife as before to press the garlic against the cutting board. Repeat until the garlic turns into a fine paste. The mashed garlic is now ready for use in your favorite recipe.

| | | |
|---|---|---|
| 1 tbsp | olive oil | 15 mL |
| 1¼ cups | chopped onions | 300 mL |
| 1 | large eggplant, trimmed and cut into 1-inch (2.5 cm) cubes | 1 |
| 1 lb | cremini or button mushrooms, halved (or quartered if large) | 500 g |
| 1½ tsp | ground cumin | 7 mL |
| 1 tsp | ground coriander | 5 mL |
| ½ tsp | ground cinnamon | 2 mL |
| ¼ tsp | cayenne pepper | 1 mL |
| 1 cup | canned diced tomatoes, with juice | 250 mL |
| ¾ cup | ready-to-use reduced-sodium vegetable broth (GF, if needed) | 175 mL |
| ½ cup | packed fresh cilantro leaves, chopped, divided | 125 mL |
| 2 tbsp | freshly squeezed lemon juice | 30 mL |
| | Fine sea salt and freshly cracked black pepper | |
| 1 | clove garlic, mashed (see tip, at left) | 1 |
| ⅓ cup | finely chopped toasted walnuts | 75 mL |
| ¾ cup | plain yogurt | 175 mL |
| 3 cups | hot cooked quinoa (see page 10) | 750 mL |

1. In a large saucepan, heat oil over medium-high heat. Add onions and cook, stirring, for 5 minutes or until starting to soften. Add eggplant, mushrooms, cumin, coriander, cinnamon, and cayenne; cook, stirring, for 5 minutes or until mushrooms release their liquid.

2. Stir in tomatoes and broth; bring to a boil. Reduce heat to low, cover and simmer, stirring occasionally, for 10 minutes. Stir in half the cilantro and the lemon juice; simmer, uncovered, stirring occasionally, for 5 minutes to heat through and blend the flavors. Season to taste with salt and black pepper.

3. Meanwhile, in a small bowl, combine garlic, the remaining cilantro, walnuts and yogurt.

4. Serve ragù over quinoa, with dollops of yogurt sauce.

# Quinoa and Eggplant Parmesan Melts

*Forget the fuss — and the heaviness — of casserole-style eggplant Parmesan. This version has all of the flavor, plus added protein from the quinoa, and is ready in no time.*

## Tip

Regular mozzarella (not packed in water) may be used in place of the water-packed mozzarella.

- **Preheat oven to 400°F (200°C)**
- **2 large rimmed baking sheets, sprayed with nonstick cooking spray (preferably olive oil)**

| | | |
|---|---|---|
| 2 | large eggplants (each about 2 lbs/1 kg), trimmed and cut crosswise into 1/2-inch (1 cm) thick slices | 2 |
| | Nonstick cooking spray (preferably olive oil) | |
| | Fine sea salt and freshly cracked black pepper | |
| 3 tbsp | prepared basil pesto | 45 mL |
| 1 1/2 cups | hot cooked quinoa (see page 10) | 375 mL |
| 4 | tomatoes, sliced | 4 |
| 1 | ball (about 8 oz/250 g) fresh mozzarella in water, drained and diced | 1 |
| 3 tbsp | freshly grated Parmesan cheese | 45 mL |

1. Lightly spray both sides of eggplant slices with cooking spray. Place on prepared baking sheets and season to taste with salt and pepper. Bake in preheated oven for 25 to 30 minutes or until softened.

2. Stir pesto into hot quinoa. Spread quinoa mixture on top of eggplant slices. Arrange tomato slices on top of quinoa. Sprinkle with mozzarella and Parmesan. Bake for 5 to 8 minutes or until cheese is melted.

# Mushroom, Kale and Quinoa Casserole

*Healthy eating, great taste and frugality were priorities in my mother's kitchen, and casseroles were one of the ways she achieved all three with ease. With this quick casserole, I follow her example on all three points.*

## Tip

Unlike other greens, kale stems are so tough they are virtually inedible. Hence, they, along with the tougher part of the center rib, must be removed before cooking. To do so, lay a leaf upside down on a cutting board and use a paring knife to cut a V shape along both sides of the rib, cutting it and the stem free from the leaf.

- **Preheat oven to 400°F (200°C)**
- **Food processor or blender**
- **8-cup (2 L) baking dish, sprayed with nonstick cooking spray**

| | | |
|---|---|---|
| 1 lb | cottage cheese (reduced-fat or regular) | 500 g |
| 1 tbsp | olive oil | 15 mL |
| 2 cups | sliced mushrooms | 500 mL |
| 1 cup | finely chopped shallots or onions | 250 mL |
| 2 tsp | dried thyme | 10 mL |
| ½ | large bunch kale, tough stems and center ribs removed, leaves chopped (about 4 cups/1 L) | ½ |
| 4 cups | hot cooked quinoa (see page 10) | 1 L |
| 1½ cups | shredded Gruyère or Swiss cheese, divided | 375 mL |
| | Fine sea salt and freshly cracked black pepper | |

1. In food processor, process cottage cheese until smooth.

2. In a large pot, heat oil over medium-high heat. Add mushrooms, shallots and thyme; cook, stirring, for 5 minutes or until mushrooms release their liquid. Add kale and cook, stirring, for 4 to 5 minutes or until slightly wilted.

3. In a large bowl, combine cottage cheese, kale mixture, quinoa and half the Gruyère. Season to taste with salt and pepper. Spoon into prepared baking dish and sprinkle with the remaining Gruyère.

4. Bake in preheated oven for 15 to 18 minutes or until heated through and top is golden.

# Quinoa Bisteeya

*This vegetarian take on the festive Moroccan dish bisteeya (pigeon pie) is transportive. The elaborate-looking phyllo topping is actually quite easy. And with a rich mushroom and quinoa filling beneath, this innovation rivals the classic.*

## Tips

If you do not have garam masala, use the following combination of spices in its place: 1 tsp (5 mL) ground cinnamon and ¼ tsp (1 mL) each ground coriander, ground nutmeg, ground cloves and freshly ground black pepper.

To make this dish gluten-free, omit the phyllo dough. After step 3, pack the quinoa mixture into an 8- or 9-inch (20 or 23 cm) square glass baking dish sprayed with nonstick cooking spray. Sprinkle with 1½ cups (375 mL) gluten-free bread crumbs and spray with cooking spray. Skip steps 4 and 5 and proceed with step 6.

- **Preheat oven to 350°F (180°C)**
- **9-inch (23 cm) springform pan, sprayed with nonstick cooking spray**

| | | |
|---|---|---:|
| 1½ cups | quinoa, rinsed | 375 mL |
| 1 tbsp | olive oil | 15 mL |
| 2 | sweet onions, thinly sliced | 2 |
| 12 oz | cremini or button mushrooms, halved (or quartered if large) | 375 g |
| 1 | can (14 to 15 oz/398 to 425 mL) diced tomatoes, drained | 1 |
| 2 tsp | garam masala | 10 mL |
| 1 tsp | ground cumin | 5 mL |
| 1 cup | packed fresh cilantro or flat-leaf (Italian) parsley leaves, chopped | 250 mL |
| ½ cup | chopped dried apricots | 125 mL |
| ½ cup | lightly salted roasted almonds, coarsely chopped | 125 mL |
| | Fine sea salt and freshly ground black pepper | |
| 4 | large eggs, lightly beaten | 4 |
| 10 | sheets phyllo dough | 10 |
| | Nonstick cooking spray (preferably olive oil) | |
| 1 tbsp | confectioners' (icing) sugar (optional) | 15 mL |

1. In a medium saucepan of boiling salted water, cook quinoa for 9 minutes. Drain and transfer to a large bowl.

2. Meanwhile, in a large skillet, heat oil over medium-high heat. Add onions and cook, stirring, for 6 minutes or until starting to soften. Add mushrooms and cook, stirring, for 5 minutes or until they release their liquid. Stir in tomatoes, garam masala and cumin; cook, stirring, for 1 minute.

3. To the quinoa, add onion mixture, cilantro, apricots and almonds. Generously season with salt and pepper. Stir in eggs.

**4.** On a work surface, layer 5 sheets of phyllo dough, turning each successive one a quarter turn so that the stack forms a large round. Spray the top sheet with cooking spray. Repeat with the 5 remaining phyllo sheets, layering them on top of the previous sheets and spraying the top sheet with cooking spray.

**5.** Lifting the layered sheets from the bottom, transfer phyllo stack to prepared pan, pressing it into the corners and letting the overhang drape over the sides. Gently pack quinoa mixture into the pan, smoothing the surface with the back of a spoon. Fold the phyllo overhang over the filling, tucking the edges into the pan. Spray top with cooking spray.

**6.** Bake in preheated oven for 55 to 60 minutes or until phyllo is deep golden and filling is set in the center. Let cool in pan on a wire rack for 15 minutes. Carefully remove the ring and slide torte onto a large serving plate. Dust with confectioners' sugar, if desired. Cut into wedges and serve warm or let cool slightly.

# Calabrese Quinoa with Mustard Greens

**Makes 4 servings**

*Calabria, Italy, is renowned for its myriad preparations of seasonal vegetables. Here, mustard greens are cooked in a traditional manner with olive oil, garlic, raisins and vinegar. The finish is what makes this simple dish unusual: the cooked greens are tossed with hot quinoa (a replacement for pasta, if you will) and finished with a sprinkle of Parmesan cheese and toasted pine nuts. Buon appetito!*

| | | |
|---|---|---|
| 2 tbsp | olive oil | 30 mL |
| 4 | cloves garlic, thinly sliced | 4 |
| 8 cups | packed chopped mustard greens | 2 L |
| 3 tbsp | raisins, chopped | 45 mL |
| ¼ tsp | hot pepper flakes | 1 mL |
| 3 cups | hot cooked quinoa (see page 10) | 750 mL |
| 1 tbsp | red wine vinegar | 15 mL |
| | Fine sea salt and freshly cracked black pepper | |
| ½ cup | freshly grated Parmesan cheese | 125 mL |
| ¼ cup | toasted pine nuts | 60 mL |

**1.** In a large skillet, heat oil over medium-high heat. Add garlic and cook, stirring, for 30 seconds. Add mustard greens, raisins and hot pepper flakes; cook, stirring, for 2 to 3 minutes or until greens are wilted.

**2.** Stir in quinoa and vinegar; cook, stirring, for 1 minute to heat through. Season to taste with salt and black pepper. Serve sprinkled with cheese and pine nuts.

# Shepherd's Pie with Sweet Potato Mash

*Drawing inspiration from the shepherd's pie my mother made (and I loved) throughout my childhood, I developed this newfangled vegetarian "pie." Meaty mushrooms and quinoa comprise the filling, and a sprinkle of sharp Cheddar cheese tops all.*

## Storage Tip

Store the pie tightly covered with foil or plastic wrap in the refrigerator for up to 2 days. Reheat individual-sized portions in the microwave on Medium (50%) for 1 1/2 to 2 minutes or until warmed through.

- **Preheat oven to 400°F (200°C)**
- **8-cup (2 L) baking dish, sprayed with nonstick cooking spray**

| | | |
|---|---|---|
| 2 tbsp | unsalted butter, divided | 30 mL |
| 1 1/4 cups | chopped onions | 300 mL |
| 12 oz | cremini or button mushrooms, halved (or quartered if large) | 375 g |
| 3 | cloves garlic, minced | 3 |
| 2 tsp | dried thyme | 10 mL |
| 1 | can (14 to 15 oz/398 to 425 mL) tomato purée | 1 |
| 1/2 cup | dry red wine | 125 mL |
| 3 cups | hot cooked quinoa (see page 10) | 750 mL |
| | Fine sea salt and freshly cracked black pepper | |
| 1 1/2 lbs | sweet potatoes, peeled and cut into chunks | 750 g |
| 1 cup | shredded white extra-sharp (extra-old) Cheddar cheese, divided | 250 mL |

1. In a large saucepan, melt half the butter over medium-high heat. Add onions and cook, stirring, for 5 minutes or until starting to soften. Add mushrooms, garlic and thyme; cook, stirring, for 5 minutes or until mushrooms release their liquid.

2. Stir in tomato purée and wine; bring to a boil. Reduce heat to low, cover and simmer, stirring occasionally, for 5 minutes. Remove from heat and stir in quinoa. Season to taste with salt and pepper. Spoon into prepared baking dish.

3. Meanwhile, place sweet potatoes in a large pot of cold water. Bring to a boil over high heat. Reduce heat to medium-high and boil for 15 to 20 minutes or until sweet potatoes are very tender. Drain, reserving 1/4 cup (60 mL) cooking water. Return sweet potatoes and reserved water to the pot, along with the remaining butter; mash until smooth. Stir in half the cheese. Season to taste with salt and pepper. Spread over quinoa mixture and sprinkle with the remaining cheese.

4. Bake in preheated oven for 15 to 20 minutes or until heated through and cheese is melted and golden brown.

# Quinoa Millet Polenta with Mushrooms

*Millet has been a staple food in many parts of the world for thousands of years, and rivals corn for its ability to create a creamy polenta (the Romans made millet polenta for centuries). Quinoa adds a nutty flavor and extra protein to the polenta, making it entrée-worthy. Top with sautéed mushrooms and a final sprinkle of cheese, and a luscious, nutritious dinner is yours.*

## Tip

When selecting mushrooms, choose those with a fresh, smooth appearance, free from major blemishes and with a dry surface. Once home, keep mushrooms refrigerated; they're best when used within a few days after purchase. When ready to use, gently wipe mushrooms with a damp cloth or soft brush to remove dirt particles. Alternatively, rinse mushrooms quickly with cold water, then immediately pat dry with paper towels.

| | | |
|---|---|---|
| ¾ cup | millet | 175 mL |
| ½ cup | quinoa, rinsed | 125 mL |
| 6 cups | ready-to-use reduced-sodium vegetable broth (GF, if needed) | 1.5 L |
| ½ cup | freshly grated Romano or Parmesan cheese, divided | 125 mL |
| 3 tbsp | minced fresh chives, divided | 45 mL |
| | Fine sea salt and freshly ground black pepper | |
| 1 tbsp | olive oil | 15 mL |
| 1 lb | cremini or button mushrooms, quartered | 500 g |
| 1 | clove garlic, minced | 1 |
| 2 tbsp | dry white wine or sherry | 30 mL |

1. In a medium saucepan, toast millet and quinoa over medium heat, stirring constantly, for 2 to 3 minutes or until grains smell toasty and begin to make a popping sound.

2. Stir in broth and bring to a boil. Reduce heat to low, cover and simmer, stirring every 5 to 6 minutes to prevent sticking, for 33 to 38 minutes or until mixture appears very creamy. Remove from heat and stir in half the cheese and 2 tbsp (30 mL) of the chives. Season to taste with salt and pepper.

3. Meanwhile, in a large skillet, heat oil over medium-high heat. Add mushrooms and cook, stirring, for 5 to 6 minutes or until golden brown. Add garlic and wine; cook, stirring, until liquid is evaporated. Season to taste with salt and pepper.

4. Spoon polenta into shallow bowls and top with mushroom mixture. Sprinkle with the remaining cheese and chives.

# Quick Quinoa-Stuffed Portobellos

*The meaty robustness of portobello mushrooms makes a delicious "crust" in this addictive spin on pizza.*

- **Preheat oven to 500°F (260°C)**
- **Large rimmed baking sheet, lined with foil and sprayed with nonstick cooking spray (preferably olive oil)**

| | | |
|---|---|---|
| 4 | extra-large portobello mushrooms | 4 |
| 2 tsp | balsamic vinegar | 10 mL |
| 3 tsp | olive oil, divided | 15 mL |
| 3 cups | packed baby spinach | 750 mL |
| 1¼ cups | hot cooked quinoa (see page 10) | 300 mL |
| 3 tbsp | chopped drained oil-packed sun-dried tomatoes | 45 mL |
| 2 tbsp | chopped pitted brine-cured black olives (such as kalamata) | 30 mL |
| | Fine sea salt and freshly cracked black pepper | |
| 3 tbsp | freshly grated Parmesan cheese | 45 mL |

1. Remove stems from mushrooms. Chop stems and set aside. Using a spoon, gently scoop out black gills on underside of mushroom caps. Discard gills. Place mushrooms, hollow side down, on prepared baking sheet. Brush vinegar and 2 tsp (10 mL) of the oil over tops of mushrooms. Bake in preheated oven for 5 to 7 minutes or until tender.

2. Meanwhile, in a large skillet, heat the remaining oil over medium-high heat. Add spinach and cook, stirring, for 1 to 2 minutes or until wilted. Add quinoa, sun-dried tomatoes and olives; cook, stirring, for 1 to 2 minutes to heat through and blend the flavors. Season to taste with salt and pepper.

3. Turn mushrooms over on baking sheet and fill caps with quinoa mixture. Sprinkle with cheese. Bake for 7 to 10 minutes or until filling is hot.

# Quinoa-Stuffed Peppers

*You can't go wrong
with stuffed peppers for
supper, especially when
they're enlivened with
fire-roasted tomatoes,
mushrooms and
Parmesan cheese. Quinoa
becomes irresistible when
it soaks up the flavors
from the pepper shells,
as well as the herbs and
sautéed mushrooms in
the stuffing.*

- **Preheat oven to 350°F (180°C)**
- **13- by 9-inch (33 by 23 cm) glass baking dish**

| | | |
|---|---|---|
| 6 | red or green bell peppers | 6 |
| 1 tsp | olive oil | 5 mL |
| 1 lb | cremini or button mushrooms, chopped | 500 g |
| 1 cup | packed fresh flat-leaf (Italian) parsley leaves, chopped | 250 mL |
| 2 tsp | dried oregano | 10 mL |
| 2½ cups | hot cooked quinoa (see page 10) | 625 mL |
| 1 | can (14 to 15 oz/398 to 425 mL) fire-roasted diced tomatoes, with juice | 1 |
| | Fine sea salt and freshly cracked black pepper | |
| ¼ cup | freshly grated Parmesan cheese | 60 mL |

1. Cut tops off bell peppers and set tops aside. Pull out and discard seeds and membranes.
2. In a large skillet, heat oil over medium-high heat. Add mushrooms and cook, stirring, for 4 to 5 minutes or until tender. Add parsley and oregano; cook, stirring, for 1 minute. Add quinoa and tomatoes with juice; cook, stirring, for 3 minutes. Season to taste with salt and pepper.
3. Spoon about ¾ cup (175 mL) quinoa mixture into each bell pepper. Top each with 2 tsp (10 mL) cheese. Place stuffed peppers in baking dish, tucking tops beside peppers.
4. Bake in preheated oven for 25 to 30 minutes or until peppers are soft. Serve, replacing pepper tops on stuffed peppers.

# Quinoa-Stuffed Poblano Chiles

*In Central America,
poblanos are typically
stuffed with rice, meat or
a combination of the two.
Here, quinoa substitutes,
which is perfectly fitting
(as well as scrumptious),
given its Andean pedigree.*

- **Preheat oven to 350°F (180°C)**
- **8- or 9-inch (20 or 23 cm) square glass baking dish**

| | | |
|---|---|---|
| ¾ cup | quinoa, rinsed | 175 mL |
| 1½ cups | ready-to-use reduced-sodium vegetable broth (GF, if needed) | 375 mL |
| 2 tsp | vegetable oil | 10 mL |
| 4 | cloves garlic, minced | 4 |
| 1 | small red bell pepper, chopped | 1 |
| 1 cup | chopped green onions | 250 mL |
| 2 tsp | minced seeded jalapeño pepper | 10 mL |
| 1½ tsp | ground cumin | 7 mL |
| ½ cup | packed fresh cilantro leaves, chopped | 125 mL |
| 2 tbsp | freshly squeezed lime juice | 30 mL |
| | Fine sea salt and freshly cracked black pepper | |
| 4 | poblano chile peppers, cut in half lengthwise and seeded | 4 |
| 2 cups | canned tomato purée | 500 mL |
| 4 oz | soft goat cheese, crumbled (about 1 cup/250 mL) | 125 g |

1. In a medium saucepan, combine quinoa and broth. Bring to a boil over medium-high heat. Reduce heat to low, cover and simmer for 12 to 15 minutes or until liquid is absorbed. Remove from heat and let stand, covered, for 5 minutes. Fluff with a fork.

2. Meanwhile, in a large skillet, heat oil over medium-high heat. Add garlic, red pepper, green onions, jalapeño and cumin; cook, stirring, for 5 to 6 minutes or until pepper is slightly softened. Remove from heat and stir in quinoa, cilantro and lime juice. Season to taste with salt and pepper.

3. Place poblano halves, cut side up, in baking dish. Spoon about ⅓ cup (75 mL) quinoa mixture into each half. Pour tomato purée into pan (do not pour on top of poblanos).

4. Cover and bake in preheated oven for 20 minutes. Sprinkle poblanos with cheese. Bake, uncovered, for 10 to 14 minutes or until tomato juice is bubbling and poblanos are softened. Serve, spooning tomato purée over poblanos.

# Delicata Squash with Quinoa Stuffing

*Delicata squash at its seasonal best lends subtle sweetness and rich, mellow flavor to a protein-, vitamin- and antioxidant-rich stuffing of quinoa, peppery arugula and tart cranberries.*

## Tip

Acorn squash may be used in place of the delicata squash.

- **Preheat oven to 350°F (180°C)**
- **Large rimmed baking sheet**

| | | |
|---|---|---|
| 2 | delicata squash (each about 1 lb/500 g), halved lengthwise and seeded | 2 |
| | Nonstick cooking spray (preferably olive oil) | |
| 1 tsp | fine sea salt, divided | 5 mL |
| 1 cup | black, red or white quinoa, rinsed | 250 mL |
| 2 cups | ready-to-use reduced-sodium vegetable broth (GF, if needed) | 500 mL |
| 1/3 cup | dried cranberries, chopped | 75 mL |
| 1/4 tsp | freshly cracked black pepper | 1 mL |
| 1 tbsp | white wine vinegar | 15 mL |
| 2 tsp | liquid honey or agave nectar | 10 mL |
| 2 cups | packed arugula, roughly chopped | 500 mL |
| 1/2 cup | packed fresh mint leaves, chopped | 125 mL |
| 1/3 cup | chopped toasted hazelnuts or almonds | 75 mL |

1. Lightly spray cut sides of squash with cooking spray. Sprinkle with half the salt. Place cut side down on baking sheet. Bake in preheated oven for 40 to 45 minutes or until tender.

2. Meanwhile, in a medium saucepan, combine quinoa and broth. Bring to a boil over medium-high heat. Reduce heat to low, cover and simmer for 10 minutes. Stir in cranberries, cover and simmer for 2 to 5 minutes or until liquid is absorbed. Let stand, covered, for 5 minutes. Fluff with a fork.

3. In a large bowl, whisk together the remaining salt, pepper, vinegar and honey. Add quinoa mixture, arugula, mint and hazelnuts, gently tossing to combine.

4. Fill squash cavities with quinoa mixture.

# Potato Masala with Toasted Coconut Quinoa

*You might expect to find russet potatoes in a sensually spiced masala such as this, but I've used yellow-fleshed potatoes, which hold their shape better after a long simmer.*

## Tips

To toast coconut, preheat oven to 300°F (150°C). Spread coconut in a thin, even layer on an ungreased baking sheet. Bake for 15 to 20 minutes, stirring every 5 minutes, until golden brown and fragrant. Transfer to a plate and let cool completely.

An equal amount of fresh mint leaves can be used in place of the cilantro.

• **Blender**

| | | |
|---|---|---|
| 3 | cloves garlic | 3 |
| 1 | 2-inch (5 cm) piece gingerroot, roughly chopped | 1 |
| 1 tbsp | mild curry powder | 15 mL |
| 1½ tsp | ground cumin | 7 mL |
| 1 tsp | garam masala | 5 mL |
| ¾ cup | light coconut milk | 175 mL |
| 2 tsp | vegetable oil | 10 mL |
| 1½ cups | chopped onions | 375 mL |
| 2 lbs | yellow-fleshed potatoes (such as Yukon gold), peeled and cut into 1-inch (2.5 cm) cubes | 1 kg |
| 1¼ cups | ready-to-use reduced-sodium vegetable broth (GF, if needed) | 300 mL |
| 1⅓ cups | frozen petite peas, thawed | 325 mL |
| ⅔ cup | unsweetened flaked coconut, toasted | 150 mL |
| 3 cups | hot cooked quinoa (see page 10) | 750 mL |
| ½ cup | packed fresh cilantro leaves, chopped | 125 mL |

1. In blender, combine garlic, ginger, curry powder, cumin, garam masala and coconut milk; purée until smooth.

2. In a large saucepan, heat oil over medium-high heat. Add onions and cook, stirring occasionally, for 5 to 6 minutes or until softened. Add garlic purée and cook, stirring, for 1 minute or until thickened. Add potatoes, reduce heat and boil gently, stirring often, for about 10 minutes or until potatoes are barely tender.

3. Stir in broth, scraping up any brown bits from bottom of pan. Increase heat to medium-high and bring to a boil. Reduce heat to medium-low, cover and simmer, stirring occasionally, for 16 to 20 minutes or until potatoes are tender. Stir in peas and simmer for 1 minute.

4. Just before serving, stir coconut into quinoa. Spoon quinoa mixture into bowls and top with potato mixture. Sprinkle with cilantro.

# Butternut Squash and Brussels Sprouts Quinoa

*This autumnal entrée is layered with bold flavors — from the maple-roasted butternut squash to the roasted Brussels sprouts and quinoa — each of which makes a real statement.*

- **Preheat oven to 475°F (240°C)**
- **Large rimmed baking sheet, lined with foil and sprayed with nonstick cooking spray (preferably olive oil)**

| | | |
|---|---|---|
| 1 | large red onion, cut into 1-inch (2.5 cm) chunks | 1 |
| 3 cups | cubed peeled butternut squash (1-inch/2.5 cm cubes) | 750 mL |
| 8 oz | Brussels sprouts, trimmed and quartered lengthwise | 250 g |
| 2 tsp | dried rubbed sage | 10 mL |
| 2 tbsp | pure maple syrup | 30 mL |
| 1 tbsp | olive oil, divided | 15 mL |
| | Fine sea salt and freshly cracked black pepper | |
| 3 cups | hot cooked quinoa (see page 10) | 750 mL |
| ½ cup | packed fresh flat-leaf (Italian) parsley leaves, chopped | 125 mL |
| ½ cup | chopped toasted pecans | 125 mL |
| ¼ cup | freshly grated Parmesan cheese (optional) | 60 mL |

1. In a large bowl, combine red onion, squash, Brussels sprouts, sage, maple syrup and oil. Season to taste with salt and pepper. Spread in a single layer on prepared baking sheet. Roast in preheated oven for 18 to 23 minutes, stirring once or twice, until vegetables are golden brown and tender.

2. In a large bowl, combine squash mixture, quinoa and parsley, tossing to combine. Season to taste with salt and pepper. Serve sprinkled with pecans and cheese (if using).

# Spaghetti Squash with Quinoa Ragù

**Makes 4 servings**

*If you are a fan of spaghetti and red sauce — an Italian classic — think of this dish as its health nut cousin. Strands of delicately sweet spaghetti squash stand in for pasta, while meaty mushrooms and quinoa enrich the ragù with good health and great depth.*

## Tip

The spaghetti squash can also be prepared in the oven. Preheat oven to 325°F (160°C) and lightly spray a small rimmed baking sheet with nonstick cooking spray (preferably olive oil). Cut squash in half lengthwise and remove seeds. Place squash, cut side down, on prepared baking sheet and bake for 35 to 40 minutes or until a knife is easily inserted. Let cool for 5 to 10 minutes, then scoop out pulp and continue with step 3.

| | | |
|---|---|---|
| 1 | spaghetti squash (about 2 lbs/1 kg) | 1 |
| 5 tsp | olive oil, divided | 25 mL |
| 8 oz | mushrooms, chopped | 250 g |
| 1½ cups | hot cooked quinoa (see page 10) | 375 mL |
| ½ cup | packed fresh basil leaves, chopped, divided | 125 mL |
| 2 cups | marinara sauce | 500 mL |
| ¼ cup | dry red wine | 60 mL |
| 1 tbsp | olive oil | 15 mL |
| | Fine sea salt and freshly cracked black pepper | |
| ¼ cup | freshly grated Parmesan cheese | 60 mL |

1. Pierce squash all over with a fork. Place on a paper towel in the microwave. Microwave on Medium-High (70%) for 13 to 15 minutes or until soft. Let cool for 5 to 10 minutes.

2. Meanwhile, in a large skillet, heat 2 tsp (10 mL) of the oil over medium-high heat. Add mushrooms and cook, stirring, for 3 to 4 minutes or until they release their liquid. Add quinoa, half the basil, marinara sauce and wine; reduce heat and simmer, stirring occasionally, for 10 minutes or until thickened.

3. Cut squash in half, remove seeds and scoop out pulp. Transfer pulp to a bowl and, using a fork, rake into strands. Add the remaining oil, tossing to coat. Season to taste with salt and pepper.

4. Divide squash among four plates and top with quinoa mixture, cheese and the remaining basil.

# Sweet Potato and Spinach Curry with Quinoa

*If you've never had sweet potatoes in a curry dish before, you'll be surprised by how well they take to bold spices. Coconut milk and quinoa act as dual complements, stealthily rounding out the interplay of sweet and umami that will have you savoring every last bite.*

| | | |
|---|---|---|
| 1 cup | quinoa, rinsed | 250 mL |
| 3½ cups | ready-to-use reduced-sodium vegetable broth (GF, if needed), divided | 875 mL |
| 2 tsp | vegetable oil | 10 mL |
| 1 | large onion, thinly sliced | 1 |
| 2 tbsp | mild curry powder | 30 mL |
| ⅛ tsp | cayenne pepper | 0.5 mL |
| 2 lbs | sweet potatoes, peeled and cut into 1-inch (2.5 cm) chunks | 1 kg |
| 1 | can (14 oz/400 mL) light coconut milk | 1 |
| 8 cups | packed baby spinach (about 6 oz/175 g) | 2 L |
| 1 tbsp | freshly squeezed lime juice | 15 mL |
| | Fine sea salt and ground black pepper | |

**1.** In a medium saucepan, combine quinoa and 2 cups (500 mL) of the broth. Bring to a boil over medium-high heat. Reduce heat to low, cover and simmer for 12 to 15 minutes or until liquid is absorbed. Remove from heat and let stand, covered, for 5 minutes. Fluff with a fork.

**2.** Meanwhile, in a large saucepan, heat oil over medium-high heat. Add onion and cook, stirring, for 6 to 8 minutes or until softened. Add curry powder and cayenne; cook, stirring, for 30 seconds.

**3.** Stir in sweet potatoes and the remaining broth; bring to a boil. Reduce heat and boil for 12 minutes. Add coconut milk, reduce heat and simmer, stirring occasionally, for 3 to 7 minutes or until sweet potatoes are tender. Stir in spinach and lime juice; simmer for 1 to 2 minutes or until spinach is wilted. Season to taste with salt and pepper. Serve over quinoa.

# Swiss Chard Quinoa with Goat Cheese

**Makes 4 servings**

*This streamlined, satisfying quinoa dish will surprise and delight you with a depth of flavor that belies its short list of ingredients.*

| | | |
|---|---|---|
| 1 | large bunch red Swiss chard | 1 |
| 1 tbsp | olive oil | 15 mL |
| 1 | large shallot, thinly sliced | 1 |
| ¼ tsp | fine sea salt | 1 mL |
| ¼ cup | Marsala or sherry | 60 mL |
| 3 cups | hot cooked quinoa (see page 10) | 750 mL |
| ½ cup | crumbled soft goat cheese | 125 mL |
| ½ cup | chopped toasted walnuts | 125 mL |

1. Trim off tough stems from Swiss chard and discard. Trim tender stems and ribs from leaves and finely chop stems and ribs. Thinly slice leaves crosswise (to measure about 5 cups/1.25 L). Set chopped stems and sliced leaves aside separately.

2. In a large saucepan, heat oil over medium-high heat. Add shallot, Swiss chard stems and salt; cook, stirring, for 6 to 7 minutes or until stems are tender and slightly browned. Stir in Swiss chard leaves and Marsala; cook, stirring, for about 2 minutes or until wilted. Stir in quinoa and cook, stirring, for 3 to 4 minutes to heat through and blend the flavors. Serve sprinkled with cheese and walnuts.

# Quinoa al Pomodoro

*In this exemplar of easy summer meal prep, the only cooking required is for the quinoa. All of the other flavor-packed ingredients — the sweetest summer tomatoes, fragrant basil, ricotta salata — are simply chopped, sliced or crumbled before being combined with the hot quinoa.*

## Tip

Ricotta salata is quite different from fresh ricotta in texture and appearance. To make it, salt is added to fresh ricotta (hence "salata"), then it is aged for 2 months, then pressed to reduce much of the moisture. The result is a somewhat dry, spongy cheese with much of the fresh, milky taste of ricotta, but a notably salty edge and a texture akin to feta cheese. You can crumble it, cube it, shave it, grate it or slice it for use in quinoa dishes, salads, pizza, fresh vegetables and so much more. It is also very affordable. Look for it in the cheese section of well-stocked supermarkets.

| | | |
|---|---|---|
| 1¼ cups | quinoa, rinsed | 300 mL |
| 2½ cups | ready-to-use reduced-sodium vegetable broth (GF, if needed) | 625 mL |
| 2 | cloves garlic, minced | 2 |
| 4 cups | chopped tomatoes | 1 L |
| 2 tbsp | extra virgin olive oil | 30 mL |
| 2 tsp | balsamic vinegar | 10 mL |
| | Fine sea salt and freshly cracked black pepper | |
| 4 oz | ricotta salata or mild feta cheese, crumbled (about 1 cup/250 mL) | 125 g |
| ⅔ cup | packed fresh basil leaves, thinly sliced | 150 mL |
| ¼ cup | toasted pine nuts (optional) | 60 mL |

1. In a medium saucepan, combine quinoa and broth. Bring to a boil over medium-high heat. Reduce heat to low, cover and simmer for 12 to 15 minutes or until liquid is absorbed. Remove from heat and let stand, covered, for 5 minutes. Fluff with a fork.

2. Meanwhile, in a medium bowl, combine garlic, tomatoes, oil and vinegar. Generously season with salt and pepper. Let stand for at least 10 minutes to blend the flavors.

3. Add tomato mixture to the quinoa, tossing to combine. Serve sprinkled with cheese, basil and pine nuts (if using).

# Quinoa Casserole with Greens and Ricotta

*A touch of nutmeg adds just the right nuance to this easily assembled quinoa casserole that is at once sophisticated and approachable.*

## Storage Tip

Store the casserole tightly covered with foil or plastic wrap in the refrigerator for up to 2 days. Reheat individual-sized portions in the microwave on Medium (50%) for 1½ to 2 minutes or until warmed through.

- **8-cup (2 L) casserole dish, sprayed with nonstick cooking spray**

| | | |
|---|---|---|
| 2 tsp | olive oil | 10 mL |
| 1 | large bunch red Swiss chard, tough stems and center ribs removed, leaves thinly sliced crosswise (about 5 cups/1.25 L) | 1 |
| 3 | cloves garlic, minced | 3 |
| ½ tsp | ground nutmeg | 2 mL |
| | Fine sea salt and freshly cracked black pepper | |
| 3 cups | cooked quinoa (see page 10), cooled | 750 mL |
| 5 | large eggs, beaten | 5 |
| 2 cups | ricotta cheese (reduced-fat or regular) | 500 mL |
| ½ cup | freshly grated Parmesan cheese, divided | 125 mL |
| 2 cups | cherry or grape tomatoes, halved | 500 mL |

1. In a large skillet, heat oil over medium-high heat. Add Swiss chard and cook, stirring, for 5 to 6 minutes or until wilted and tender. Add garlic and cook, stirring, for 1 minute. Remove from heat. Press chard against side of pan with a wooden spoon to release juices. Drain and discard juices. Stir in nutmeg and season to taste with salt and pepper. Let cool to room temperature.

2. Preheat oven to 400°F (200°C).

3. In a medium bowl, combine quinoa, eggs, ricotta and half the Parmesan. Stir in Swiss chard mixture. Spread evenly in prepared casserole dish. Scatter tomatoes evenly over top. Sprinkle with the remaining Parmesan.

4. Bake for 15 to 20 minutes or until golden and set at the center. Let cool on a wire rack for at least 10 minutes before cutting. Serve warm or let cool completely.

# Quinoa with Wilted Watercress and Blue Cheese

**Makes 4 servings**

*This all-purpose quinoa dish is a friend to busy cooks when spring and summer commence. It's simple, scrumptious and requires virtually no time investment.*

## Tips

An equal amount of arugula, roughly torn or chopped, may be used in place of the watercress.

To toast sliced almonds, place up to 1/2 cup (125 mL) almonds in a medium skillet set over medium heat. Cook, shaking the skillet, for 2 to 3 minutes or until almonds are golden brown and fragrant. Let cool completely before use.

| | | |
|---|---|---|
| 1½ tbsp | olive oil | 22 mL |
| 1 cup | thinly sliced leeks (white and light green parts only) | 250 mL |
| 2 | cloves garlic, thinly sliced | 2 |
| 1 cup | black, red or white quinoa, rinsed | 250 mL |
| 2 cups | ready-to-use reduced-sodium vegetable broth (GF, if needed) | 500 mL |
| 4 cups | packed tender watercress sprigs | 1 L |
| | Fine sea salt and freshly ground black pepper | |
| 1 | firm-ripe Hass avocado, diced | 1 |
| ½ cup | crumbled blue cheese | 125 mL |
| ½ cup | sliced almonds, toasted (see tip, at left) | 125 mL |
| 2 tsp | white wine vinegar | 10 mL |

1. In a large skillet, heat oil over medium-high heat. Add leeks and garlic; cook, stirring, for 1 to 2 minutes or until leeks are slightly softened.

2. Stir in quinoa and broth; bring to a boil. Reduce heat to low, cover and simmer for 12 to 15 minutes or until liquid is absorbed. Remove from heat and let stand, covered, for 5 minutes.

3. Add watercress to the quinoa mixture, tossing to combine. Season to taste with salt and pepper. Serve sprinkled with avocado, cheese, almonds and vinegar.

# Roasted Vegetables with Basil Quinoa

*On their own, roasted vegetables have a fantastic caramelized sweetness, but this recipe goes a step further and jazzes them up by serving them over a blanket of basil quinoa. Tossing the vegetables with garlic before the roast allows the flavor to penetrate every morsel.*

## Tip

When selecting mushrooms, choose those with a fresh, smooth appearance, free from major blemishes and with a dry surface. Once home, keep mushrooms refrigerated; they're best when used within a few days after purchase. When ready to use, gently wipe mushrooms with a damp cloth or soft brush to remove dirt particles. Alternatively, rinse mushrooms quickly with cold water, then immediately pat dry with paper towels.

- **Preheat oven to 450°F (230°C)**
- **Large roasting pan, lined with foil and sprayed with nonstick cooking spray (preferably olive oil)**

| | | |
|---|---|---|
| 3 | cloves garlic, minced | 3 |
| 1 | small red onion, cut into 1-inch (2.5 cm) chunks | 1 |
| 12 oz | cremini mushrooms, trimmed and thickly sliced | 375 g |
| 12 oz | asparagus, trimmed and cut into 1-inch (2.5 cm) pieces | 375 g |
| 1 tbsp | olive oil | 15 mL |
| | Fine sea salt and freshly cracked black pepper | |
| 2 cups | cherry or grape tomatoes | 500 mL |
| 1 cup | quinoa, rinsed | 250 mL |
| 2 cups | ready-to-use reduced-sodium vegetable broth (GF, if needed) | 500 mL |
| ½ cup | packed fresh basil leaves, chopped | 125 mL |
| ½ cup | dry white wine | 125 mL |

1. In a large bowl, combine garlic, red onion, mushrooms, asparagus and oil. Season to taste with salt and pepper. Spread in a single layer in prepared roasting pan. Roast in preheated oven for 18 to 21 minutes, stirring occasionally, until mushrooms and onions begin to brown. Add tomatoes and roast for 7 to 10 minutes or until tomatoes begin to burst and shrivel. Return vegetables to large bowl. Reserve roasting pan.

2. Meanwhile, in a medium saucepan, combine quinoa and broth. Bring to a boil over medium-high heat. Reduce heat to low, cover and simmer for 12 to 15 minutes or until liquid is absorbed. Remove from heat and let stand, covered, for 5 minutes. Fluff with a fork. Gently stir in basil. Season to taste with salt and pepper.

3. Add wine to the roasting pan, scraping up any browned bits from bottom of pan. Place pan over medium heat and simmer for 2 to 3 minutes (or return pan to oven for 5 minutes if pan is not stovetop-safe), until liquid is reduced by half.

4. Spoon quinoa into shallow bowls and top with roasted vegetables. Drizzle pan liquid over top.

# Quinoa Koshari

*Koshari is to Egyptians
what chili is to
Americans. Made of
lentils, rice, tomato sauce
and a kick of spice, it is
a fast-food staple offered
by street vendors in cities
such as Cairo. Here, I've
given it an Andean spin
by replacing the rice
with quinoa. Variations
of koshari are unlimited,
so tweak to your heart's
content to make this basic
recipe your own.*

## Tips

If you are not following a
gluten-free diet, feel free
to use whole wheat or
multigrain macaroni.

Feta cheese is similar to
the Egyptian cheese gibna
beida, a traditional topping
for koshari.

| | | |
|---|---|---|
| 1 cup | dried brown lentils, rinsed | 250 mL |
| 3 cups | water | 750 mL |
| 1 cup | quinoa macaroni (see tip, at left) | 250 mL |
| 3 cups | hot cooked quinoa (see page 10) | 750 mL |
| 1 tbsp | ground cumin | 15 mL |
| ¼ tsp | cayenne pepper | 1 mL |
| 1 | jar (26 oz/700 mL) chunky marinara sauce | 1 |

**Suggested Accompaniments**

Chopped fresh mint

Chopped fresh parsley

Crumbled feta cheese

1. In a large saucepan, combine lentils and water. Bring to a boil over medium-high heat. Reduce heat to low, cover, leaving lid ajar, and simmer, stirring occasionally, for 40 to 45 minutes or until very tender. Drain, then return lentils to the pan.

2. Meanwhile, in a large pot of boiling water, cook macaroni for 7 to 9 minutes or until al dente. Drain and add to lentils.

3. To the lentil mixture, stir in quinoa, cumin, cayenne and marinara sauce; simmer, stirring occasionally, for 10 minutes to heat through and blend flavors.

4. Serve in bowls, with any of the suggested accompaniments, as desired.

# Ras el Hanout Red Lentils and Quinoa

*An ample dose of ras el hanout, an ubiquitous spice blend used throughout Morocco, amplifies the rustic flavors of spinach, lentils and quinoa in this exotic, yet comforting, dish.*

## Tip

A 10-oz (300 g) package of frozen chopped spinach, thawed and squeezed dry, may be used in place of the fresh spinach.

| | | |
|---|---|---|
| 2 tsp | olive oil | 10 mL |
| 3 cups | chopped onions | 750 mL |
| 3 | cloves garlic, minced | 3 |
| 1 tbsp | ras el hanout (see recipe, opposite) | 15 mL |
| 1 tbsp | red wine vinegar | 15 mL |
| ⅔ cup | dried red lentils, rinsed | 150 mL |
| 2 cups | water | 500 mL |
| 1 cup | quinoa, rinsed | 250 mL |
| 2 cups | ready-to-use reduced-sodium vegetable broth (GF, if needed) | 500 mL |
| 8 cups | packed baby spinach (about 6 oz/175 g) | 2 L |
| | Fine sea salt and freshly cracked black pepper | |
| ½ cup | crumbled feta cheese | 125 mL |

1. In a large skillet, heat oil over medium-high heat. Add onions, garlic and ras el hanout. Reduce heat to medium-low, cover and cook, stirring occasionally, for 20 to 25 minutes or until onions are very tender and golden. Remove from heat and stir in vinegar.

2. Meanwhile, in a medium saucepan, combine lentils and water. Bring to a boil over medium-high heat. Reduce heat and simmer for about 22 minutes or until very tender but not mushy. Drain and add to onion mixture.

3. In a large saucepan, combine quinoa and broth. Bring to a boil over medium-high heat. Reduce heat to low, cover and simmer for 12 to 15 minutes or until liquid is absorbed. Remove from heat and let stand, covered, for 5 minutes. Fluff with a fork.

4. To the quinoa, add lentil mixture and spinach. Cook over medium-low heat, tossing to combine, for 1 minute or until spinach is just wilted. Season to taste with salt and pepper. Serve sprinkled with cheese.

# Ras el Hanout

**Makes about 2½ tbsp (37 mL)**

*Literally translating as "top of the shop," ras el hanout is a Moroccan spice blend that can contain upwards of two dozen different spices. This streamlined version includes the main spices of the traditional mixture.*

| | | |
|---|---|---|
| 1½ tsp | ground cumin | 7 mL |
| 1¼ tsp | fine sea salt | 6 mL |
| 1 tsp | ground ginger | 5 mL |
| 1 tsp | freshly ground black pepper | 5 mL |
| ¾ tsp | ground cinnamon | 3 mL |
| ¾ tsp | ground coriander | 3 mL |
| ½ tsp | ground allspice | 2 mL |
| ¼ tsp | ground cloves | 1 mL |

1. In a small bowl, whisk together cumin, salt, ginger, pepper, cinnamon, coriander, allspice and cloves until blended. Store in an airtight container in a cool, dark place for up to 6 months.

# Red Curry Tempeh with Pineapple

**Makes 4 servings**

*You'll love the many textures and flavors in this spicy coconut curry with tempeh, pineapple and quinoa.*

| | | |
|---|---|---|
| 1 cup | light coconut milk | 250 mL |
| 1½ tbsp | Thai red curry paste | 22 mL |
| 1 tbsp | vegetable oil | 15 mL |
| 8 oz | tempeh, cut into ½-inch (1 cm) strips | 250 g |
| 2 cups | diced pineapple or mango | 500 mL |
| 1 cup | packed fresh basil leaves, chopped | 250 mL |
| 1 tbsp | freshly squeezed lime juice | 15 mL |
| | Fine sea salt and freshly ground black pepper | |
| 4 cups | hot cooked quinoa (see page 10) | 1 L |

1. In a small bowl, whisk together coconut milk and curry paste.
2. In a large skillet, heat oil over medium-high heat. Add tempeh and cook, stirring, for 2 to 3 minutes or until browned. Add coconut milk mixture and pineapple; cook, stirring, for 3 to 4 minutes or until heated through. Stir in basil and lime juice. Season to taste with salt and pepper. Serve over quinoa.

# Okra and Black-Eyed Pea Jambalaya

**Makes 4 servings**

*Stir-frying okra until it's crisp and brown before simmering it with spicy tomatoes and black-eyed peas unlocks its succulence.*

| | | |
|---|---|---|
| 4 tsp | olive oil, divided | 20 mL |
| 1 lb | fresh or thawed frozen okra, trimmed and cut into ½-inch (1 cm) slices | 500 g |
| | Fine sea salt and freshly ground black pepper | |
| 1 | large green bell pepper, chopped | 1 |
| 1¼ cups | chopped onions | 300 mL |
| 4 | cloves garlic, minced | 4 |
| 2 tsp | paprika | 10 mL |
| 1 tsp | dried thyme | 5 mL |
| ½ tsp | dried oregano | 2 mL |
| ¼ tsp | cayenne pepper | 1 mL |
| 1 cup | packed fresh flat-leaf (Italian) parsley leaves, chopped, divided | 250 mL |
| 1 | can (14 to 15 oz/398 to 425 mL) diced tomatoes, with juice | 1 |
| 1 | can (14 to 19 oz/398 to 540 mL) black-eyed peas, drained and rinsed | 1 |
| ½ cup | ready-to-use reduced-sodium vegetable broth (GF, if needed) | 125 mL |
| 3 cups | hot cooked quinoa (see page 10) | 750 mL |

1. In a large saucepan, heat half the oil over medium-high heat. Add okra and cook, stirring, for 12 to 15 minutes or until browned. Transfer to a plate and season to taste with salt and black pepper.

2. In the same pan, heat the remaining oil over medium-high heat. Add green pepper and onions; cook, stirring, for 6 to 8 minutes or until softened. Add garlic, paprika, thyme, oregano and cayenne; cook, stirring, for 30 seconds.

3. Stir in half the parsley, tomatoes with juice, peas and broth; bring to a boil. Reduce heat to medium-low, cover, leaving lid ajar, and simmer, stirring once or twice, for 10 minutes. Return okra to the pan and simmer for 3 minutes to heat through and blend the flavors. Season to taste with salt and black pepper. Serve over quinoa, sprinkled with the remaining parsley.

# Zucchini Chickpea Tagine with Cilantro Quinoa

**Makes 4 servings**

*A hearty yet refined mingling of sweet and spicy, this easy Moroccan-inspired meal is reason enough to keep peas on hand — both protein-rich chickpeas and vitamin-packed spring peas.*

## Tip

Other varieties of tender squash, such as yellow crookneck or a small pattypan, may be used in place of the zucchini.

| | | |
|---|---|---|
| 1 cup | quinoa, rinsed | 250 mL |
| 3 cups | ready-to-use reduced-sodium vegetable broth (GF, if needed), divided | 750 mL |
| 1/2 cup | packed fresh cilantro leaves, chopped | 125 mL |
| 1 tbsp | olive oil | 15 mL |
| 2 cups | chopped onions | 500 mL |
| 2 tsp | ground cumin | 10 mL |
| 1 tsp | ground cinnamon | 5 mL |
| 1 tsp | ground coriander | 5 mL |
| 3 | small zucchini, trimmed and diced | 3 |
| 1 | can (14 to 15 oz/398 to 425 mL) diced tomatoes, with juice | 1 |
| 1 | can (14 to 19 oz/398 to 540 mL) chickpeas, drained and rinsed | 1 |
| 1/4 cup | golden or dark raisins | 60 mL |
| 1 cup | frozen petite peas, thawed | 250 mL |

1. In a medium saucepan, combine quinoa and 2 cups (500 mL) of the broth. Bring to a boil over medium-high heat. Reduce heat to low, cover and simmer for 12 to 15 minutes or until liquid is absorbed. Remove from heat and let stand, covered, for 5 minutes. Fluff with a fork, then gently stir in cilantro.

2. Meanwhile, in a large saucepan, heat oil over medium-high heat. Add onions and cook, stirring, for 6 to 8 minutes or until softened. Add cumin, cinnamon and coriander; cook, stirring, for 30 seconds.

3. Stir in zucchini, tomatoes with juice, chickpeas, raisins and the remaining broth; bring to a boil. Reduce heat to medium-low, cover and simmer, stirring occasionally, for 10 minutes or until zucchini is tender. Stir in peas and simmer for 1 minute. Serve over quinoa.

# Zucchini, Carrot and Butter Bean Quinoa

*When zucchini is
abundant in the garden,
reach for this recipe.
And if you think butter
beans are an expensive,
hard-to-find ingredient,
think again: these creamy,
buttery, beige beauties
are simply mature
lima beans. You'll find
them alongside other
canned beans at your
local supermarket for
roughly the same price
as black beans, chickpeas
and pintos.*

## Tip

Canned white beans (any
variety) or chickpeas may
be substituted for the
butter beans.

| | | |
|---|---|---|
| 1 tbsp | olive oil | 15 mL |
| 2½ cups | shredded zucchini | 625 mL |
| 1½ cups | shredded carrots | 375 mL |
| 3 | cloves garlic, minced | 3 |
| 1 | can (14 to 19 oz/398 to 540 mL) butter beans, drained and rinsed | 1 |
| ½ cup | dry white wine | 125 mL |
| 3 cups | hot cooked quinoa (see page 10) | 750 mL |
| ½ cup | freshly grated Romano, manchego or Parmesan cheese, divided | 125 mL |
| 3 tbsp | minced fresh chives, divided | 45 mL |
| | Fine sea salt and freshly cracked black pepper | |

**1.** In a large skillet, heat oil over medium-low heat. Add zucchini and carrots; cook, stirring, for 2 to 3 minutes or until softened. Add garlic and cook, stirring, for 30 seconds. Add beans and wine; cook, stirring, for 1 minute. Add quinoa, half the cheese and 2 tbsp (30 mL) of the chives, gently tossing to combine. Cook, stirring, for 1 to 2 minutes to blend the flavors. Season to taste with salt and pepper. Serve sprinkled with the remaining cheese and chives.

# Andalusian Beans, Spinach and Quinoa

*The round, rich taste of white beans perfectly complements fresh, grassy spinach in this spicy, Spanish-inspired main dish.*

## Tip

For the white beans, you could use Great Northern beans, cannellini (white kidney) beans or white pea (navy) beans.

| | | |
|---|---|---|
| 1 tbsp | olive oil | 15 mL |
| 1½ cups | thinly sliced red onions | 375 mL |
| 2 | cloves garlic, thinly sliced | 2 |
| 1 tsp | hot or sweet smoked paprika | 5 mL |
| 8 cups | packed baby spinach (about 6 oz/175 g) | 2 L |
| 1 | can (14 to 19 oz/398 to 540 mL) white beans, drained and rinsed | 1 |
| ¼ cup | dry sherry | 60 mL |
| 1 tsp | sherry vinegar or white wine vinegar | 5 mL |
| | Fine sea salt and freshly cracked black pepper | |
| ¼ cup | chopped drained oil-packed sun-dried tomatoes | 60 mL |
| 3 cups | hot cooked quinoa (see page 10) | 750 mL |

1. In a large skillet, heat oil over medium-high heat. Add red onions and cook, stirring, for 6 to 8 minutes or until golden. Add garlic and paprika; cook, stirring, for 30 seconds. Stir in spinach, beans and sherry; reduce heat to medium, cover and cook, stirring occasionally, for 4 to 5 minutes or until spinach is wilted. Stir in vinegar. Season to taste with salt and pepper.

2. Stir sun-dried tomatoes into hot quinoa. Season to taste with salt and pepper. Divide among four shallow bowls and top with spinach mixture.

# Quinoa Chilaquiles Casserole

*In its simplest form, chilaquiles consists of salsa and tortillas. Beans or eggs are sometimes added, and occasionally leftover chicken or pork. Here, the dish is prepared as a hearty, delicious casserole with added south-of-the border ingredients, namely quinoa, pinto beans and queso fresco.*

## Storage Tip

Store the casserole tightly covered with foil or plastic wrap in the refrigerator for up to 2 days. Reheat individual-sized portions in the microwave on Medium (50%) for 1½ to 2 minutes or until warmed through.

- Preheat oven to 450°F (230°C)
- 8- or 9-inch (20 or 23 cm) square glass baking dish, sprayed with nonstick cooking spray (preferably olive oil)

| | | |
|---|---|---|
| 1 tsp | vegetable oil | 5 mL |
| 1 cup | thinly sliced onion | 250 mL |
| 2 cups | hot cooked quinoa (see page 10) | 500 mL |
| 4 | cloves garlic, minced | 4 |
| 2 tsp | ground cumin | 10 mL |
| 1 | can (14 to 19 oz/398 to 540 mL) pinto beans, drained and rinsed | 1 |
| 1 | can (10 oz/284 mL) diced tomatoes with chiles, with juice | 1 |
| 1 cup | ready-to-use reduced-sodium vegetable broth (GF, if needed) | 250 mL |
| 15 | 6-inch (15 cm) corn tortillas (GF, if needed), cut into 1-inch (2.5 cm) strips | 15 |
| 1 cup | crumbled queso fresco or feta cheese | 250 mL |

1. In a large skillet, heat oil over medium-high heat. Add onion and cook, stirring, for 5 to 6 minutes or until softened. Add quinoa, garlic and cumin; cook, stirring, for 1 minute. Remove from heat and stir in beans.
2. In a medium bowl, combine tomatoes with juice and broth.
3. Arrange half the tortilla strips in bottom of prepared baking dish. Layer half the quinoa mixture over tortillas. Top with the remaining tortillas, then the remaining quinoa mixture. Pour tomato mixture evenly over top. Sprinkle with cheese.
4. Bake in preheated oven for 12 to 15 minutes or until tortillas are lightly browned and cheese is melted.

# Cumin-Scented Black Beans and Quinoa

*Black beans, quinoa and cumin are the perfect trio for a quick dinner dish: delicious, easy and healthy. Gussy up with assorted accompaniments to your palate's content.*

| 2 tsp | vegetable oil | 10 mL |
|---|---|---|
| 1 | red bell pepper, chopped | 1 |
| 1½ cups | chopped onions | 375 mL |
| 1 cup | quinoa, rinsed | 250 mL |
| 2 tsp | ground cumin | 10 mL |
| ½ tsp | chipotle chile powder | 2 mL |
| 2 cups | ready-to-use reduced-sodium vegetable broth (GF, if needed) | 500 mL |
| 1 | can (14 to 19 oz/398 to 540 mL) black beans, drained and rinsed | 1 |

**Suggested Accompaniments**

Tomato or tomatillo salsa

Fresh cilantro leaves

Chopped radishes

Plain Greek yogurt

Crumbled queso fresco or feta cheese

1. In a medium saucepan, heat oil over medium-high heat. Add red pepper and onions; cook, stirring, for 5 to 6 minutes or until slightly softened.

2. Stir in quinoa, cumin, chipotle chile powder and broth; bring to a boil. Reduce heat to medium-low, cover and simmer for 12 to 15 minutes or until quinoa is barely tender. Remove from heat and stir in beans. Let stand, covered, for 5 minutes. Fluff with a fork. Serve topped with any of the suggested accompaniments, as desired.

# Black Quinoa with Miso and Edamame

*The Japanese flavors at work — nutty, slightly sweet miso, buttery edamame, minty shiso and peppery radishes — add stylishness and exoticism to a quick and easy quinoa bowl.*

## Tip

Shiso is the Japanese name for the herb perilla; it is also called Japanese basil. It is related to mint and, like mint, comes in many different varieties. Shiso leaves come in red and green (the latter are more commonly available) and are used much like fresh mint and basil leaves: typically raw, and sliced or chopped in everything from soups to salads to sushi. Shiso leaves are available at Asian grocery stores and well-stocked supermarkets.

| | | |
|---|---|---|
| 1 cup | black or white quinoa, rinsed | 250 mL |
| 1 tsp | ground ginger | 5 mL |
| 2¼ cups | water | 550 mL |
| 1½ tbsp | yellow or white miso | 22 mL |
| 1 tbsp | liquid honey | 15 mL |
| 2 cups | frozen shelled edamame | 500 mL |
| 2 tsp | toasted sesame oil | 10 mL |
| ¾ cup | chopped green onions | 175 mL |
| | Fine sea salt and freshly cracked black pepper | |
| ¼ cup | packed fresh shiso or mint leaves, thinly sliced | 60 mL |
| ½ cup | chopped radishes | 125 mL |
| ¾ cup | lightly salted roasted almonds, coarsely chopped | 175 mL |

1. In a medium saucepan, combine quinoa, ginger, water, miso and honey. Bring to a boil over high heat. Reduce heat to low, cover and simmer for 8 minutes. Stir in edamame, cover and simmer for 5 to 7 minutes or until most (but not all) of the liquid is absorbed. Remove from heat and let stand, covered, for 5 minutes. Fluff with a fork.

2. In a large skillet, heat oil over medium-high heat. Add green onions and cook, stirring, for 1 to 2 minutes or until wilted. Add quinoa mixture and cook, stirring, for 1 to 2 minutes to heat through and blend the flavors. Season to taste with salt and pepper. Serve topped with shiso, radishes and almonds.

# Chimichurri Tempeh and Quinoa Bowls

| **Makes 4 servings** | | |
|---|---|---|

*Chimichurri, a quick blended sauce of olive oil, fresh herbs, acid (such as lemon juice or vinegar) and a touch of heat, is the national condiment of both Uruguay and Argentina. Although it is renowned for pairing up with grilled steak, it also plays well in this vegetarian tempeh dish.*

### Blender or food processor

| 2 | cloves garlic | 2 |
|---|---|---|
| 1 cup | packed fresh cilantro leaves | 250 mL |
| ¼ tsp | hot pepper flakes | 1 mL |
| 5 tbsp | extra virgin olive oil, divided | 75 mL |
| 2 tbsp | red wine vinegar | 30 mL |
| | Fine sea salt and freshly ground black pepper | |
| 1 | red bell pepper, sliced | 1 |
| 8 oz | tempeh, cut into 1-inch (2.5 cm) cubes | 250 g |
| 3 cups | hot cooked quinoa (see page 10) | 750 mL |

### Suggested Accompaniments

Crumbled queso fresco

Diced mango or pineapple

Thinly sliced red jalapeño pepper

1. In blender, combine garlic, cilantro, hot pepper flakes, 4 tbsp (60 mL) of the oil and vinegar; purée until smooth. Season to taste with salt and black pepper.

2. In a large nonstick skillet, heat the remaining oil over medium-high heat. Add red pepper and cook, stirring, for 5 minutes. Add tempeh and cook, stirring, for 1 to 2 minutes or until pepper is softened.

3. Stir half the cilantro mixture (chimichurri) into hot quinoa. Divide among four bowls and top with tempeh mixture. Serve drizzled with the remaining chimichurri and topped with any of the suggested accompaniments, as desired.

# Hoisin Bok Choy and Tempeh

*Asian chili-garlic sauce brings pungent notes to this dish, tempered by cool, crisp baby bok choy, nutty quinoa and salty-sweet hoisin sauce.*

## Tip

To toast sesame seeds, place up to 3 tbsp (45 mL) seeds in a medium skillet set over medium heat. Cook, shaking the skillet, for 3 to 5 minutes or until seeds are golden brown and fragrant. Let cool completely before use.

| | | |
|---|---|---|
| 2 tsp | vegetable oil | 10 mL |
| 8 oz | tempeh (GF, if needed), cut into 1/2-inch (1 cm) strips | 250 g |
| 1/2 cup | thinly sliced green onions | 125 mL |
| 1 tbsp | minced gingerroot | 15 mL |
| 1 tsp | Asian chili-garlic sauce | 5 mL |
| 1 lb | bok choy, trimmed and cut crosswise into 1/2-inch (1 cm) slices | 500 g |
| 1/4 cup | ready-to-use reduced-sodium vegetable broth (GF, if needed) | 60 mL |
| 3 tbsp | hoisin sauce (GF, if needed) | 45 mL |
| 3 cups | hot cooked quinoa (see page 10) | 750 mL |
| 2 tbsp | toasted sesame seeds (see tip, at left) | 30 mL |

1. In a large skillet, heat oil over medium-high heat. Add tempeh, green onions, ginger and chili-garlic sauce; cook, stirring, for 1 to 2 minutes or until tempeh is heated through. Add bok choy, broth and hoisin sauce; cover and cook for 1 to 2 minutes or until bok choy is wilted.

2. Divide quinoa among four deep bowls and top with tempeh mixture. Sprinkle with sesame seeds.

# Tofu and Eggplant Fried Quinoa

*This quick-to-the-table tofu and eggplant dish couldn't be simpler or more satisfying.*

## Tips

An equal amount of fresh cilantro leaves may be used in place of the basil.

| | | |
|---|---|---|
| 4 tsp | vegetable oil, divided | 20 mL |
| 16 oz | extra-firm tofu, drained, cut into 1-inch (2.5 cm) cubes and patted dry | 500 g |
| 1 lb | eggplant, trimmed and cut into 3- by 1-inch (7.5 by 2.5 cm) strips | 500 g |
| 1 | red bell pepper, sliced | 1 |
| 3 | cloves garlic, minced | 3 |
| 3 cups | cooked quinoa (see page 10), chilled | 750 mL |
| 1/4 cup | hoisin sauce (GF, if needed) | 60 mL |
| 1/4 cup | ready-to-use reduced-sodium vegetable broth (GF, if needed) | 60 mL |
| 1/4 cup | packed fresh basil leaves, thinly sliced | 60 mL |

1. In a large skillet, heat half the oil over medium-high heat. Add tofu and cook, stirring, for 4 to 6 minutes or until browned. Using a slotted spoon, transfer tofu to a plate.

2. In the same skillet, heat the remaining oil over medium-high heat. Add eggplant, red pepper and garlic; cook, stirring, for 8 to 10 minutes or until softened. Return tofu to the pan and add quinoa, hoisin sauce and broth; cook, stirring, for 3 to 4 minutes or until heated through. Remove from heat and stir in basil.

# Thai Tofu Green Curry

**Makes
4 servings**

*Here, store-bought Thai green curry paste turns a weeknight tofu dish into something special. The complex curry flavors mingle with creamy coconut milk and fresh cilantro and basil to make an addictive sauce for the tofu and vegetables on top and the quinoa beneath.*

| | | |
|---|---|---|
| 4 tsp | vegetable oil, divided | 20 mL |
| 16 oz | extra-firm tofu, drained, cut into ½-inch (1 cm) cubes and patted dry | 500 g |
| 1 | large red bell pepper, cut into thin strips | 1 |
| 1½ cups | thinly sliced onions | 375 mL |
| ½ cup | packed fresh cilantro leaves, chopped | 125 mL |
| 2 tsp | natural cane sugar or packed light brown sugar | 10 mL |
| 1 | can (14 oz/400 mL) light coconut milk | 1 |
| 2 tbsp | Thai green curry paste | 30 mL |
| 1 tbsp | tamari or soy sauce (GF, if needed) | 15 mL |
| ½ cup | packed fresh basil leaves, thinly sliced | 125 mL |
| 2 tbsp | freshly squeezed lime juice | 30 mL |
| | Fine sea salt and freshly ground black pepper | |
| 3 cups | hot cooked black, red or white quinoa (see page 10) | 750 mL |

1. In a large skillet, heat half the oil over medium-high heat. Add tofu and cook, stirring, for 4 to 6 minutes or until browned. Using a slotted spoon, transfer tofu to a plate.

2. In the same skillet, heat the remaining oil over medium-high heat. Add red pepper and onions; cook, stirring for 5 to 6 minutes or until softened. Return tofu to the pan and add cilantro, sugar, coconut milk, curry paste and tamari; bring to a boil. Reduce heat and simmer for 5 minutes. Stir in basil and lime juice. Season to taste with salt and pepper.

3. Divide quinoa among four bowls and top with tofu mixture.

# Quick Quinoa and Tofu Stir-Fry

*Here, quinoa is studded with assorted vegetables, tofu and sesame seeds, creating a substantial stir-fry worthy of its billing as a main course.*

## Tip

To toast sesame seeds, place up to 3 tbsp (45 mL) seeds in a medium skillet set over medium heat. Cook, shaking the skillet, for 3 to 5 minutes or until seeds are golden brown and fragrant. Let cool completely before use.

| | | |
|---|---|---|
| 4 tsp | vegetable oil, divided | 20 mL |
| 12 oz | extra-firm tofu, drained, cut into 1-inch (2.5 cm) cubes and patted dry | 375 g |
| 12 oz | frozen stir-fry vegetables, thawed and patted dry | 375 g |
| 3 | cloves garlic, minced | 3 |
| 1 tbsp | minced gingerroot | 15 mL |
| 3 cups | cooked quinoa (see page 10), chilled | 750 mL |
| 1/3 cup | thinly sliced green onions | 75 mL |
| 1/4 cup | teriyaki sauce (GF, if needed) | 60 mL |
| 1 tbsp | toasted sesame seeds (see tip, at left) | 15 mL |

1. In a large skillet, heat half the oil over medium-high heat. Add tofu and cook, stirring, for 3 to 4 minutes or until golden. Using a slotted spoon, transfer tofu to a plate.

2. In the same skillet, heat the remaining oil over medium-high heat. Add stir-fry vegetables and cook, stirring, for 2 minutes. Add garlic and ginger; cook, stirring, for 30 seconds. Return tofu to the pan and add quinoa, green onions and teriyaki sauce; cook, stirring, for 2 to 3 minutes or until well coated and warmed through. Serve sprinkled with sesame seeds.

# Spicy Quinoa and Tofu Kedgeree

*Kedgeree, which typically comprises rice, eggs, flaked fish and spices, is a British dish dating back to colonial India. Although more traditionally served for breakfast, it makes a smashing supper on busy weeknights. Here it has a vegetarian spin, with tofu in place of the fish and quinoa in place of the rice.*

## Tip

To hard-cook eggs, place eggs in a saucepan large enough to hold them in a single layer. Add enough cold water to cover eggs by 1 inch (2.5 cm). Heat over high heat until water is just boiling. Remove from heat and cover pan. Let stand for about 12 minutes for large eggs (9 minutes for medium eggs; 15 minutes for extra-large eggs). Drain eggs and cool completely under cold running water or in a bowl of ice water. Refrigerate until ready to eat.

| | | |
|---|---|---|
| 4 tsp | vegetable oil, divided | 20 mL |
| 12 oz | extra-firm tofu, drained, cut into ½-inch (1 cm) cubes and patted dry | 375 g |
| 1½ cups | chopped onions | 375 mL |
| 2 tsp | ground cumin | 10 mL |
| 1 tsp | ground coriander | 5 mL |
| ¾ tsp | mild curry powder | 3 mL |
| ½ tsp | hot pepper flakes | 2 mL |
| 3 cups | hot cooked black, red or white quinoa (see page 10) | 750 mL |
| ¾ cup | packed fresh cilantro leaves, chopped, divided | 175 mL |
| 2 tsp | finely grated lime zest | 10 mL |
| 2 tbsp | freshly squeezed lime juice | 30 mL |
| 3 | hard-cooked large eggs (see tip, at left), peeled and quartered lengthwise | 3 |

1. In a large skillet, heat half the oil over medium-high heat. Add tofu and cook, stirring, for 4 to 6 minutes or until browned. Using a slotted spoon, transfer tofu to a plate.

2. In the same skillet, heat the remaining oil over medium-high heat. Add onions and cook, stirring, for 5 to 6 minutes or until golden. Add cumin, coriander, curry powder and hot pepper flakes; cook, stirring, for 1 minute. Return tofu to the pan, reduce heat to medium and cook, stirring occasionally, for 1 to 2 minutes or until heated through.

3. Stir in quinoa, half the cilantro, lime zest and lime juice; cook, stirring, for 1 to 2 minutes or until heated through. Serve topped with eggs and sprinkled with the remaining cilantro.

# Punjabi Cauliflower and Quinoa Scramble

*Hearty and satisfying, my Indian-spiced scramble has a newfangled twist with the addition of quinoa. The fresh flavors of spinach and lemon make it an excellent meal for the transition from winter to spring, but it crosses over beautifully to a fall menu, too.*

## Tip

For a milder dish, use an equal amount of mild curry powder in place of the hot curry powder.

| | | |
|---|---|---|
| 12 oz | firm tofu, drained and crumbled | 375 g |
| 2 tsp | vegetable oil | 10 mL |
| 2 cups | small cauliflower florets | 500 mL |
| 2 | cloves garlic, minced | 2 |
| 1 tbsp | minced gingerroot | 15 mL |
| 2 tsp | hot or medium curry powder | 10 mL |
| 1½ tsp | garam masala | 7 mL |
| 1½ cups | hot cooked quinoa (see page 10) | 375 mL |
| ½ cup | ready-to-use reduced-sodium vegetable broth (GF, if needed) | 125 mL |
| | Fine sea salt and freshly cracked black pepper | |
| 8 cups | packed baby spinach (about 6 oz/175 g) | 2 L |
| | Fresh lemon wedges | |

1. Spread tofu on paper towels and let drain for 15 minutes.
2. Meanwhile, in a large saucepan, heat oil over medium-high heat. Add cauliflower and cook, stirring, for 10 to 12 minutes or until browned. Add garlic, ginger, curry powder and garam masala; cook, stirring, for 30 seconds.
3. Stir in drained tofu, quinoa and broth; cook, stirring, for 2 minutes or until heated through. Season to taste with salt and pepper. Add spinach and cook, stirring, for 2 to 3 minutes or until wilted. Serve with lemon wedges.

# Kale Quinoa with Eggs and Za'atar

*I have no doubt that
you'll return to this recipe
again and again: it's easy,
healthy and fabulously
delicious. If you hard-
cook the eggs, trim the
kale and make the za'atar
blend in advance, the
last-minute assembly will
be that much swifter.*

## Tips

Sumac is available at
Middle Eastern grocers
and from online spice
purveyors. If you can't
find it, omit it from the
za'atar blend and increase
the lemon juice to 4 tsp
(20 mL).

Unlike other greens, kale
stems are so tough they
are virtually inedible.
Hence, they, along with
the tougher part of
the center rib, must be
removed before cooking.
To do so, lay a leaf upside
down on a cutting board
and use a paring knife to
cut a V shape along both
sides of the rib, cutting it
and the stem free from
the leaf.

- **Steamer basket**

### Za'atar

| | | |
|---|---|---|
| 2 tbsp | toasted sesame seeds (see tip, page 291) | 30 mL |
| 1 tsp | minced fresh thyme | 5 mL |
| 1 tsp | ground sumac (see tip, at left) | 5 mL |
| ½ tsp | coarse sea salt | 2 mL |

### Sautéed Kale

| | | |
|---|---|---|
| 1 | large bunch kale, tough stems and center ribs removed, leaves very thinly sliced crosswise (about 6 cups/1.5 L) | 1 |
| 1 tbsp | olive oil | 15 mL |
| 1 cup | thinly sliced red onion | 250 mL |
| 2 | cloves garlic, minced | 2 |
| ¼ tsp | hot pepper flakes | 1 mL |
| 1 tbsp | freshly squeezed lemon juice | 15 mL |
| 3 cups | hot cooked quinoa (see page 10) | 750 mL |
| 3 | hard-cooked large eggs (see tip, page 292), peeled and chopped | 3 |

1. *Za'atar:* In a small bowl, combine sesame seeds, thyme, sumac and salt.
2. *Kale:* Place kale in a steamer basket set over a large pot of boiling water. Cover and steam for 8 to 10 minutes or until tender.
3. In a large skillet, heat oil over medium-high heat. Add red onion and cook, stirring, for 6 to 8 minutes or until golden. Add garlic and hot pepper flakes; cook, stirring, for 1 minute. Add kale, reduce heat to medium and cook, stirring occasionally, for 1 to 2 minutes or until heated through. Remove from heat and stir in lemon juice.
4. Stir half the za'atar into hot quinoa. Divide among four shallow bowls or dinner plates and top with kale mixture and eggs. Sprinkle with the remaining za'atar.

# Quinoa Ratatouille with Poached Eggs

*Only in summer, when vegetables are so full of flavor, could a one-dish dinner like ratatouille seem so special. A gentle simmer, fresh basil and a small amount of olive oil are all that's needed to enhance the vegetables' natural goodness. But adding quinoa and poached eggs to the mix, to make the dish entrée-worthy, is a fine idea, too.*

## Tip

When selecting an eggplant, choose one with firm, shiny, blemish-free skin and a mostly green (not brown) stem top. The eggplant should feel heavier than it looks; the greater the moisture, the fresher the eggplant.

| | | |
|---|---|---|
| 2 tsp | olive oil | 10 mL |
| 1 | large red bell pepper, coarsely chopped | 1 |
| 1½ cups | chopped onions | 375 mL |
| 3 | cloves garlic, minced | 3 |
| 2 tsp | dried herbes de Provence or Italian seasoning | 10 mL |
| 2 | small zucchini, cut into 1-inch (2.5 cm) cubes | 2 |
| 1 | eggplant (about 1½ lbs/750 g), trimmed and cut into 1-inch (2.5 cm) cubes | 1 |
| 1 | can (14 to 15 oz/398 to 425 mL) diced tomatoes, with juice | 1 |
| 2 cups | ready-to-use reduced-sodium vegetable broth (GF, if needed) | 500 mL |
| ½ cup | quinoa, rinsed | 125 mL |
| 2 tsp | balsamic vinegar | 10 mL |
| 4 | large eggs | 4 |
| ⅛ tsp | freshly ground black pepper | 0.5 mL |
| ¾ cup | packed fresh basil leaves, torn | 175 mL |

1. In a large skillet, heat oil over medium-high heat. Add red pepper, onions, garlic and herbes de Provence; cook, stirring, for 6 to 8 minutes or until onions are softened. Add zucchini and eggplant; cook, stirring, for 5 minutes or until softened.

2. Stir in tomatoes with juice and broth; bring to a boil. Reduce heat to low, cover and simmer, stirring occasionally, for 20 minutes. Stir in quinoa and simmer, uncovered, stirring occasionally, for 12 to 15 minutes or until quinoa is tender. Stir in vinegar.

3. Using the back of a spoon, make four holes for the eggs in the ratatouille. Crack an egg into each hole and season with pepper. Cover and cook for 2 to 5 minutes or until eggs are set as desired. Serve sprinkled with basil.

# Tunisian Chickpeas, Quinoa and Poached Eggs

*This North African–
sauced chickpea dish
gets brilliant color and
lively flavor from an
easy tomato topping.
Gently poached eggs add
to the succulence, while
quinoa makes a perfect
foundation for soaking up
every drop of flavor.*

**• Blender or food processor**

| | | |
|---|---|---|
| 1 cup | packed fresh cilantro leaves, divided | 250 mL |
| 1½ tsp | ground cumin | 7 mL |
| ½ tsp | ground cinnamon | 2 mL |
| ¼ tsp | ground coriander | 1 mL |
| ¼ tsp | ground ginger | 1 mL |
| ⅛ tsp | ground cloves | 0.5 mL |
| ⅛ tsp | cayenne pepper | 0.5 mL |
| 1 | can (14 to 15 oz/398 to 425 mL) diced tomatoes, with juice | 1 |
| 2 tbsp | freshly squeezed lemon juice | 30 mL |
| | Fine sea salt and freshly cracked black pepper | |
| 2 tsp | olive oil | 10 mL |
| 1 | can (14 to 19 oz/398 to 540 mL) chickpeas, drained and rinsed | 1 |
| 4 | large eggs | 4 |
| 3 cups | hot cooked quinoa (see page 10) | 750 mL |

1. In blender, combine half the cilantro, cumin, cinnamon, coriander, ginger, cloves, cayenne, tomatoes with juice and lemon juice; purée until smooth. Season to taste with salt and black pepper.

2. In a large skillet, heat oil over medium-high heat. Add tomato purée and chickpeas; cook, stirring, for 4 to 5 minutes or until warmed through.

3. Using the back of a spoon, make four holes for the eggs in the tomato mixture. Crack an egg into each hole and season with pepper. Cover and cook for 2 to 5 minutes or until eggs are set as desired.

4. Stir the remaining cilantro into hot quinoa. Season to taste with salt and pepper. Divide among four shallow bowls and top with tomato mixture and eggs.

# Browned Butter Cauliflower Quinoa Omelet

*Here, quinoa and manchego cheese are matched with the fresh, grassy flavor of parsley to bring out cauliflower's best, turning this otherwise simple weeknight omelet into a fine-dining experience.*

| | | |
|---|---|---|
| 6 | large eggs | 6 |
| ½ tsp | fine sea salt | 2 mL |
| ¼ tsp | freshly cracked black pepper | 1 mL |
| 1 tbsp | unsalted butter | 15 mL |
| 2 cups | coarsely chopped cauliflower florets | 500 mL |
| 1½ cups | cooked quinoa (see page 10), cooled | 375 mL |
| 2 | cloves garlic, minced | 2 |
| ½ cup | grated manchego, Romano or Parmesan cheese | 125 mL |
| ¼ cup | packed fresh flat-leaf (Italian) parsley leaves, chopped | 60 mL |

1. In a large bowl, whisk together eggs, salt and pepper. Set aside.
2. In a large skillet, melt butter over medium-high heat. Add cauliflower and cook, stirring, for 7 to 10 minutes or until browned and tender. Reduce heat to medium and add quinoa and garlic; cook, stirring, for 1 minute.
3. Pour egg mixture over quinoa mixture. Cook, lifting edges to allow uncooked eggs to run underneath and shaking skillet occasionally to loosen omelet, for 4 to 5 minutes or until almost set. Slide out onto a large plate.
4. Invert skillet over omelet and, using pot holders, firmly hold plate and skillet together. Invert omelet back into skillet and cook for 1 to 2 minutes to set eggs. Slide out onto plate and sprinkle with cheese and parsley.

# Quinoa, Pepper and Green Onion Frittata

*In this redesigned version
of an Italian classic,
nutty quinoa joins salty
Parmesan and roasted red
peppers, lending the eggs
a satisfying undercurrent
of umami.*

- **Preheat oven to 350°F (180°C)**
- **8-inch (20 cm) square glass baking dish, sprayed with
  nonstick cooking spray (preferably olive oil)**

| | | |
|---|---|---|
| 6 | large eggs | 6 |
| ½ tsp | fine sea salt | 2 mL |
| ¼ tsp | freshly ground black pepper | 1 mL |
| 2 tsp | olive oil | 10 mL |
| 1½ cups | chopped green onions | 375 mL |
| 1 cup | drained roasted red bell peppers, chopped | 250 mL |
| 1½ cups | cooked quinoa (see page 10), cooled | 375 mL |
| ¼ cup | freshly grated Parmesan cheese | 60 mL |

1. In a large bowl, whisk together eggs, salt and pepper.
   Set aside.
2. In a large skillet, heat oil over medium-high heat. Add
   green onions and roasted peppers; cook, stirring, for
   1 to 2 minutes or until onions are slightly softened.
   Stir in quinoa and cook, stirring, for 1 minute. Spread
   mixture in prepared baking dish.
3. Pour egg mixture over quinoa mixture. Sprinkle
   with cheese.
4. Bake in preheated oven for 23 to 28 minutes or
   until golden and set. Let cool on a wire rack for at
   least 10 minutes before cutting. Serve warm or let
   cool completely.

# Caramelized Onion Quinoa Tart

**Makes
6 servings**

*Adding quinoa to an already richly flavored onion tart sets this version apart from all others.*

## Tip

Adding sugar to the onions hastens their caramelization.

- **10-inch (25 cm) tart pan or pie plate, sprayed with nonstick cooking spray**

| | | |
|---|---|---:|
| 1 tbsp | unsalted butter | 15 mL |
| 4 cups | sliced onions (about 3 large) | 1 L |
| 1 tbsp | natural cane sugar or packed brown sugar | 15 mL |
| | Fine sea salt and freshly cracked black pepper | |
| 3 | large eggs | 3 |
| 3 cups | cooked quinoa (see page 10), cooled | 750 mL |
| ¾ cup | freshly grated Parmesan cheese | 175 mL |
| 1 tsp | chopped fresh rosemary | 5 mL |
| 1½ cups | shredded smoked Gouda cheese | 375 mL |
| ¾ cup | chopped pecans | 175 mL |

1. In a large skillet, melt butter over medium-low heat. Add onions and sugar; cook, stirring, for about 25 minutes or until deep golden brown. Season to taste with salt and pepper.
2. Preheat oven to 400°F (200°C).
3. In a medium bowl, whisk eggs. Stir in quinoa, Parmesan and rosemary. Season to taste with salt and pepper. Press mixture into bottom of prepared pan.
4. Spread caramelized onions over quinoa mixture. Sprinkle with Gouda and pecans.
5. Bake in preheated oven for 12 to 15 minutes or until pecans are toasted.

# Cheese Quinoa Soufflé

*I suspect soufflés earned their fussbudget reputation in the days before oven windows: anxious home cooks, tempted by the intoxicating scents of baking cheese and butter, couldn't help but take a peek (or two, or three) at the rising puff, and then plop! Down it fell. It's high time that all such notions of temperamentality be cast aside, as soufflés are really quite easy to prepare. And this quinoa-and cheese-packed one is hearty enough for dinner, too.*

## Tip

Other semi-firm cheeses, such as Cheddar or Gouda, may be used in place of the Gruyère.

- **8-cup (2 L) soufflé dish, lightly greased**

| | | |
|---|---|---|
| 1²⁄₃ cups | milk | 400 mL |
| 3 cups | cooked quinoa (see page 10), cooled | 750 mL |
| 1 cup | freshly grated Parmesan cheese | 250 mL |
| 1 cup | shredded Gruyère or Swiss cheese | 250 mL |
| ½ cup | unsalted butter, cut into small pieces | 125 mL |
| | Fine sea salt and freshly cracked black pepper | |
| 6 | large eggs, separated | 6 |

1. In a medium saucepan, heat milk over medium-high heat until hot but not boiling.
2. In a large bowl, combine hot milk, quinoa, Parmesan, Gruyère and butter, stirring until cheeses are melted. Season to taste with salt and pepper. Let cool to room temperature.
3. Preheat oven to 350°F (180°C).
4. In a small bowl, whisk egg yolks. Stir into cooled quinoa mixture.
5. In a large bowl, using an electric mixer on high speed, beat egg whites until stiff peaks form. Gently fold into quinoa mixture. Spoon into prepared soufflé dish.
6. Bake for 30 minutes. With soufflé still in oven, increase heat to 450°F (230°C). Bake for 7 to 10 minutes or until top is dry and golden brown. Serve immediately.

# Seared Haloumi with Chickpea Salsa and Herbed Quinoa

*Haloumi, a firm, mild
Cypriot cheese popular in
Greece — and becoming
increasingly so in the
U.S. and Canada — can
be cooked directly on a
grill or in a skillet. The
outside will get brown
and crisp; the inside will
be soft and melted.*

| | | |
|---|---|---|
| 1 cup | quinoa, rinsed | 250 mL |
| 2 cups | ready-to-use reduced-sodium vegetable broth (GF, if needed) | 500 mL |
| ½ cup | packed fresh mint leaves, chopped | 125 mL |
| ½ cup | packed fresh cilantro leaves, chopped | 125 mL |
| 1 | can (14 to 19 oz/398 to 540 mL) chickpeas, drained and rinsed | 1 |
| 1½ cups | cherry or grape tomatoes, quartered | 375 mL |
| ¼ tsp | cayenne pepper | 1 mL |
| 4 tsp | extra virgin olive oil, divided | 20 mL |
| 2 tsp | sherry vinegar or red wine vinegar | 10 mL |
| 8 oz | haloumi cheese, cut into 4 thick slices | 250 g |

1. In a medium saucepan, combine quinoa and broth. Bring to a boil over medium-high heat. Reduce heat and simmer for 12 to 15 minutes or until liquid is absorbed. Remove from heat and let stand, covered, for 5 minutes. Fluff with a fork, then gently stir in mint and cilantro.

2. Meanwhile, in a medium bowl, combine chickpeas, tomatoes, cayenne, half the oil and vinegar.

3. In a large skillet, heat the remaining oil over medium-high heat. Add cheese and cook, turning once, for 2 to 3 minutes per side or until golden brown on both sides.

4. Divide quinoa among four plates and top with grilled cheese and chickpea salsa.

# Zucchini Quinoa Lasagna

**Makes 6 to
8 servings**

*Forget the noodles: this
lovely lasagna eschews
pasta, favoring long strips
of zucchini in its place.
Quinoa adds protein and
umami flavor, while the
herbal freshness of pesto
enlivens the layers.*

## Storage Tip

Store the lasagna tightly
covered with foil or plastic
wrap in the refrigerator
for up to 2 days. Reheat
individual-sized portions in
the microwave on Medium
(50%) for 1½ to 2 minutes
or until warmed through.

- **13- by 9-inch (33 by 23 cm) glass baking dish, sprayed
with nonstick cooking spray**

| | | |
|---|---|---|
| 5 | zucchini | 5 |
| 1 tsp | fine sea salt | 5 mL |
| 3 cups | cooked quinoa (see page 10), cooled | 750 mL |
| ⅓ cup | basil pesto | 75 mL |
| 1 | jar (26 oz/700 mL) marinara sauce, divided | 1 |
| 2 cups | ricotta cheese (reduced-fat or regular) | 500 mL |
| 2 cups | shredded mozzarella cheese | 500 mL |

1. Using a sharp knife, thinly slice zucchini lengthwise.
   Sprinkle slices with salt and place in colander to drain
   for 20 minutes. Pat dry with paper towels.
2. Meanwhile, in a medium bowl, combine quinoa
   and pesto.
3. Preheat oven to 375°F (190°C).
4. Spread ½ cup (125 mL) of the marinara sauce in
   prepared baking dish. Cover with zucchini slices,
   cutting to fit as necessary. Gently spread one-third of
   the ricotta over zucchini, then spread with one-third of
   the remaining sauce. Sprinkle one-third of the quinoa
   over sauce, then top with one-third of the mozzarella.
   Repeat layers two more times, starting with zucchini
   and ending with mozzarella. Cover dish with foil.
5. Bake in preheated oven for 35 to 40 minutes or until
   bubbling. Remove foil and bake for 5 minutes or
   until cheese is golden brown. Let cool for 10 minutes
   before cutting.

# Ricotta Quinoa Lasagna Rolls

**Makes
6 servings**

*I predict you'll have this so-easy recipe committed to memory in no time. Add as few or as many additional fillings as you like, such as cooked mushrooms, chopped fresh herbs or black olives.*

## Tip

Make sure to use fine sea salt in the water you use to cook the pasta. Conventional table salt contains chemicals and additives, whereas sea salt contains an abundance of naturally occurring trace minerals.

## Storage Tip

Store the lasagna rolls tightly covered with foil or plastic wrap in the refrigerator for up to 2 days. Reheat individual-sized portions (1 or 2 rolls) in the microwave on Medium (50%) for 1½ to 2 minutes or until warmed through.

- **Preheat oven to 400°F (200°C)**
- **8- or 9-inch (20 or 23 cm) square glass baking dish, sprayed with nonstick cooking spray**

| | | |
|---|---|---|
| 12 | lasagna noodles with ruffled edges (GF, if needed) | 12 |
| 1 cup | cooked quinoa (see page 10), cooled | 250 mL |
| 1 cup | ricotta cheese (reduced-fat or regular) | 250 mL |
| ¼ cup | freshly grated Parmesan cheese | 60 mL |
| | Fine sea salt and freshly cracked black pepper | |
| 2 cups | marinara sauce | 500 mL |
| 3 cups | packed baby spinach | 750 mL |
| 1 cup | shredded mozzarella cheese | 250 mL |

1. In a large pot of boiling salted water (see tip, at left), cook noodles according to package directions until al dente. Drain and gently pat noodles dry with paper towels.
2. In a small bowl, combine quinoa, ricotta and Parmesan. Season to taste with salt and pepper.
3. Lay noodles flat on a work surface. Spread about 3 tbsp (45 mL) ricotta mixture, 2 tbsp (30 mL) marinara sauce and a layer of spinach over each noodle. Starting at a short end, tightly roll up noodles. Place seam side down in prepared baking dish. Pour the remaining marinara sauce over rolls and sprinkle with cheese.
4. Bake in preheated oven for 20 to 24 minutes or until cheese is browned and bubbly.

## Variation

*Vegan Lasagna Rolls:* Replace the ricotta cheese with 8 oz (250 g) firm tofu, well drained and mashed with a fork, then seasoned with salt and pepper. Omit the Parmesan and replace the mozzarella with an equal amount of non-dairy cheese alternative.

# Lentil, Sweet Potato and Quinoa Cakes

**Makes
6 servings**

*Warning: these satisfying
patties may incite
"vegetarian envy" among
carnivorous guests.
Leftovers are fantastic
piled in a pita or wrap for
lunch the following day.*

## Tip

Whenever possible, use
whole-grain bread crumbs.

## Storage Tip

Store the quinoa cakes
wrapped in foil or in
an airtight container in
the refrigerator for up
to 2 days. Reheat in the
microwave on Medium
(50%) for 45 to 60 seconds
or until warmed through.

- **Large rimmed baking sheet, lined with foil and sprayed with nonstick cooking spray (preferably olive oil)**

| | | |
|---|---|---|
| ¾ cup | dried red lentils, rinsed | 175 mL |
| 4 cups | water | 1 L |
| ¾ cup | quinoa, rinsed | 175 mL |
| 1 tbsp | olive oil | 15 mL |
| 1 cup | finely chopped onion | 250 mL |
| 1½ cups | finely shredded peeled sweet potatoes | 375 mL |
| 3 | cloves garlic, minced | 3 |
| 2 tsp | ground cumin | 10 mL |
| ¾ tsp | fine sea salt | 3 mL |
| ⅛ tsp | cayenne pepper | 0.5 mL |
| ¾ cup | fresh bread crumbs (GF, if needed) | 175 mL |
| ¾ cup | packed fresh cilantro leaves, divided | 175 mL |
| 2 | large eggs, lightly beaten | 2 |
| | Nonstick cooking spray (preferably olive oil) | |
| 1 cup | plain yogurt | 250 mL |
| 1 tbsp | freshly squeezed lemon juice | 15 mL |
| 8 cups | packed arugula or baby spinach | 2 L |

1. In a medium saucepan, combine lentils and water. Bring to a boil over medium-high heat. Reduce heat and simmer for about 10 minutes. Stir in quinoa and simmer for 12 to 14 minutes or until lentils are very tender but not mushy. Drain and let cool completely.

2. Preheat broiler, with rack set 4 to 6 inches (10 to 15 cm) from the heat source.

3. In a large skillet, heat oil over medium-high heat. Add onion and cook, stirring, for 5 to 6 minutes or until softened. Add sweet potatoes and cook, stirring, for 2 to 3 minutes or until softened. Add garlic, cumin, salt and cayenne; cook, stirring, for 30 seconds. Let cool.

4. In a large bowl, combine cooled lentil mixture, onion mixture, bread crumbs, half the cilantro and eggs. Form into 12 balls. Place balls on prepared baking sheet. Using a spatula, flatten balls to ½-inch (1 cm) thickness. Spray tops with cooking spray.

5. Broil, turning once, for 3 to 4 minutes per side or until golden brown on both sides and hot in the center.

6. Meanwhile, in a small bowl, whisk together the remaining cilantro, yogurt and lemon juice.

7. Divide arugula among six plates and top with patties. Dollop with yogurt sauce.

# Quinoa Vegetable Cakes

**Makes 4 servings**

*This vegetarian showstopper will bowl you over with its layers of flavor. One bite of the crispy cakes, forked up with some of the tangy yogurt sauce, is enough to understand why quinoa is causing such a sensation.*

**Tip**

If you prefer, an equal amount of chopped fresh cilantro, basil or flat-leaf (Italian) parsley may be used in place of the dill.

**Storage Tip**

Store the quinoa cakes wrapped in foil or in an airtight container in the refrigerator for up to 2 days. Reheat in the microwave on Medium (50%) for 45 to 60 seconds or until warmed through.

- Preheat oven to 400°F (200°C)
- Large rimmed baking sheet, sprayed with nonstick cooking spray (preferably olive oil)

| | | |
|---|---|---|
| 2 | cloves garlic, minced | 2 |
| 1 | package (10 oz/300 g) frozen chopped spinach, thawed and squeezed dry | 1 |
| 3 cups | cooked quinoa (see page 10), cooled | 750 mL |
| ¾ cup | finely shredded carrots | 175 mL |
| ½ cup | finely chopped green onions | 125 mL |
| ¼ cup | quinoa flour | 60 mL |
| 1 tbsp | dried Italian seasoning | 15 mL |
| 1 tsp | baking powder | 5 mL |
| | Fine sea salt and freshly cracked black pepper | |
| 2 | large eggs, lightly beaten | 2 |
| 1 tbsp | chopped fresh dill | 15 mL |
| 1 cup | plain yogurt | 250 mL |
| 1 tbsp | freshly squeezed lemon juice | 15 mL |

1. In a large bowl, combine garlic, spinach, quinoa, carrots, green onions, quinoa flour, Italian seasoning, baking powder, ½ tsp (2 mL) salt, ½ tsp (2 mL) pepper and eggs.

2 Scoop 8 equal mounds of quinoa mixture onto prepared baking sheet. Using a spatula, flatten mounds to ½-inch (1 cm) thickness.

3. Bake in preheated oven for 15 minutes. Turn cakes over and bake for 8 to 12 minutes or until golden brown and hot in the center.

4. Meanwhile, in a small bowl, whisk together dill, yogurt and lemon juice. Season to taste with salt and pepper.

5. Serve warm quinoa cakes with yogurt sauce drizzled on top or served alongside.

# French Potato Quinoa Croquettes

*Everyone goes crazy for crisp potatoes, but when they combine with quinoa and flavorful cheeses to become a healthy main dish, brace yourself for stampedes to the dinner table.*

## Tip

You can make the patties half the size and serve them as an appetizer.

- **Rimmed baking sheet**

| | | |
|---|---|---|
| 1 | large russet potato (about 12 oz/375 g) | 1 |
| 6 tsp | olive oil, divided | 30 mL |
| 1 cup | thinly sliced green onions | 250 mL |
| ½ cup | packed fresh flat-leaf (Italian) parsley leaves, chopped | 125 mL |
| 2 tsp | dried thyme | 10 mL |
| 4 | cloves garlic, minced | 4 |
| 3 cups | cooked quinoa (see page 10), cooled | 750 mL |
| 1 cup | shredded Gruyère or Swiss cheese | 250 mL |
| ½ cup | cottage cheese (reduced-fat or regular) | 125 mL |
| | Fine sea salt and freshly cracked black pepper | |
| 1 | large egg, lightly beaten | 1 |
| 1 cup | panko or dry bread crumbs (GF, if needed) | 250 mL |
| 1½ cups | marinara sauce, warmed | 375 mL |

1. Using a fork, pierce potato all over. Loosely wrap potato in a paper towel. Microwave on High for 3 minutes. Turn potato over and microwave for 3 to 4 minutes or until easily pierced with a fork. Wrap potato in a clean kitchen towel and let stand for 5 minutes. Peel and mash potato.

2. In a large nonstick skillet, heat 1 tsp (5 mL) of the oil over medium-high heat. Add green onions, parsley, thyme and garlic; cook, stirring, for 1 minute or until softened.

3. In a large bowl, combine potato, onion mixture, quinoa, Gruyère and cottage cheese until well blended. Season generously with salt and pepper. Form into twelve ½-inch (1 cm) thick patties.

4. Place egg and panko in separate shallow dishes. Carefully dip each patty in egg, then in panko, turning to coat. Place on baking sheet. Cover and place in freezer for 15 minutes.

5. In a large nonstick skillet, heat 2½ tsp (12 mL) oil over medium heat. Add patties, in batches as necessary, and cook for 2 to 3 minutes per side or until golden brown. Transfer to plate and loosely cover with foil to keep warm. Repeat with the remaining oil and patties, adjusting heat as necessary between batches. Serve warm, with marinara sauce.

# Sunflower Seed and Quinoa Burgers

*These veggie burgers have great texture, thanks to a combination of quinoa, sunflower seeds and red kidney beans. They get a power-up from hot smoked paprika and cumin, offset by luscious Greek yogurt, peppery arugula and sweet tomato.*

## Tip

Whenever possible, use whole-grain or multigrain hamburger buns.

- **Food processor**

| | | |
|---|---|---|
| 1½ cups | cooked quinoa (see page 10), cooled | 375 mL |
| 3 | cloves garlic, coarsely chopped | 3 |
| 1 cup | rinsed drained canned red kidney beans | 250 mL |
| ¾ cup | lightly salted roasted sunflower seeds | 175 mL |
| ½ cup | packed fresh cilantro leaves | 125 mL |
| 2 tsp | ground cumin | 10 mL |
| ¾ tsp | hot smoked paprika or chipotle chile powder | 3 mL |
| ½ tsp | fine sea salt | 2 mL |
| 2 tsp | olive oil | 10 mL |
| 4 | hamburger buns (GF, if needed), split and toasted | 4 |
| 4 | large tomato slices | 4 |
| 2 cups | packed arugula or baby spinach | 500 mL |
| ⅓ cup | plain Greek yogurt | 75 mL |

1. In food processor, combine quinoa, garlic, beans, sunflower seeds, cilantro, cumin, paprika and salt; pulse until blended but still chunky. Form into four ¾-inch (2 cm) thick patties.

2. In a large skillet, heat oil over medium heat. Add patties and cook for 4 minutes. Turn patties over and cook for 3 to 5 minutes or until crispy on the outside and hot in the center.

3. Transfer patties to toasted buns. Top with tomato, spinach and dollops of yogurt.

# Black Bean Quinoa Burgers

**Makes
4 servings**

*Black beans are a natural
choice for vegetarian
burgers. Their meaty
texture stands up to being
shaped into patties that
take deliciously to all
of the favorite burger
trappings. The Tex-Mex
flavorings can be swapped
out for the seasonings of
your choice.*

## Tips

If you can only find larger
19-oz (540 mL) cans of
beans, you will need about
1$\frac{1}{2}$ cans (3 cups/750 mL
drained).

Whenever possible, use
whole-grain or multigrain
hamburger buns.

● **Food processor**

| | | |
|---|---|---|
| 1 cup | cooked quinoa (see page 10), cooled | 250 mL |
| $\frac{1}{4}$ cup | finely chopped fresh cilantro | 60 mL |
| 2 tsp | ground cumin | 10 mL |
| 1 tsp | dried oregano | 5 mL |
| $\frac{1}{4}$ tsp | cayenne pepper | 1 mL |
| 2 | cans (each 14 to 15 oz/398 to 425 mL) black beans, drained and rinsed, divided | 2 |
| 1 | large egg | 1 |
| 1 tbsp | olive oil | 15 mL |
| 4 | hamburger buns (GF, if needed), split and toasted | 4 |

**Suggested Accompaniments**

Plain Greek yogurt

Salsa

Spinach leaves

1. In food processor, combine quinoa, cilantro, cumin, oregano, cayenne, half the beans and egg; pulse until a chunky purée forms.

2. Transfer purée to a medium bowl and stir in the remaining beans. Form into four $\frac{3}{4}$-inch (2 cm) thick patties.

3. In a large skillet, heat oil over medium heat. Add patties and cook for 4 minutes. Turn patties over and cook for 3 to 4 minutes or until crispy on the outside and hot in the center.

4. Transfer patties to toasted buns. Top with any of the suggested accompaniments, as desired.

## Variation

For vegan burgers, use 3 tbsp (45 mL) vegan mayonnaise alternative in place of the egg.

# California Quinoa Club Sandwich

*Here's a modern and very delicious throwback to 1970s vegetarian fare.*

## Tip

Whenever possible, use whole-grain or multigrain sandwich bread.

| | | |
|---|---|---|
| ½ cup | cooked quinoa (see page 10), cooled | 125 mL |
| ⅓ cup | hummus | 75 mL |
| 1 | small firm-ripe Hass avocado, sliced | 1 |
| 2 tsp | freshly squeezed lemon juice | 10 mL |
| | Fine sea salt and freshly cracked black pepper | |
| 3 | slices seeded sandwich bread (GF, if needed) | 3 |
| 1 | plum (Roma) tomato, sliced crosswise | 1 |
| 1 cup | quinoa sprouts (see page 13) or alfalfa sprouts | 250 mL |

1. In a small bowl, combine quinoa and hummus.
2. Sprinkle avocado slices with lemon juice. Season to taste with salt and pepper.
3. Spread one side of each bread slice with quinoa mixture. Top one slice with half each of the avocado, tomato and sprouts. Cover with another slice of bread, quinoa mixture up. Top with the remaining avocado, tomato and sprouts. Cover with the third bread slice, quinoa mixture down, pressing down gently. Cut sandwich in half.

# Avocado, Mango and Quinoa Pitas

*These so-easy sandwiches
are so very good, you'll
find yourself counting the
minutes until lunchtime.*

**Tip**

Whenever possible,
use whole-grain or
multigrain pitas.

| | | |
|---|---|---|
| 1½ cups | cooked quinoa (see page 10), cooled | 375 mL |
| 1 | firm-ripe Hass avocado, diced | 1 |
| 1 cup | chopped mango | 250 mL |
| 1 cup | diced peeled jicama | 250 mL |
| 1 tsp | ground cumin | 5 mL |
| 2 tbsp | freshly squeezed lime juice | 30 mL |
| 1 tsp | chipotle pepper sauce | 5 mL |
| ⅓ cup | lightly salted roasted cashews, coarsely chopped | 75 mL |
| | Fine sea salt and freshly cracked black pepper | |
| 2 | 6-inch (15 cm) pitas (GF, if needed), tops split open | 2 |

1. In a medium bowl, combine quinoa, avocado, mango, jicama, cumin, lime juice and chipotle pepper sauce, gently tossing to coat. Season to taste with salt and pepper. Gently stir in cashews. Stuff pitas with quinoa mixture, dividing evenly.

# Greek Quinoa Salad Pitas

*Chopped radishes add
speckles of scarlet and
a pleasant, peppery bite
to these unusual Greek
salad pitas.*

**Tip**

Whenever possible,
use whole-grain or
multigrain pitas.

| | | |
|---|---|---|
| ¼ tsp | fine sea salt | 1 mL |
| ⅛ tsp | freshly cracked black pepper | 0.5 mL |
| 1 tbsp | extra virgin olive oil | 15 mL |
| 1 tbsp | red wine vinegar | 15 mL |
| 1½ cups | cooked quinoa (see page 10), cooled | 375 mL |
| 1 | small red bell pepper, finely chopped | 1 |
| 1¼ cups | halved cherry or grape tomatoes | 300 mL |
| 1 cup | diced seeded peeled cucumber | 250 mL |
| 1 cup | chopped radishes | 250 mL |
| ½ cup | packed fresh mint leaves, chopped | 125 mL |
| ½ cup | crumbled feta cheese | 125 mL |
| 4 | 6-inch (15 cm) pitas (GF, if needed), tops split open | 4 |

1. In a medium bowl, whisk together salt, pepper, oil and vinegar. Stir in quinoa, red pepper, tomatoes, cucumber, radishes, mint and cheese, gently tossing to coat. Stuff pitas with quinoa mixture, dividing evenly.

# Mushroom, Quinoa and Kale Burritos

**Makes
4 servings**

*In this unconventional
take on a Mexican
favorite, the deep, rich
ensemble of mushrooms,
quinoa and kale is topped
with gently assertive goat
cheese and spicy salsa.
Olé!*

## Tip

Unlike other greens, kale stems are so tough they are virtually inedible. Hence, they, along with the tougher part of the center rib, must be removed before cooking. To do so, lay a leaf upside down on a cutting board and use a paring knife to cut a V shape along both sides of the rib, cutting it and the stem free from the leaf.

| | | |
|---|---|---|
| 2 tsp | olive oil | 10 mL |
| 1 | large bunch kale, tough stems and center ribs removed, leaves very thinly sliced crosswise (about 6 cups/1.5 L) | 1 |
| 1 lb | cremini or button mushrooms, sliced | 500 g |
| 2 tsp | ground cumin | 10 mL |
| 1½ cups | hot cooked quinoa (see page 10) | 375 mL |
| ¾ cup | salsa | 175 mL |
| 4 | 10-inch (25 cm) multigrain tortillas (GF, if needed), warmed | 4 |
| 4 oz | soft mild goat cheese, crumbled (about 1 cup/250 mL) | 125 g |

1. In a large pot, heat oil over medium-high heat. Add kale, mushrooms and cumin; cook, stirring, for 5 minutes. Reduce heat to medium-low and cook, stirring, for 12 to 15 minutes or until kale is very wilted and mushrooms are browned. Add quinoa and salsa; cook, stirring, for 3 minutes or until heated through.

2. Spoon quinoa mixture down the center of each warmed tortilla, leaving a 2-inch (5 cm) border. Sprinkle with cheese. Roll up like burritos, enclosing filling, or like jelly rolls (ends open).

# Pinto Bean, Quinoa and Spinach Burritos

*Who needs meat? This cumin- and cilantro-scented bean and quinoa filling is hearty, satisfying and incredibly easy to prepare.*

## Tip

To streamline preparation time, use thawed frozen chopped onions in place of fresh. They are inexpensive and are available in the frozen foods section of most supermarkets.

- **Preheat oven to 350°F (180°C)**

| | | |
|---|---|---|
| 2 tsp | vegetable oil | 10 mL |
| 1 cup | chopped onion | 250 mL |
| 1½ cups | hot cooked quinoa (see page 10) | 375 mL |
| 1 | can (14 to 19 oz/398 to 540 mL) pinto beans, drained and rinsed | 1 |
| 2 tsp | ground cumin | 10 mL |
| ¼ tsp | fine sea salt | 1 mL |
| ⅓ cup | packed fresh cilantro leaves | 75 mL |
| 4 | 10-inch (25 cm) multigrain tortillas (GF, if needed), warmed | 4 |
| 4 cups | packed baby spinach | 1 L |
| 1 cup | crumbled queso fresco or feta cheese | 250 mL |
| 1 cup | salsa | 250 mL |

1. In a large skillet, heat oil over medium-high heat. Add onion and cook, stirring, for 5 to 6 minutes or until softened. Add quinoa, beans, cumin and salt; cook, stirring, for 1 minute. Stir in cilantro.

2. Top warmed tortillas with bean mixture, spinach and cheese, dividing evenly. Roll up like burritos, enclosing filling. Wrap tortillas individually in foil.

3. Bake in preheated oven for 20 minutes. Unwrap, cut in half and serve with salsa.

# Broccoli and Quinoa Enchiladas

*This California-inspired
variation of classic
Mexican fare is my idea
of rich, delicious comfort
food at its best. Broccoli
and quinoa are the perfect
ingredients for balancing
the tangy cheese and
hearty tortillas.*

- **Preheat oven to 350°F (180°C)**
- **8- or 9-inch (20 or 23 cm) square glass baking dish or metal baking pan, sprayed with nonstick cooking spray**

| | | |
|---|---|---|
| 2 tsp | olive oil | 10 mL |
| 1¼ cups | chopped onions | 300 mL |
| 2 cups | finely chopped broccoli florets | 500 mL |
| 1 tsp | ground cumin | 5 mL |
| 1½ cups | picante sauce, divided | 375 mL |
| 1½ cups | cooked quinoa (see page 10), cooled | 375 mL |
| 1 cup | cottage or ricotta cheese (reduced-fat or regular) | 250 mL |
| 1 cup | shredded sharp (old) white Cheddar cheese, divided | 250 mL |
| 8 | 8-inch (20 cm) multigrain tortillas (GF, if needed), warmed | 8 |

1. In a large skillet, heat oil over medium heat. Add onions and cook, stirring, for 6 to 8 minutes or until softened. Add broccoli, cumin and ⅓ cup (75 mL) of the picante sauce; cook, stirring, for 1 minute. Remove from heat and stir in quinoa, cottage cheese and ⅓ cup (75 mL) of the Cheddar.

2. Spoon about ⅓ cup (75 mL) of the quinoa mixture down the center of each warmed tortilla. Roll up like a cigar and place, seam side down, in prepared baking dish. Spoon the remaining picante sauce over top.

3. Cover and bake in preheated oven for 20 to 25 minutes or until heated through. Sprinkle with the remaining Cheddar. Bake, uncovered, for 5 minutes or until cheese is bubbling.

# Pumpkin and Quinoa Enchiladas

*This dish takes
everyday canned
pumpkin purée and,
with little effort, turns
it into an unexpectedly
sophisticated and
delicious enchilada filling.*

## Tip

For the white beans, you
could use Great Northern
beans, cannellini (white
kidney) beans or white pea
(navy) beans.

- **Preheat oven to 350°F (180°C)**
- **13- by 9-inch (33 by 23 cm) glass baking dish, sprayed
  with nonstick cooking spray (preferably olive oil)**

| | | |
|---|---|---|
| 1 cup | hot cooked quinoa (see page 10) | 250 mL |
| 1 cup | rinsed drained canned white beans | 250 mL |
| 1 cup | canned pumpkin purée (not pie filling) | 250 mL |
| 2 tsp | ground cumin, divided | 10 mL |
| 1½ cups | chipotle salsa, divided | 375 mL |
| 1½ cups | tomato juice | 375 mL |
| 12 | 6-inch (15 cm) corn tortillas (GF, if needed), warmed | 12 |
| 4 oz | mild goat cheese, crumbled (about 1 cup/250 mL) | 125 g |
| ½ cup | thinly sliced green onions | 125 mL |

1. In a medium saucepan, combine quinoa, beans, pumpkin, half the cumin and ½ cup (125 mL) of the salsa. Using a fork, coarsely mash some of the beans. Cook, stirring, over medium heat for 5 to 6 minutes to heat through and blend the flavors.

2. In a medium bowl, whisk together tomato juice, the remaining salsa and the remaining cumin. Spread 1 cup (250 mL) of the sauce in bottom of prepared baking dish.

3. Spoon about ¼ cup (60 mL) of the quinoa mixture down the center of each warmed tortilla. Roll up like a cigar and place, seam side down, in baking dish. Top with the remaining sauce.

4. Cover and bake in preheated oven for 20 minutes. Sprinkle with cheese and green onions. Bake, uncovered, for 10 to 15 minutes or until cheese is melted and sauce is bubbling.

# Mushroom-Jack Quinoa Quesadillas

**Makes
4 servings**

*A squeeze of lime unites all the flavors in these newfangled quesadillas.*

## Tip

When selecting mushrooms, choose those with a fresh, smooth appearance, free from major blemishes and with a dry surface. Once home, keep mushrooms refrigerated; they're best when used within a few days after purchase. When ready to use, gently wipe mushrooms with a damp cloth or soft brush to remove dirt particles. Alternatively, rinse mushrooms quickly with cold water, then immediately pat dry with paper towels.

- **Preheat oven to 400°F (200°C)**
- **Large rimmed baking sheet, sprayed with nonstick cooking spray (preferably olive oil)**

| | | |
|---|---|---|
| 2 tsp | vegetable oil | 10 mL |
| 8 oz | cremini or button mushrooms, thinly sliced | 250 g |
| 1 cup | chopped green onions | 250 mL |
| 1 cup | hot cooked quinoa (see page 10) | 250 mL |
| 1 tbsp | chili powder | 15 mL |
| 1 tbsp | freshly squeezed lime juice | 15 mL |
| | Fine sea salt and freshly cracked black pepper | |
| 4 | 8-inch (20 cm) multigrain tortillas (GF, if needed) | 4 |
| 2 cups | shredded pepper Jack cheese | 500 mL |
| | Nonstick cooking spray (preferably olive oil) | |
| | Salsa (optional) | |

1. In a large skillet, heat oil over medium-high heat. Add mushrooms and green onions; cook, stirring occasionally, for 4 to 5 minutes or until mushrooms are tender. Add quinoa, chili powder and lime juice; cook, stirring, for 1 minute or until warmed through. Season to taste with salt and pepper.

2. Place 2 tortillas on prepared baking sheet. Divide quinoa mixture between tortillas, spreading to cover. Sprinkle with cheese. Top with the remaining tortillas, pressing down gently. Spray lightly with cooking spray.

3. Bake in preheated oven for 10 to 12 minutes or until cheese is melted and tortillas are golden brown. Transfer to cutting board and cut each quesadilla into quarters. Serve with salsa, if desired.

# Chipotle Quinoa and Black Bean Tacos

**Makes
4 servings**

*Long on flavor and short
on time consumption, this
superfast, superfood spin
on a fast-food favorite
provides ample amounts
of lean protein, fiber and
antioxidants, all with
about 10 minutes of effort
from start to finish.*

| | | |
|---|---|---|
| 1 cup | hot cooked quinoa (see page 10) | 250 mL |
| 1 cup | rinsed drained canned black beans | 250 mL |
| 1½ cups | chipotle salsa | 375 mL |
| 1 tsp | ground cumin | 5 mL |
| ½ cup | plain Greek yogurt | 125 mL |
| 1 tbsp | freshly squeezed lime juice | 15 mL |
| 8 | 6-inch (15 cm) corn tortillas (GF, if needed), warmed | 8 |
| 2 cups | shredded coleslaw mix (shredded cabbage and carrots) | 500 mL |
| ½ cup | packed fresh cilantro leaves | 125 mL |
| ½ cup | crumbled queso fresco | 125 mL |

1. In a large skillet, combine quinoa, beans and salsa. Using a fork, partially mash beans. Cook, stirring, over medium heat for 4 to 5 minutes or until heated through.
2. Meanwhile, in a small bowl, whisk together cumin, yogurt and lime juice.
3. Fill warmed tortillas with quinoa mixture, coleslaw, cilantro, queso fresco and dollops of lime yogurt.

# Seafood, Poultry and Lean Meat Main Dishes

# Grilled Cod with North African Quinoa

*This dish combines a number of sensations: buttery fish and an accompanying side dish of such flavorful depth — think quinoa, olives, herbs and Moroccan spices — you'll hardly believe it was so simple to prepare.*

## Tip

Sea bass, halibut, tilapia or any other firm white fish fillets may be used in place of the cod.

- Preheat broiler, with rack set 4 to 6 inches (10 to 15 cm) from heat source
- Broiler pan, sprayed with nonstick cooking spray (preferably olive oil)

| | | |
|---|---|---|
| 4 tsp | olive oil, divided | 20 mL |
| 1 tsp | ground cumin | 5 mL |
| 3/4 tsp | ground cinnamon | 3 mL |
| 1/4 tsp | cayenne pepper | 1 mL |
| 1 cup | quinoa, rinsed | 250 mL |
| 2 cups | ready-to-use reduced-sodium vegetable or chicken broth (GF, if needed) | 500 mL |
| 2/3 cup | chopped drained roasted red bell peppers | 150 mL |
| 1/3 cup | finely chopped red onion | 75 mL |
| 1/4 cup | chopped pitted brine-cured black olives (such as kalamata) | 60 mL |
| 1/4 cup | packed fresh mint leaves, chopped | 60 mL |
| 3 tbsp | golden raisins, chopped | 45 mL |
| 2 tbsp | freshly squeezed lemon juice, divided | 30 mL |
| | Fine sea salt and freshly cracked black pepper | |
| 4 | skin-on black cod (sablefish) fillets (each about 5 oz/150 g) | 4 |

1. In a medium saucepan, heat half the oil over medium heat. Add cumin, cinnamon and cayenne; cook, stirring, for about 30 seconds or until fragrant. Stir in quinoa and broth; increase heat to medium-high and bring to a boil. Reduce heat to low, cover and simmer for 12 to 15 minutes or until liquid is absorbed. Remove from heat and stir in roasted peppers, red onion, olives, mint, raisins and half the lemon juice. Cover and let stand for 5 minutes. Fluff with a fork, then season to taste with salt and black pepper.

2. Meanwhile, place fish, skin side down, on prepared pan. Sprinkle top with the remaining lemon juice, then brush with the remaining oil. Sprinkle with salt and black pepper. Broil for 6 to 8 minutes or until fish is opaque and flakes easily when tested with a fork. Serve with quinoa mixture.

# Ginger Soy Cod with Scallion Quinoa

*Here, fresh ginger gives sprightliness to meaty cod fillets, while scallions and chili-garlic sauce do the same for mellow quinoa. The result is an ultra-easy weeknight dish that manages to be both substantial and refreshing.*

## Tip

Sea bass, halibut, tilapia or any other firm white fish fillets may be used in place of the cod.

| | | |
|---|---|---|
| 1 cup | quinoa, rinsed | 250 mL |
| 2 cups | ready-to-use reduced-sodium vegetable or chicken broth (GF, if needed) | 500 mL |
| 2 tsp | Asian chili-garlic sauce | 10 mL |
| ¾ cup | thinly sliced green onions (scallions), divided | 175 mL |
| 2 tbsp | minced gingerroot | 30 mL |
| 3 tbsp | unseasoned rice vinegar | 45 mL |
| 2 tbsp | tamari or soy sauce (GF, if needed) | 30 mL |
| 4 | skinless Pacific cod fillets (each about 5 oz/150 g) | 4 |

1. In a medium saucepan, combine quinoa, broth and chili-garlic sauce. Bring to a boil over medium-high heat. Reduce heat to low, cover and simmer for 12 to 15 minutes or until liquid is absorbed. Remove from heat and let stand, covered, for 5 minutes. Fluff with a fork, then gently stir in ½ cup (125 mL) of the green onions.

2. Meanwhile, in a large, deep skillet, combine ginger, vinegar and tamari. Add fish and bring to a boil over medium-high heat. Reduce heat to low, cover and simmer for 5 to 7 minutes or until fish is almost opaque. Scatter remaining green onions over fish. Cover and simmer for 1 to 2 minutes or until fish is opaque and flakes easily when tested with a fork. Serve fish with quinoa mixture.

# Tapenade Cod with Lemon Quinoa

*Poaching is one of the easiest ways to cook fish; poaching cod in a tapenade-flavored broth is one of the most delicious. Partnered with a vibrant lemon-herb quinoa, it's a smashing supper.*

## Tip

Sea bass, halibut, tilapia or any other firm white fish fillets may be used in place of the cod.

| | | |
|---|---|---|
| 1 cup | quinoa, rinsed | 250 mL |
| 2½ cups | ready-to-use reduced-sodium chicken or vegetable broth (GF, if needed), divided | 625 mL |
| ⅓ cup | packed fresh flat-leaf (Italian) parsley leaves, chopped | 75 mL |
| 1 tsp | finely grated lemon zest | 5 mL |
| 1 tbsp | freshly squeezed lemon juice | 15 mL |
| | Fine sea salt and freshly cracked black pepper | |
| 1 | can (14 to 15 oz/398 to 425 mL) diced tomatoes with Italian seasonings, with juice | 1 |
| ⅓ cup | chopped pitted brine-cured black olives (such as kalamata) | 75 mL |
| ½ tsp | hot pepper flakes | 2 mL |
| ¾ cup | dry white wine | 175 mL |
| 4 | skinless Pacific cod fillets (each about 6 oz/175 g) | 4 |

1. In a medium saucepan, combine quinoa and 2 cups (500 mL) of the broth. Bring to a boil over medium-high heat. Reduce heat to low, cover and simmer for 12 to 15 minutes or until liquid is absorbed. Remove from heat and let stand, covered, for 5 minutes. Fluff with a fork, then gently stir in parsley, lemon zest and lemon juice. Season to taste with salt and pepper.
2. Meanwhile, in a large skillet, combine tomatoes with juice, olives, hot pepper flakes, wine and the remaining broth. Bring to a boil over medium-high heat. Reduce heat and simmer, stirring occasionally, for 2 minutes.
3. Season both sides of fish with salt and pepper. Add fish to skillet, reduce heat to low, cover and simmer for 5 to 6 minutes or until fish is opaque and flakes easily when tested with a fork.
4. Divide quinoa mixture among four shallow bowls and top with fish and broth.

# Bistro Salmon with Arugula Quinoa Salad

*This dish showcases both salmon and quinoa with unmistakable French style.*

## Tips

According to the Monterey Bay Aquarium Seafood Watch, some of the best choices for wild salmon are those caught in Alaska, British Columbia, California, Oregon and Washington State. Compared with salmon caught in other regions, these options are abundant, well managed and caught in an environmentally friendly way.

If wild salmon is unavailable, look for North American–farmed salmon (such as Coho, Sake or Silver), which is farmed in an environmentally friendly way.

| | | |
|---|---|---|
| ¾ cup | quinoa, rinsed | 175 mL |
| 1½ cups | ready-to-use reduced-sodium chicken or vegetable broth (GF, if needed) | 375 mL |
| 2 tbsp | extra virgin olive oil, divided | 30 mL |
| 1½ tbsp | red wine vinegar | 22 mL |
| 2 tsp | Dijon mustard | 10 mL |
| 1 tsp | liquid honey | 5 mL |
| | Fine sea salt and freshly cracked black pepper | |
| 4 | skinless wild salmon fillets (each about 5 oz/150 g) | 4 |
| 3 cups | packed arugula, roughly chopped | 750 mL |
| ⅓ cup | finely chopped red onion | 75 mL |

1. In a medium saucepan, combine quinoa and broth. Bring to a boil over medium-high heat. Reduce heat to low, cover and simmer for 12 to 15 minutes or until liquid is absorbed. Remove from heat and let stand, covered, for 5 minutes. Fluff with a fork.

2. In a medium bowl, combine quinoa, half the oil, vinegar, mustard and honey. Season to taste with salt and pepper. Let cool slightly.

3. Meanwhile, sprinkle both sides of fish with salt and pepper. In a large skillet, heat the remaining oil over medium-high heat. Add fish and cook, turning once, for 3 to 4 minutes per side or until fish is opaque and flakes easily when tested with a fork.

4. To the quinoa mixture, add arugula and red onion, gently tossing to combine. Serve with salmon.

# Mustard Maple Salmon with Watercress Quinoa

*With a nod to the Pacific Northwest, this super-quick mustard and maple glaze keeps the salmon fillets incredibly moist. A peppery bed of fresh watercress quinoa balances and brightens all.*

## Tips

According to the Monterey Bay Aquarium Seafood Watch, some of the best choices for wild salmon are those caught in Alaska, British Columbia, California, Oregon and Washington State. Compared with salmon caught in other regions, these options are abundant, well managed and caught in an environmentally friendly way.

If wild salmon is unavailable, look for North American–farmed salmon (such as Coho, Sake or Silver), which is farmed in an environmentally friendly way.

• **Preheat barbecue grill to medium-high**

| | | |
|---|---|---|
| ¾ cup | quinoa, rinsed | 175 mL |
| 1½ cups | ready-to-use reduced-sodium chicken or vegetable broth (GF, if needed) | 375 mL |
| 1 tbsp | cider vinegar | 15 mL |
| 1 tbsp | pure maple syrup | 15 mL |
| 1 tbsp | extra virgin olive oil | 15 mL |
| 2 tsp | whole-grain Dijon mustard | 10 mL |
| 4 | skinless wild salmon fillets (each about 5 oz/150 g) | 4 |
| | Nonstick cooking spray | |
| | Fine sea salt and freshly cracked black pepper | |
| 3 cups | packed watercress sprigs | 750 mL |

1. In a medium saucepan, combine quinoa and broth. Bring to a boil over medium-high heat. Reduce heat to low, cover and simmer for 12 to 15 minutes or until liquid is absorbed. Remove from heat and let stand, covered, for 5 minutes. Fluff with a fork.

2. In a small bowl, whisk together vinegar, maple syrup, oil and mustard. Set aside.

3. Lightly spray both sides of fish with cooking spray, then sprinkle with salt and pepper. Grill on preheated barbecue, turning once, for 3 to 4 minutes per side or until fish is opaque and flakes easily when tested with a fork.

4. To the quinoa, add watercress, gently tossing to combine. Season to taste with salt and pepper. Serve salmon atop quinoa mixture, with maple mixture drizzled over fish.

# Seared Salmon with Pineapple Mint Quinoa

*Orange marmalade might seem like an odd addition here, but it's a handy ingredient that can perform amazing feats even when used in small amounts.*

## Tip

A pineapple is ripe enough to eat when a leaf is easily pulled from the top. To prepare it, cut off the leafy top and a small layer of the base, then slice off the tough skin and "eyes." Cut the flesh into slices, then remove the chewy central core from each slice. Cut each slice into dice.

| | | |
|---|---|---|
| 1 cup | diced fresh pineapple | 250 mL |
| 2 tbsp | chopped fresh mint | 30 mL |
| 2 tsp | minced gingerroot | 10 mL |
| 2 tbsp | orange marmalade | 30 mL |
| 1 tbsp | freshly squeezed lime juice | 15 mL |
| 1½ cups | cooked quinoa (see page 10), cooled | 375 mL |
| 4 | skinless wild salmon fillets (each about 5 oz/150 g) | 4 |
| 2 tsp | vegetable oil | 10 mL |
| ¼ tsp | fine sea salt | 1 mL |
| ⅛ tsp | cayenne pepper | 0.5 mL |

1. In a medium bowl, combine pineapple, mint, ginger, orange marmalade and lime juice. Add quinoa, gently tossing to combine. Cover and refrigerate until ready to use.

2. Brush both sides of fish with oil and sprinkle with salt and cayenne. Heat a large skillet over medium-high heat. Add fish and cook, turning once, for 3 to 4 minutes per side or until fish is opaque and flakes easily when tested with a fork. Serve with pineapple quinoa.

# Oven-BBQ Salmon with Corn and Basil Quinoa

**Makes 4 servings**

*Roasting salmon on a piece of foil eliminates any chance of it sticking to the baking sheet. Once the barbecue sauce has caramelized on the fish and the flesh flakes easily, simply slide a spatula between skin and flesh and serve. Cleanup is equally easy: crumple, toss, done.*

## Tips

According to the Monterey Bay Aquarium Seafood Watch, some of the best choices for wild salmon are those caught in Alaska, British Columbia, California, Oregon and Washington State. Compared with salmon caught in other regions, these options are abundant, well managed and caught in an environmentally friendly way.

If wild salmon is unavailable, look for North American–farmed salmon (such as Coho, Sake or Silver), which is farmed in an environmentally friendly way.

- **Preheat oven to 500°F (260°C)**
- **Small rimmed baking sheet, lined with foil and sprayed with nonstick cooking spray**

| | | |
|---|---|---|
| 4 | skin-on wild salmon fillets (each about 5 oz/150 g) | 4 |
| ¼ cup | barbecue sauce | 60 mL |
| 1 tsp | vegetable oil | 5 mL |
| 1 cup | fresh or thawed frozen corn kernels | 250 mL |
| ¼ cup | finely chopped red onion | 60 mL |
| 2 cups | hot cooked quinoa (see page 10) | 500 mL |
| ¼ cup | packed fresh basil leaves, chopped | 60 mL |
| 1 tbsp | freshly squeezed lemon juice | 15 mL |
| | Fine sea salt and freshly cracked black pepper | |

1. Place fish, skin side down, on prepared baking sheet. Generously brush with barbecue sauce. Bake in preheated oven for 7 to 11 minutes or until fish is opaque and flakes easily when tested with a fork.

2. Meanwhile, in a large, deep skillet, heat oil over medium-high heat. Add corn and red onion; cook, stirring, for 3 minutes. Stir in quinoa, basil and lemon juice. Season to taste with salt and pepper. Serve with salmon.

# Salmon and Quinoa Chirashi

*Prepare for chirashi (also
called chirashizushi)
to become one of
your favorite go-to
meals. Chirashi means
"scattered" in Japanese
and typically refers to
a big bowl of sushi rice
topped with assorted
vegetables, sashimi (or
cooked fish), sesame
seeds, hard-cooked
eggs — you name it. In
essence, it's a big bowl of
sushi. Here, I've replaced
the rice with quinoa
for fun and flavor. The
toppings should be seen
as suggestions only;
substitute whatever you
prefer (or whatever
is lurking in the
refrigerator).*

- **Preheat broiler, with rack positioned 6 inches (15 cm) from heat source**
- **Broiler pan, lined with foil and sprayed with nonstick cooking spray**

| | | |
|---|---|---|
| 1 cup | white, red or black quinoa, rinsed | 250 mL |
| 2 cups | water | 500 mL |
| 1 lb | skinless wild salmon fillets, cut into 4 pieces | 500 g |
| 3 tsp | toasted sesame oil, divided | 15 mL |
| | Fine sea salt and freshly ground black pepper | |
| 1 | Haas avocado, diced | 1 |
| 1 | sheet toasted nori, torn or snipped into small pieces | 1 |
| 1 cup | diced seeded peeled cucumber | 250 mL |
| 1/3 cup | thinly sliced green onions | 75 mL |
| 2 tbsp | toasted sesame seeds (see tip, page 254) | 30 mL |
| 2 tbsp | wasabi powder | 30 mL |
| 1/4 cup | soy sauce (GF, if needed) | 60 mL |
| 1 tbsp | liquid honey or brown rice syrup | 15 mL |
| 1 tsp | unseasoned rice vinegar or cider vinegar | 5 mL |

1. In a medium saucepan, combine quinoa and water. Bring to a boil over medium-high heat. Reduce heat to low, cover and simmer for 12 to 15 minutes or until water is absorbed. Remove from heat and let stand, covered, for 5 minutes. Fluff with a fork.

2. Meanwhile, brush both sides of fish with 2 tsp (10 mL) of the oil and sprinkle with salt and pepper. Place on prepared broiler pan. Broil for 6 to 8 minutes or until fish is opaque and flakes easily when tested with a fork.

3. Divide quinoa among four serving bowls. Lay a piece of salmon on each. Top with avocado, nori, cucumber, green onions and sesame seeds.

4 In a small bowl, whisk together wasabi powder, soy sauce, honey, vinegar and the remaining oil. Drizzle over salmon and quinoa.

# Quinoa-Crusted Salmon with Maple Mustard Vinaigrette

**Makes 4 servings**

*The quinoa in this recipe is initially cooked until just barely tender so that it still has a bit of a bite to it. Add a quick maple mustard dressing, and this becomes a powerhouse salmon dish.*

## Tip

Make sure to use fine sea salt in the water you use to cook the quinoa. Conventional table salt contains chemicals and additives, whereas sea salt contains an abundance of naturally occurring trace minerals.

| | | |
|---|---|---|
| 1/3 cup | cooked white, red or black quinoa (see page 10), chilled | 75 mL |
| | Fine sea salt and freshly cracked black pepper | |
| 1 | large egg | 1 |
| 4 | skinless wild salmon fillets (each about 6 oz/175 g) | 4 |
| 3 tbsp | extra virgin olive oil, divided | 45 mL |
| 1½ tbsp | pure maple syrup | 22 mL |
| 1½ tbsp | cider vinegar | 22 mL |
| 2 tsp | whole-grain Dijon mustard | 10 mL |
| 4 cups | packed watercress sprigs or arugula | 1 L |

1. In a medium saucepan of boiling salted water, cook quinoa for 9 minutes. Drain and rinse under cold water until cool. Transfer to a shallow dish and season to taste with salt and pepper.

2. In another shallow dish, beat egg. Season fish with salt and pepper. Dip top sides of fish in egg, shaking off excess, then in quinoa, pressing to adhere. Discard any excess quinoa and egg.

3. In a large, deep skillet, heat 1 tbsp (15 mL) of the oil over medium-high heat. Add fish, top side down, and cook, turning once, for about 3 to 4 minutes per side or until fish is opaque and flakes easily when tested with a fork.

4. In a small bowl, whisk together remaining oil, maple syrup, vinegar and mustard. Season to taste with salt and pepper.

5. Divide watercress among four dinner plates and top with salmon. Drizzle fish and watercress with vinaigrette.

# Salmon Quinoa Cakes with Lemon Yogurt

*Move over bread crumbs: toasted quinoa flakes add a nutty taste and texture — without heaviness — to these quick salmon cakes.*

| | | |
|---|---|---|
| ½ cup | quinoa flakes | 125 mL |
| 6 tbsp | finely chopped green onions, divided | 90 mL |
| ¾ cup | plain Greek yogurt | 175 mL |
| 4 tsp | Dijon mustard, divided | 20 mL |
| 1 tbsp | freshly squeezed lemon juice | 15 mL |
| | Fine sea salt and freshly ground black pepper | |
| 1 | can (15 oz/425 g) wild Alaskan salmon, drained and flaked (skin removed, if necessary) | 1 |
| 1 | large egg, beaten | 1 |
| 4 tsp | olive oil, divided | 20 mL |
| 6 cups | packed baby spinach, arugula or mesclun | 1.5 L |

1. Heat a large, deep skillet over medium-high heat. Add quinoa flakes and toast, stirring occasionally, for 1 to 2 minutes or until golden brown and just beginning to pop. Transfer to a plate and let cool.

2. In a small bowl, combine 2 tbsp (30 mL) of the green onions, yogurt, half the mustard and lemon juice. Season to taste with salt and pepper. Cover and refrigerate until ready to use.

3. In a large bowl, gently combine quinoa flakes, the remaining green onions, salmon, egg and the remaining mustard. Generously season with salt and pepper. Form into eight ¾-inch (2 cm) thick patties.

4. In the same large, deep skillet, heat half the oil over medium-high heat. Add half the patties and cook, turning once, for 5 to 6 minutes per side or until golden brown on both sides and hot in the center. Transfer to a plate and tent with foil to keep warm. Repeat with the remaining oil and patties.

5. Divide spinach among four dinner plates and top each with 2 salmon cakes. Dollop with yogurt mixture. Serve remaining yogurt mixture alongside.

# Quinoa Flake–Crusted Fish Sticks

**Makes 4 servings**

*Many fish partisans turn their noses up at fish sticks, but they'll clamor for these. The coating bakes up crisp and crunchy, light and golden, keeping the fish moist and flaky beneath.*

## Tips

Other mild, lean white fish, such as orange roughy, snapper, cod, tilefish or striped bass may be used in place of the tilapia.

The fish sticks can be prepared through step 1 and frozen. Wrap the fish sticks in plastic wrap, then foil, completely enclosing them, and freeze for up to 3 months. When ready to bake, unwrap the frozen fish sticks (do not thaw), place on prepared baking sheet and bake at 450°F (230°C) for 18 to 22 minutes, turning once halfway through, until coating is golden brown and fish is opaque and flakes easily when tested with a fork.

- **Preheat oven to 425°F (220°C)**
- **Large rimmed baking sheet, lined with foil, wire rack set on top**

| | | |
|---|---|---|
| 1 cup | quinoa flakes | 250 mL |
| 1/4 cup | ground flax seeds (flaxseed meal) | 60 mL |
| 1 tbsp | Old Bay seasoning | 15 mL |
| 2 | large eggs | 2 |
| | Fine sea salt and freshly ground black pepper | |
| 1 1/2 lbs | skinless farmed tilapia fillets, cut into 3- by 1 1/2-inch (7.5 by 4 cm) strips | 750 g |
| | Nonstick cooking spray (preferably olive oil) | |

1. In a shallow dish, combine quinoa flakes, flax seeds and Old Bay seasoning. In another shallow dish, beat eggs; sprinkle with salt and pepper. Dip fish strips in egg, shaking off excess, then in quinoa mixture, pressing to adhere and shaking off excess. Place on rack on prepared baking sheet and lightly spray with cooking spray. Discard any excess quinoa mixture and egg.

2. Bake in preheated oven for 12 to 16 minutes or until coating is golden brown and fish is opaque and flakes easily when tested with a fork.

# Mediterranean Grilled Tilapia and Quinoa

**Makes 4 servings**

*Aromatic without being spicy, this tilapia dish has a touch of the exotic but will please traditionalists, too. The quinoa hits notes of earthy, briny, sweet and salty, and the tilapia is wonderfully delicious with a bit of char from the grill.*

## Tips

According to the Monterey Bay Aquarium Seafood Watch, U.S.- and Canadian-farmed tilapia are the best choices because the supplies are abundant, well managed and farmed in an environmentally friendly way. A good alternative is tilapia farmed in Brazil, Costa Rica, Honduras or Ecuador.

Other mild, lean white fish, such as orange roughy, snapper, cod, tilefish or striped bass may be used in place of the tilapia.

| | | |
|---|---|---|
| 2 | cloves garlic, minced | 2 |
| 1 tsp | minced fresh rosemary | 5 mL |
| 2 tbsp | freshly squeezed lemon juice | 30 mL |
| 1 tbsp | olive oil | 15 mL |
| | Fine sea salt and freshly cracked black pepper | |
| 4 | skinless farmed tilapia fillets (each about 6 oz/175 g) | 4 |
| 1 cup | white, red or black quinoa, rinsed | 250 mL |
| 2 cups | ready-to-use reduced-sodium vegetable or chicken broth (GF, if needed) | 500 mL |
| 1/3 cup | packed fresh flat-leaf (Italian) parsley leaves, chopped | 75 mL |
| 1/4 cup | chopped drained oil-packed sun-dried tomatoes | 60 mL |
| 3 tbsp | minced pitted brine-cured black olives (such as kalamata) | 45 mL |

1. In a shallow dish, whisk together garlic, rosemary, lemon juice and oil. Generously season with salt and pepper. Add fish and turn to coat. Let stand for 15 minutes.
2. Meanwhile, preheat barbecue grill to medium-high.
3. In a medium saucepan, combine quinoa and broth. Bring to a boil over medium-high heat. Reduce heat to low, cover and simmer for 12 to 15 minutes or until liquid is absorbed. Remove from heat and let stand, covered, for 5 minutes. Fluff with fork, then gently stir in parsley, tomatoes and olives. Season to taste with salt and pepper.
4. Grill fish for 2 to 3 minutes per side or until fish is opaque and flakes easily when tested with a fork. Serve with quinoa mixture.

# Grilled Tilapia with Wasabi Kiwi Quinoa

*Too often, kiwis are relegated to fruit salads and tarts. Here, they take a dramatic turn as a tart-sweet complement to quinoa. Add hits of wasabi and ginger, and you have a perfect side dish for smoky grilled tilapia.*

## Tip

Other mild, lean white fish, such as orange roughy, snapper, cod, tilefish or striped bass may be used in place of the tilapia.

- **Preheat barbecue grill to medium-high**

| | | |
|---|---|---|
| 1½ tsp | wasabi powder | 7 mL |
| ½ tsp | ground ginger | 2 mL |
| 3 tbsp | freshly squeezed lemon juice | 45 mL |
| 1 tbsp | agave nectar or liquid honey | 15 mL |
| 1½ cups | cooked quinoa (see page 10), cooled | 375 mL |
| 1½ cups | diced kiwifruit | 375 mL |
| ¾ cup | diced seeded peeled cucumber | 175 mL |
| | Fine sea salt and freshly cracked black pepper | |
| 4 | skinless farmed tilapia fillets (each about 6 oz/175 g) | 4 |
| | Nonstick cooking spray | |

1. In a large bowl, whisk together wasabi powder, ginger, lemon juice and agave nectar. Add quinoa, kiwi and cucumber, gently tossing to combine. Season to taste with salt and pepper. Cover and refrigerate until ready to use.

2. Lightly spray both sides of fish with cooking spray and season with salt and pepper. Grill on preheated barbecue, turning once, for 2 to 3 minutes per side or until fish is opaque and flakes easily when tested with a fork. Serve with quinoa mixture.

# Shiitake Ginger Tilapia with Quinoa

*Shiitake mushrooms and
fresh ginger give a deep,
round intensity to budget-
friendly tilapia fillets.
The addition of grassy-
earthy quinoa makes each
forkful a hit.*

## Tips

Other mild, lean white fish,
such as orange roughy,
snapper, cod, tilefish or
striped bass may be used
in place of the tilapia.

Other mushrooms, such
as button or cremini, may
be used in place of the
shiitake mushrooms.

- Preheat oven to 400°F (200°C)
- Large rimmed baking sheet, lined with foil and
  sprayed with nonstick cooking spray (preferably
  olive oil)

| | | |
|---|---|---|
| 4 | skinless farmed tilapia fillets (each about 6 oz/175 g) | 4 |
| | Fine sea salt and freshly cracked black pepper | |
| 3 | cloves garlic, thinly sliced | 3 |
| 8 oz | shiitake mushrooms, stems removed, caps thinly sliced | 250 g |
| ½ cup | thinly sliced green onions | 125 mL |
| 2 tsp | minced gingerroot | 10 mL |
| 4 tsp | tamari or soy sauce (GF, if needed) | 20 mL |
| 2 tsp | toasted sesame oil | 10 mL |
| 3 cups | hot cooked quinoa (see page 10) | 750 mL |

1. Place fish on prepared baking sheet and sprinkle with salt and pepper.
2. In a medium bowl, combine garlic, mushrooms, green onions, ginger, tamari and oil. Spoon over fish.
3. Bake in preheated oven for 15 to 18 minutes or until fish is opaque and flakes easily when tested with a fork.
4. Divide quinoa among four shallow bowls and top with fish, mushroom mixture and accumulated juices.

# Tilapia Tacos with Quinoa and Mango

*Tilapia is a mild-tasting fish, so it tastes best accompanied by strong flavors, such as the mango, quinoa, lime and spices in these thoroughly modern tacos. Tilapia's firm, moist nature makes it an ideal fish for broiling.*

## Tips

According to the Monterey Bay Aquarium Seafood Watch, U.S.- and Canadian-farmed tilapia are the best choices because the supplies are abundant, well managed and farmed in an environmentally friendly way. A good alternative is tilapia farmed in Brazil, Costa Rica, Honduras or Ecuador.

Other mild, lean white fish, such as orange roughy, snapper, cod, tilefish or striped bass may be used in place of the tilapia.

If you are not following a gluten-free diet, try using whole wheat or multigrain tortillas.

- **Preheat broiler, with rack set 4 to 6 inches (10 to 15 cm) from heat source**
- **Broiler pan, sprayed with nonstick cooking spray**

| | | |
|---|---|---|
| ⅔ cup | black, red or white quinoa, rinsed | 150 mL |
| ½ cup | packed fresh cilantro leaves, chopped | 125 mL |
| 1½ tsp | ground cumin | 7 mL |
| 1 tsp | chili powder | 5 mL |
| ½ tsp | fine sea salt | 2 mL |
| 2 tbsp | freshly squeezed lime juice | 30 mL |
| 4 tsp | vegetable oil | 10 mL |
| 4 | skinless farmed tilapia fillets (each about 6 oz/175 g) | 4 |
| 4 | 8-inch (20 cm) quinoa tortillas or other GF tortillas (see tip, at left), warmed | 4 |
| 1½ cups | shredded purple or green cabbage | 375 mL |
| 1 cup | chopped fresh or thawed frozen mango | 250 mL |
| ½ cup | salsa | 125 mL |

1. In a medium saucepan of boiling salted water, cook quinoa for 12 minutes. Drain and rinse under cold water until cool. Transfer to a small bowl and add cilantro, gently tossing to combine.

2. Meanwhile, in a small bowl, whisk together cumin, chili powder, salt, lime juice and oil. Season to taste with salt and pepper. Drizzle half the dressing over quinoa and gently stir to combine.

3. Place fish on prepared pan and brush both sides with the remaining dressing, coating evenly. Broil for 4 to 6 minutes or until fish is opaque and flakes easily when tested with a fork. Flake fish into small pieces.

4. Fill warmed tortillas with fish, quinoa mixture, cabbage, mango and salsa.

# Skillet Tuna Quinoa "Casserole"

**Makes
4 servings**

*This version of tuna casserole is anything but traditional (technically, it is not even a casserole), but fresh vegetables, marinated artichoke hearts and quinoa bring the flavors together in a most satisfying way.*

| | | |
|---|---|---|
| 2 | cans (each 6 oz/170 g) oil-packed tuna | 2 |
| 1 | red bell pepper, chopped | 1 |
| 1 cup | chopped carrots | 250 mL |
| 1 cup | chopped onion | 250 mL |
| 2 | cloves garlic, minced | 2 |
| 1 cup | quinoa, rinsed | 250 mL |
| 1 tbsp | dried Italian seasoning | 15 mL |
| 2 cups | ready-to-use reduced-sodium vegetable or chicken broth (GF, if needed) | 500 mL |
| 3 cups | packed arugula or spinach leaves, roughly chopped | 750 mL |
| ½ cup | drained marinated artichoke hearts, 2 tbsp (30 mL) marinade reserved, hearts coarsely chopped | 125 mL |
| | Fine sea salt and freshly cracked black pepper | |

**1.** Drain tuna, reserving 1 tbsp (15 mL) oil. Flake tuna with a fork and set aside.

**2.** In a large, deep skillet, heat the reserved tuna oil over medium heat. Add red pepper, carrots and onion; cook, stirring, for 6 to 8 minutes or until softened. Add garlic, quinoa and Italian seasoning; cook, stirring, for 1 minute.

**3.** Stir in broth and bring to a boil. Reduce heat to low, cover and simmer for 12 to 15 minutes or until quinoa is tender. Stir in tuna, arugula, artichoke hearts and reserved marinade. Cover and let stand for 5 minutes or until arugula is wilted and mixture is warmed through. Season to taste with salt and pepper.

# Tuna, Olive and Golden Raisin Quinoa

*Here, I use Italian tuna packed in oil, which is darker and more strongly flavored than regular supermarket tuna, for a simple, yet robust weeknight supper. The briny tuna, piquant olives and bright-sweet golden raisins make a perfect accent to the earthiness of the quinoa.*

| | | |
|---|---|---|
| 2 | cans (each 6 oz/170 g) oil-packed tuna | 2 |
| 1¼ cups | chopped onions | 300 mL |
| 3 | cloves garlic, minced | 3 |
| 3 cups | hot cooked quinoa (see page 10) | 750 mL |
| ⅓ cup | pitted brine-cured black olives (such as kalamata), roughly chopped | 75 mL |
| ⅓ cup | golden raisins | 75 mL |
| 3 tbsp | water | 45 mL |
| ½ cup | packed fresh flat-leaf (Italian) parsley leaves, chopped | 125 mL |
| | Fine sea salt and freshly cracked black pepper | |

1. Drain tuna, reserving 1 tbsp (15 mL) oil. Flake tuna with a fork and set aside.

2. In a large, deep skillet, heat the reserved tuna oil over medium heat. Add onions and garlic; cook, stirring, for 6 to 8 minutes or until onions are golden. Stir in tuna, quinoa, olives, raisins and water; cook, stirring, for 1 to 2 minutes to blend the flavors. Stir in parsley. Season to taste with salt and pepper.

## Variation

Substitute 1½ cups (375 mL) diced cooked chicken or turkey for the tuna and use 1 tbsp (15 mL) olive oil in step 2.

# Baked Quinoa with Clams and Chorizo

**Makes 4 servings**

*My father and sister adore seafood, and the less adorned, the better. This minimalist quinoa dish featuring briny-sweet littleneck clams is right up their alley.*

## Tip

Clams are easy to cook, but they do require some essential prepping. First off, purchase clams that are not open, chipped, broken or damaged in any way. Once home, immediately unwrap the clams, allowing them to breathe, then store them in the refrigerator. Shortly before cooking, soak clams in clean, fresh water for 20 minutes. As the clams breathe, they will filter the fresh water, pushing the salt water and sand out of their shells. Remove clams from the water with a slotted spoon, leaving behind the sand in the bowl. Finally, scrub the clams with a firm brush to remove any remaining sand and sediment on the shell.

- **Preheat oven to 400°F (200°C)**
- **Large cast-iron or other ovenproof skillet**

| | | |
|---|---|---|
| 1 tbsp | olive oil | 15 mL |
| 1 cup | finely chopped onion | 250 mL |
| 3 oz | cured chorizo or smoked sausage, diced | 90 g |
| 3 | cloves garlic, minced | 3 |
| 1¼ cups | quinoa, rinsed | 300 mL |
| ½ cup | dry white wine | 125 mL |
| 2 cups | ready-to-use reduced-sodium chicken or vegetable broth (GF, if needed) | 500 mL |
| 16 | littleneck clams, scrubbed well (see tip, at left) | 16 |
| 2 tbsp | chopped fresh flat-leaf (Italian) parsley | 30 mL |

1. In cast-iron skillet, heat oil over medium-high heat. Add onion and cook, stirring, for 5 minutes. Add chorizo and garlic; cook, stirring, for 1 to 2 minutes or until onion is softened. Add quinoa and cook, stirring to coat, for 1 minute. Add wine and bring to a boil. Boil, stirring, until wine is almost evaporated. Stir in broth and return to a boil.

2. Transfer skillet to oven and bake for 5 minutes. Add clams, cover and bake for 8 to 10 minutes or until clams have opened and quinoa has absorbed all the liquid. Discard any clams that did not open. Let stand, covered, for 10 minutes. Fluff quinoa with a fork, then sprinkle with parsley.

# Shrimp Quinoa with Fennel and Orange

*Crisp, licorice-scented fennel punctuates the natural sweetness of shrimp and orange, resulting in an immensely satisfying weeknight dish.*

## Tip

To toast sliced almonds, place up to ½ cup (125 mL) almonds in a medium skillet set over medium heat. Cook, shaking the skillet, for 2 to 3 minutes or until almonds are golden brown and fragrant. Let cool completely before use.

| | | |
|---|---|---|
| 1 cup | white, red or black quinoa, rinsed | 250 mL |
| 2 cups | ready-to-use reduced-sodium vegetable or chicken broth (GF, if needed) | 500 mL |
| 1 tbsp | olive oil | 15 mL |
| 2 cups | chopped fennel bulb (about 1 large bulb), fronds reserved | 500 mL |
| 4 | cloves garlic, minced | 4 |
| 8 oz | medium shrimp, peeled and deveined | 250 g |
| ¼ cup | golden raisins, chopped | 60 mL |
| 1½ tsp | ground cumin | 7 mL |
| 1 tsp | finely grated orange zest | 5 mL |
| ⅓ cup | freshly squeezed orange juice | 75 mL |
| ¼ cup | sliced almonds, toasted (see tip, at left) | 60 mL |

1. In a medium saucepan, combine quinoa and broth. Bring to a boil over medium-high heat. Reduce heat to low, cover and simmer for 12 to 15 minutes or until liquid is absorbed. Remove from heat and let stand, covered, for 5 minutes.

2. In a large, deep skillet, heat oil over medium-high heat. Add fennel and garlic; cook, stirring, for 5 minutes. Add shrimp and cook, stirring, for 1 to 2 minutes or until fennel is tender-crisp. Stir in quinoa, raisins, cumin, orange zest and orange juice; cook, stirring, for 2 minutes or until shrimp are pink, firm and opaque.

3. Chop enough of the reserved fennel fronds to measure ¼ cup (60 mL). Stir into quinoa mixture. Serve sprinkled with almonds.

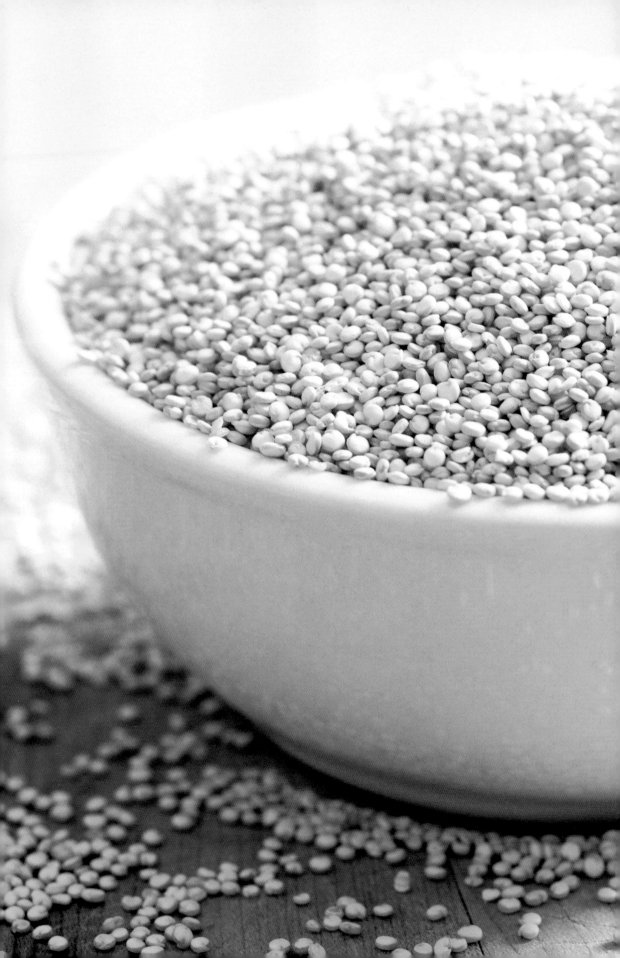

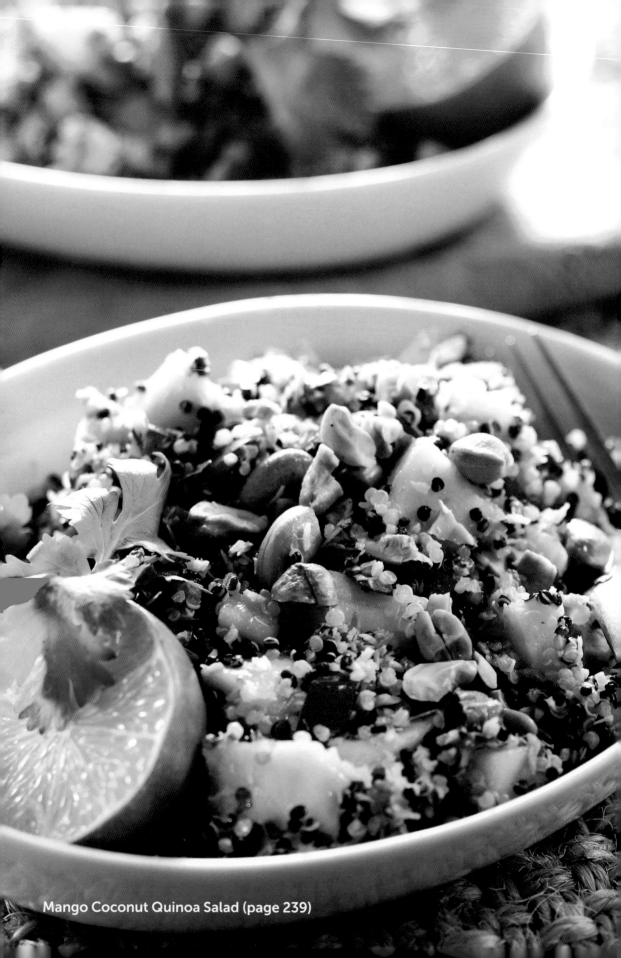

Mango Coconut Quinoa Salad (page 239)

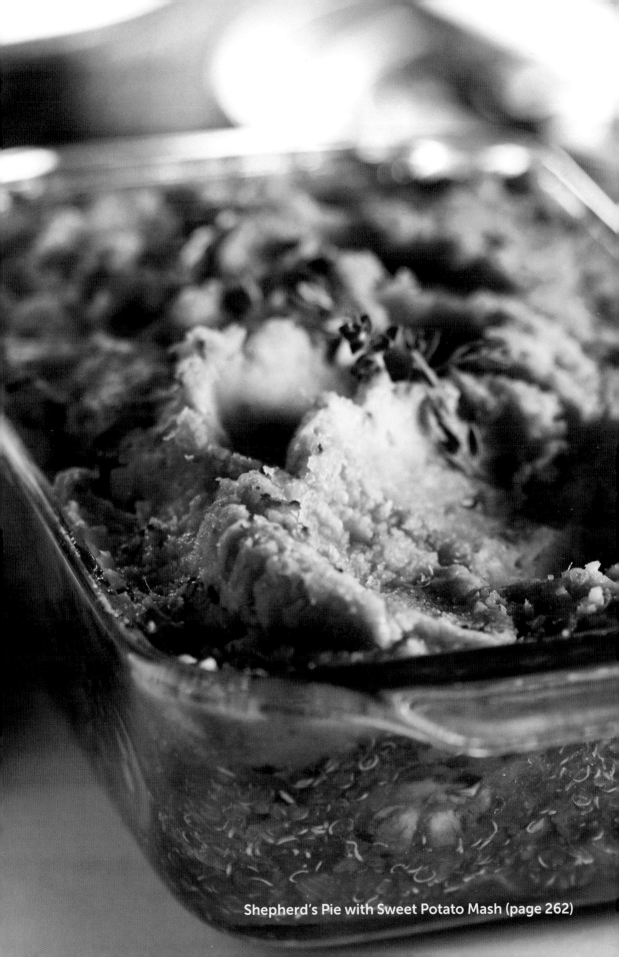
Shepherd's Pie with Sweet Potato Mash (page 262)

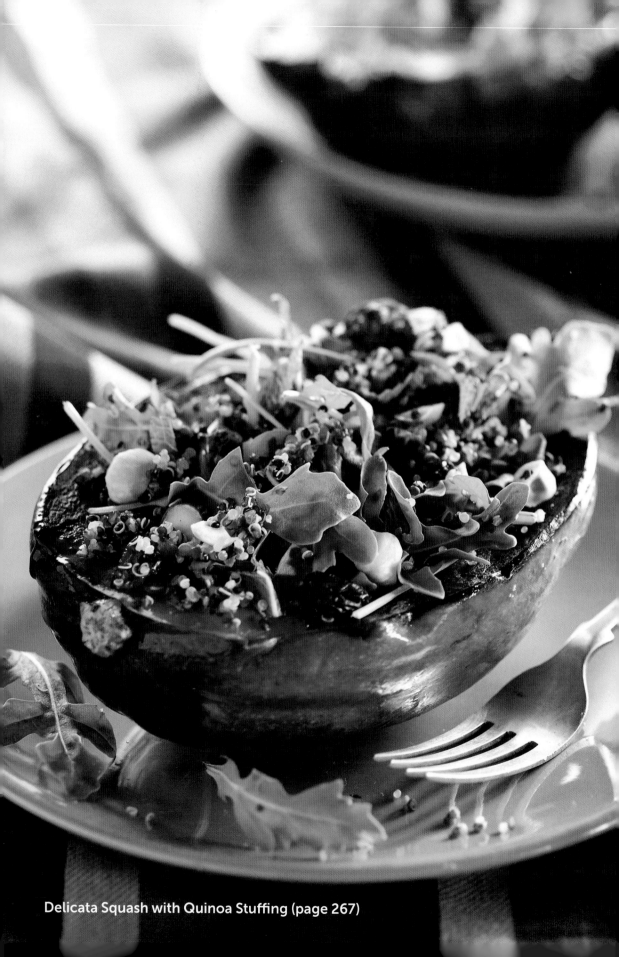

Delicata Squash with Quinoa Stuffing (page 267)

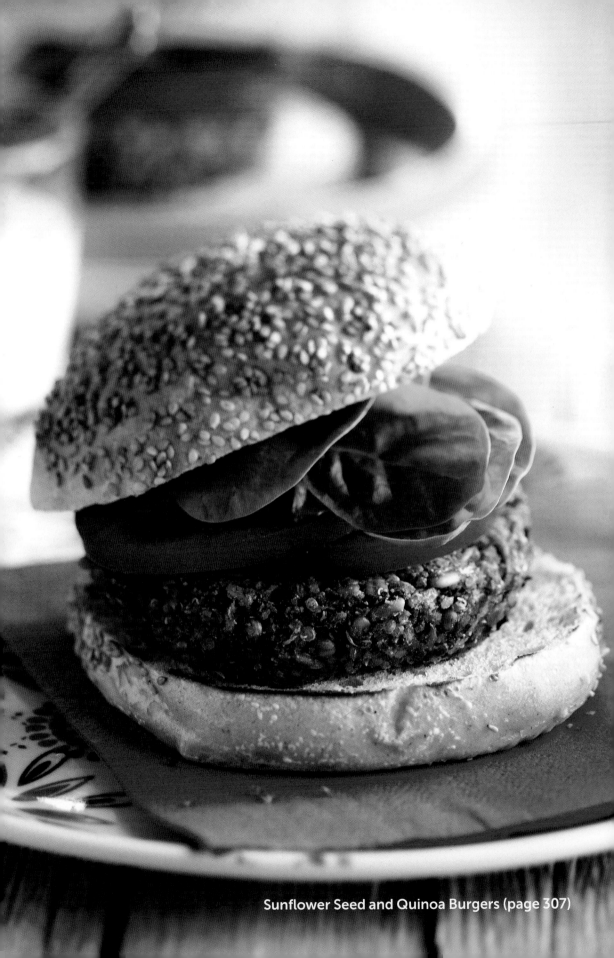

Sunflower Seed and Quinoa Burgers (page 307)

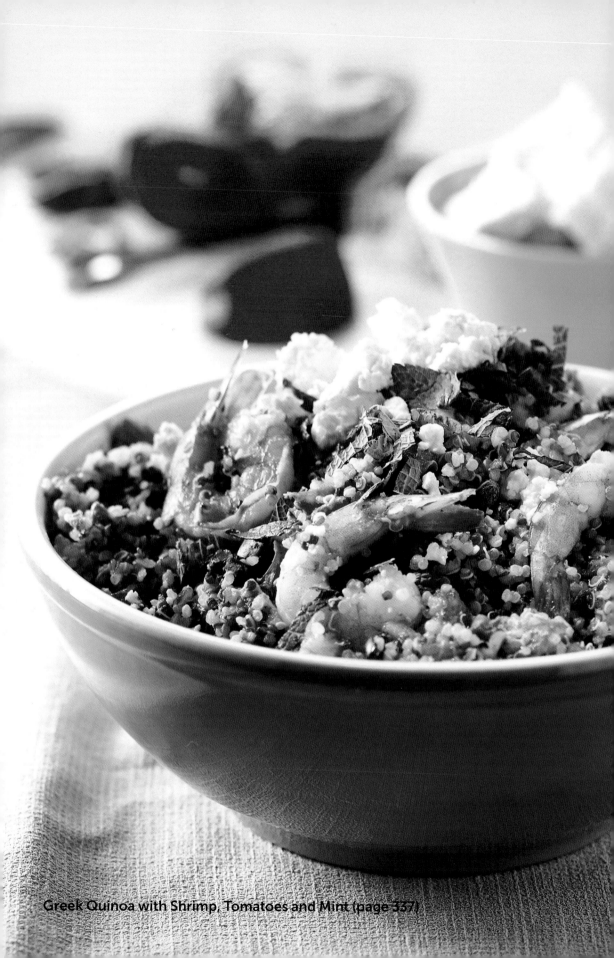

Greek Quinoa with Shrimp, Tomatoes and Mint (page 337)

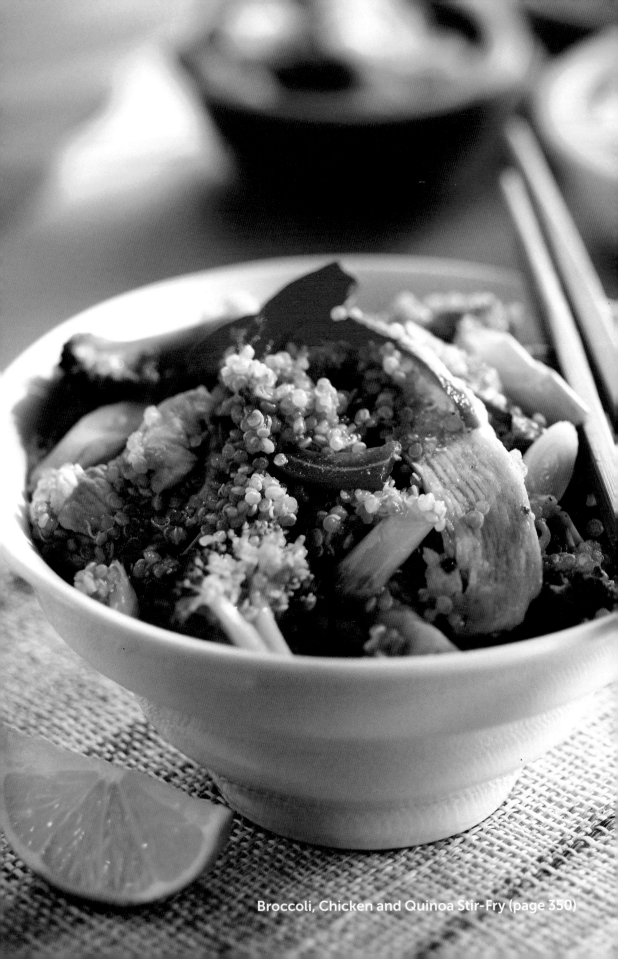

Broccoli, Chicken and Quinoa Stir-Fry (page 350)

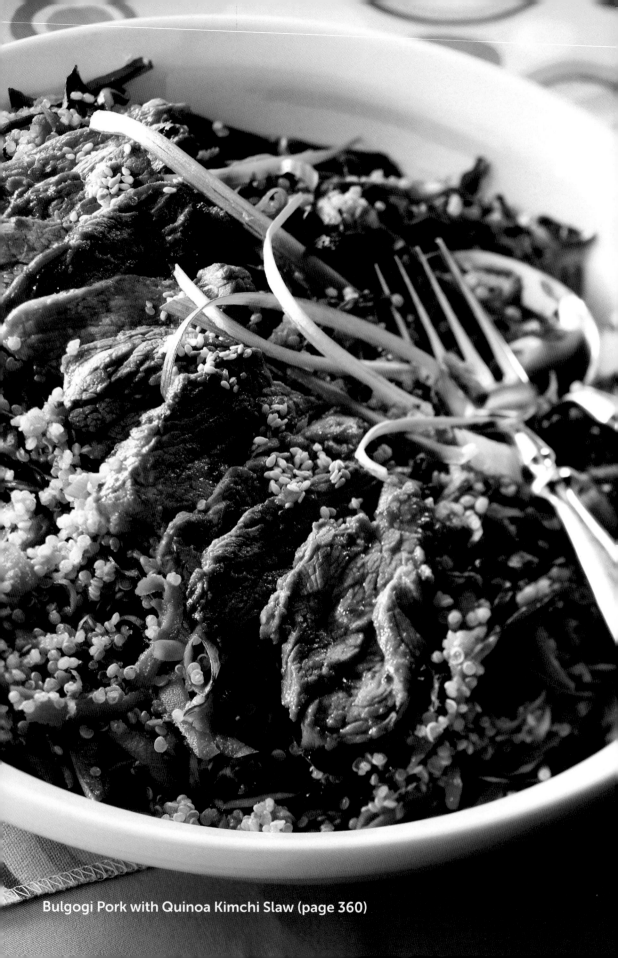

Bulgogi Pork with Quinoa Kimchi Slaw (page 360)

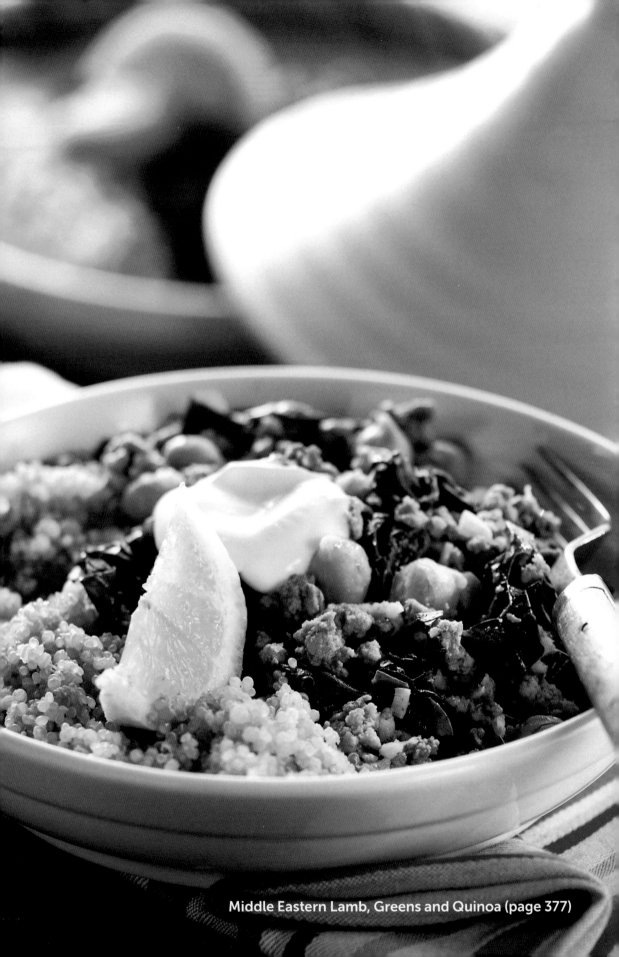

Middle Eastern Lamb, Greens and Quinoa (page 377)

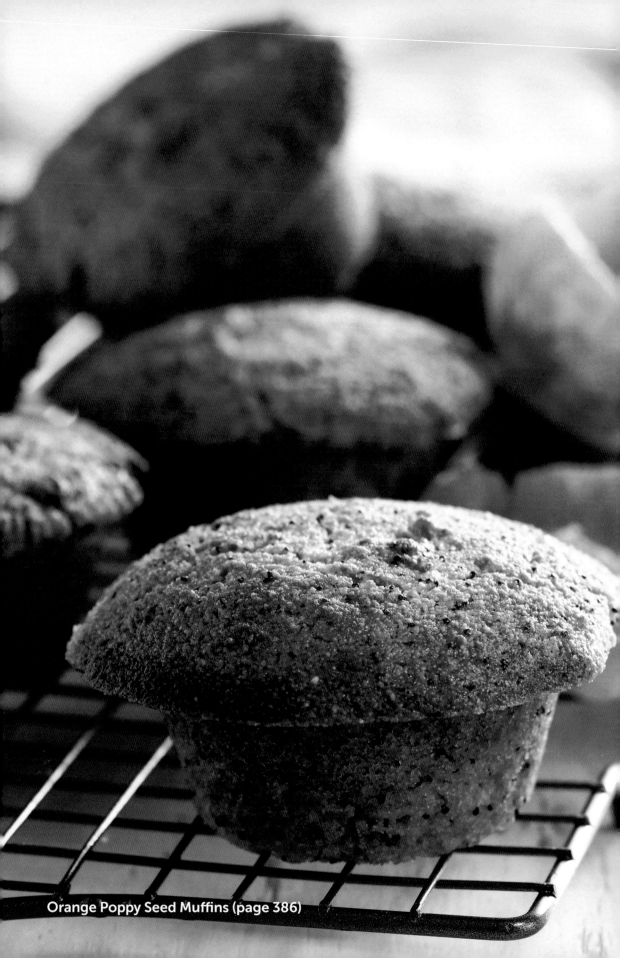

Orange Poppy Seed Muffins (page 386)

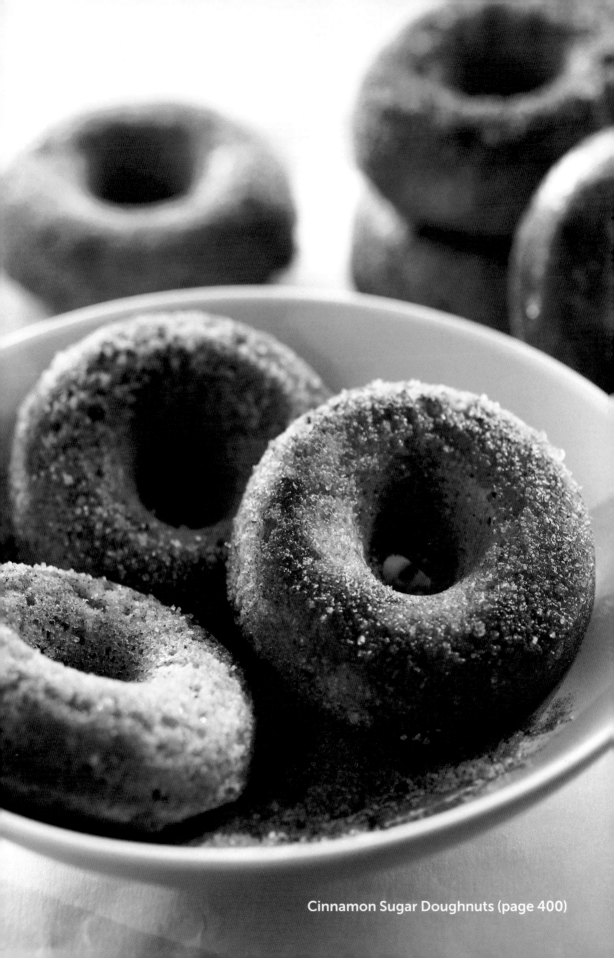

Cinnamon Sugar Doughnuts (page 400)

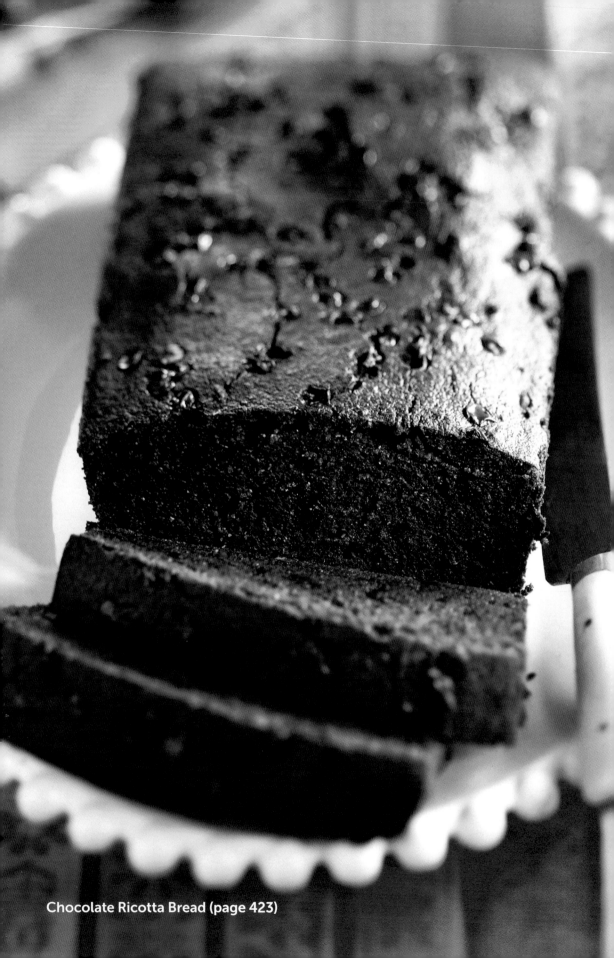

Chocolate Ricotta Bread (page 423)

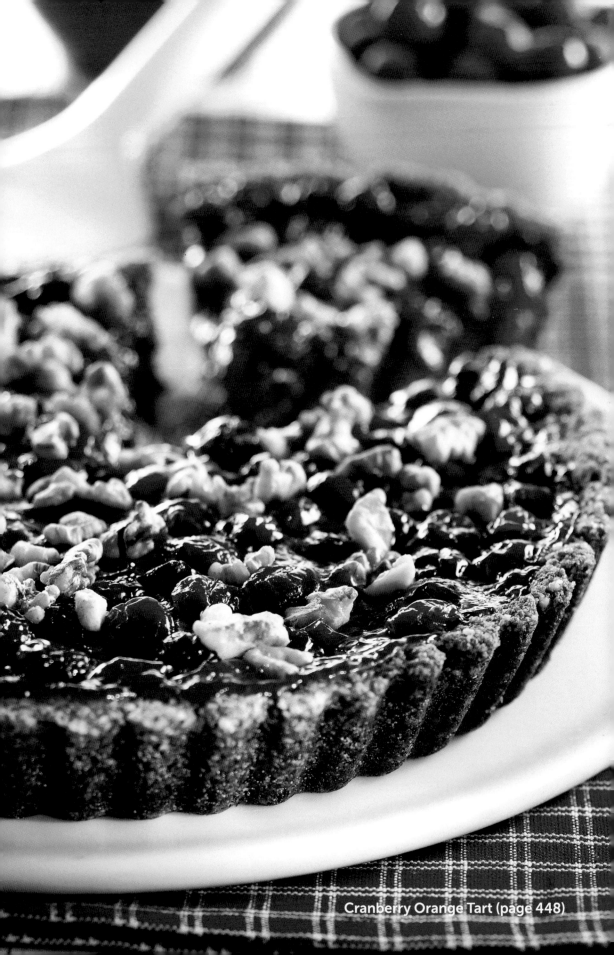

Cranberry Orange Tart (page 448)

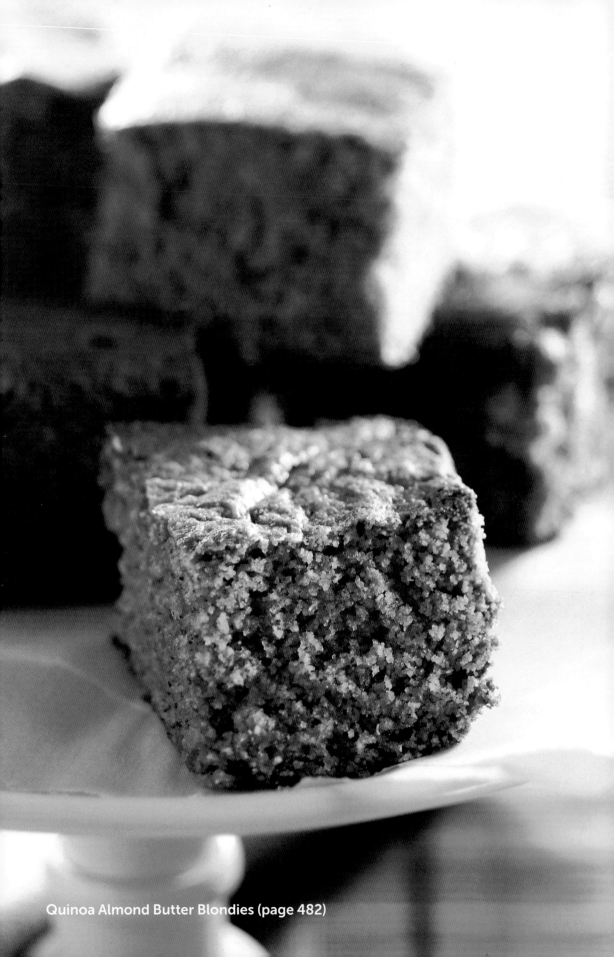

Quinoa Almond Butter Blondies (page 482)

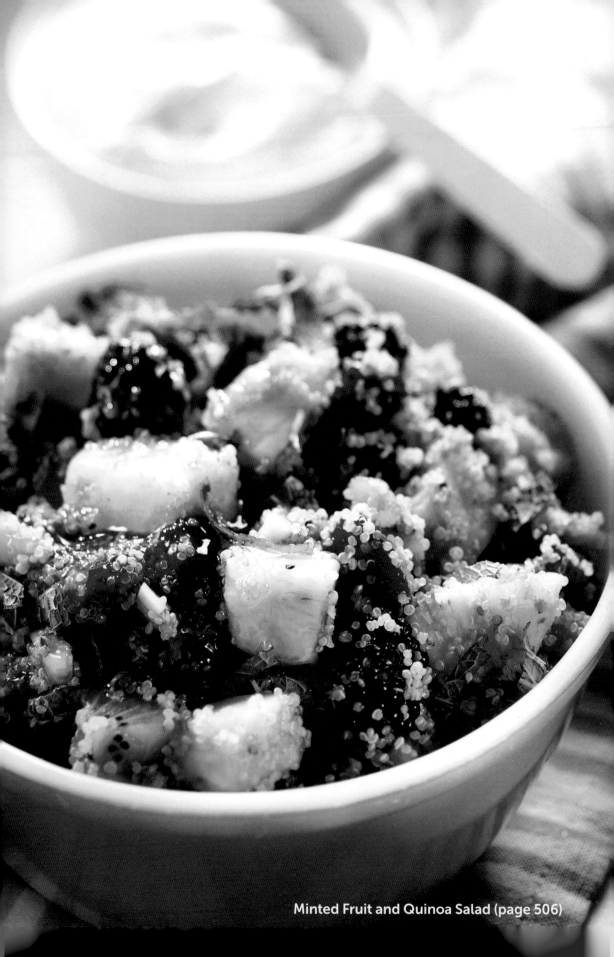

Minted Fruit and Quinoa Salad (page 506)

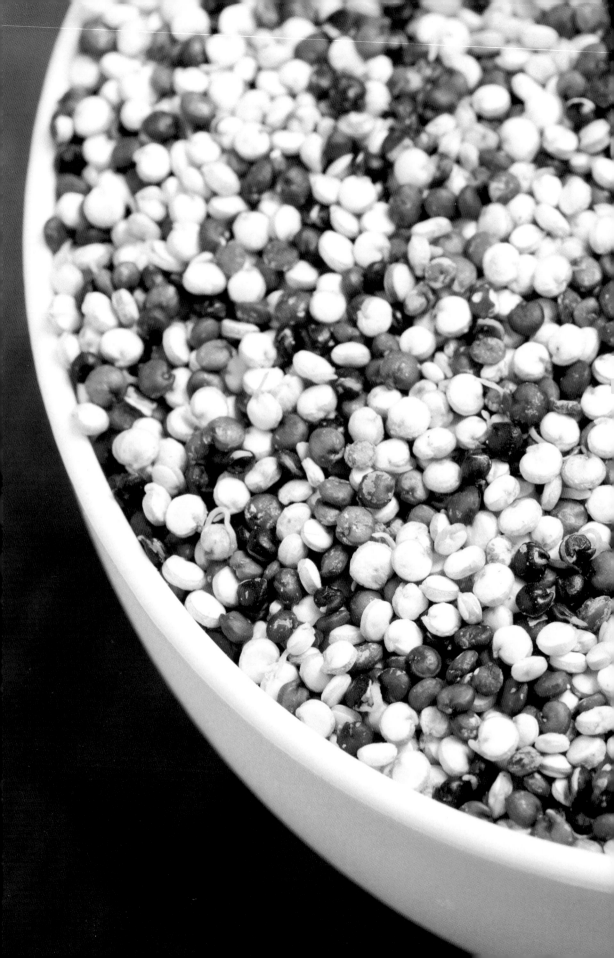

# Greek Quinoa with Shrimp, Tomatoes and Mint

*From the olives to the feta to the tomatoes, this quinoa dish is a celebration of the classic flavors of Greece — in an easy, elegant presentation. If you like, you can pile the ensemble into pitas for a handheld meal with style.*

| | | |
|---|---|---|
| 1 cup | black, white or red quinoa, rinsed | 250 mL |
| 2 cups | ready-to-use reduced-sodium vegetable or chicken broth (GF, if needed) | 500 mL |
| 2 tsp | olive oil | 10 mL |
| 8 oz | medium shrimp, peeled and deveined | 250 g |
| 2 | cloves garlic, minced | 2 |
| 2 cups | chopped tomatoes | 500 mL |
| 1/4 cup | pitted brine-cured black olives (such as kalamata), chopped | 60 mL |
| 2 tbsp | drained capers | 30 mL |
| | Fine sea salt and freshly cracked black pepper | |
| 1/2 cup | packed fresh mint leaves, thinly sliced | 125 mL |
| 1/4 cup | crumbled feta cheese | 60 mL |

1. In a medium saucepan, combine quinoa and broth. Bring to a boil over medium-high heat. Reduce heat to low, cover and simmer for 12 to 15 minutes. Let stand, covered, for 5 minutes. Fluff with a fork.

2. In a large, deep skillet, heat oil over medium-high heat. Add shrimp and garlic; cook, stirring, for 30 seconds. Add tomatoes, reduce heat and simmer, stirring occasionally, for 3 minutes or until thickened. Stir in quinoa, olives and capers; cook, stirring, for 1 minute or until shrimp are pink, firm and opaque. Season to taste with salt and pepper. Serve sprinkled with mint and cheese.

# Shrimp, Spinach and Feta Quinoa

*The sweetness of the golden raisins in this dish beautifully balances the earthy-grassy flavors of the spinach and quinoa and the briny-sweet essence of the shrimp. The combination, although simple, captures the flavors of the Mediterranean.*

| | | |
|---|---|---|
| 1 cup | quinoa, rinsed | 250 mL |
| 2 cups | ready-to-use reduced-sodium vegetable or chicken broth (GF, if needed) | 500 mL |
| 1 tbsp | olive oil | 15 mL |
| 1 | red bell pepper, thinly sliced | 1 |
| 8 cups | packed baby spinach (about 6 oz/175 g) | 2 L |
| 1 lb | cooked deveined peeled medium shrimp, thawed if frozen | 500 g |
| 1 cup | crumbled feta cheese | 250 mL |
| ½ cup | golden raisins | 125 mL |
| ¼ cup | toasted pine nuts | 60 mL |

1. In a medium saucepan, combine quinoa and broth. Bring to a boil over medium-high heat. Reduce heat to low, cover and simmer for 12 to 15 minutes or until liquid is absorbed. Remove from heat and let stand, covered, for 5 minutes. Fluff with a fork.

2. Meanwhile, in a large nonstick skillet, heat oil over medium-high heat. Add red pepper and cook, stirring, for 1 minute. Add spinach and shrimp; cook, stirring, for about 2 minutes or until spinach is just wilted and shrimp are warmed through. Stir in quinoa, cheese and raisins. Serve sprinkled with pine nuts.

# Moroccan-Spiced Shrimp and Quinoa

**Makes 4 servings**

*Here, shrimp is emboldened with warm Moroccan spices, tart citrus and sweet currants.*

| | | |
|---|---|---|
| 2 tsp | olive oil | 10 mL |
| 1 | red bell pepper, chopped | 1 |
| 1¼ cups | chopped onions | 300 mL |
| 2 tsp | ground cumin | 10 mL |
| 1 tsp | ground cinnamon | 5 mL |
| ⅛ tsp | cayenne pepper | 0.5 mL |
| 1 | can (28 oz/796 mL) whole tomatoes, drained and roughly chopped | 1 |
| ¼ cup | dried currants or chopped raisins | 60 mL |
| 1 lb | large shrimp, peeled and deveined | 500 g |
| 2 tbsp | freshly squeezed lemon juice | 30 mL |
| | Fine sea salt and freshly cracked black pepper | |
| 3 cups | hot cooked quinoa (see page 10) | 750 mL |
| ½ cup | packed fresh cilantro or flat-leaf (Italian) parsley leaves, chopped | 125 mL |

1. In a large, deep skillet, heat oil over medium-high heat. Add red pepper and onions; cook, stirring, for 6 to 8 minutes or until softened. Add cumin, cinnamon and cayenne; cook, stirring, for 30 seconds.

2. Stir in tomatoes and currants; bring to a boil. Add shrimp, reduce heat and simmer, stirring occasionally, for 2 to 3 minutes or until shrimp are pink, firm and opaque. Stir in lemon juice. Season to taste with salt and black pepper.

3. Divide quinoa among four shallow bowls and top with shrimp mixture. Sprinkle with cilantro.

# Shrimp Fried Quinoa

*A simple tamari sauce
shows off both the quinoa
and the briny shrimp in
this quinoa interpretation
of fried rice.*

| | | |
|---|---|---|
| 3 tbsp | tamari or soy sauce (GF, if needed) | 45 mL |
| 5 tsp | unseasoned rice vinegar | 25 mL |
| 1 tbsp | toasted sesame oil | 15 mL |
| 2 tsp | brown rice syrup or liquid honey | 10 mL |
| 2 tbsp | vegetable oil | 30 mL |
| 12 oz | medium shrimp, peeled and deveined | 375 g |
| 1 cup | sliced mushrooms | 250 mL |
| ¾ cup | diced carrots | 175 mL |
| ½ cup | frozen petite peas | 125 mL |
| 3 cups | thinly sliced bok choy (both green and white portions) | 750 mL |
| 2 | large eggs, lightly beaten | 2 |
| 3 cups | cooked quinoa (see page 10), chilled | 750 mL |
| 1 cup | chopped green onions | 250 mL |
| | Fine sea salt and freshly ground black pepper | |

1. In a small bowl, whisk together tamari, vinegar, sesame oil and brown rice syrup.

2. In a large, deep skillet, heat vegetable oil over medium-high heat. Add shrimp and cook, stirring, for 1 minute. Add mushrooms, carrots, peas and bok choy; cook, stirring, for 2 to 3 minutes or until just tender. Add eggs and scramble just until set. Stir in quinoa, green onions and tamari mixture; cook, stirring, for 1 to 2 minutes or until quinoa is heated through and shrimp are firm, pink and opaque. Season to taste with salt and pepper.

# Sesame Shrimp and Asparagus Quinoa

*You're going to love this stir-fry, with its salty-sweet shrimp, crisp vegetables and accompanying sesame quinoa — so much so, you may swear off takeout.*

## Tip

To toast sesame seeds, place up to 3 tbsp (45 mL) seeds in a medium skillet set over medium heat. Cook, shaking the skillet, for 3 to 5 minutes or until seeds are golden brown and fragrant. Let cool completely before use.

| | | |
|---|---|---|
| 1 cup | quinoa, rinsed | 250 mL |
| 2¼ cups | ready-to-use reduced-sodium vegetable or chicken broth (GF, if needed), divided | 550 mL |
| 1 tbsp | toasted sesame seeds (see tip, at left) | 15 mL |
| 2 tbsp | toasted sesame oil, divided | 30 mL |
| 2 | cloves garlic, minced | 2 |
| 1½ tsp | ground ginger | 7 mL |
| ½ tsp | cornstarch | 2 mL |
| 3 tbsp | mirin or sherry | 45 mL |
| 3 tbsp | tamari or soy sauce (GF, if needed) | 45 mL |
| 2 tbsp | brown rice syrup or liquid honey | 30 mL |
| 1 | small red bell pepper, cut into 1-inch (2.5 cm) pieces | 1 |
| 12 oz | asparagus, trimmed and cut into 1-inch (2.5 cm) pieces | 375 g |
| ¼ tsp | hot pepper flakes | 1 mL |
| 6 | green onions, trimmed and cut into 1-inch (2.5 cm) pieces | 6 |
| 1 lb | medium-large shrimp, peeled and deveined | 500 g |
| | Fine sea salt and freshly cracked black pepper | |

1. In a medium saucepan, combine quinoa and 2 cups (500 mL) of the broth. Bring to a boil over medium-high heat. Reduce heat to low, cover and simmer for 12 to 15 minutes or until liquid is absorbed. Let stand, covered, for 5 minutes. Fluff with a fork, then gently stir in sesame seeds and 2 tsp (10 mL) of the oil.

2. Meanwhile, in a small bowl, whisk together garlic, ginger, cornstarch, mirin, tamari, brown rice syrup and the remaining oil.

3. In a large, deep skillet, heat garlic mixture over medium-high heat. Add red pepper, asparagus and hot pepper flakes; cook, stirring, for 2 minutes or until vegetables are slightly softened. Add green onions, shrimp and the remaining broth; cook, stirring, for 2 to 3 minutes or until shrimp are pink, firm and opaque. Season to taste with salt and black pepper. Serve immediately, with sesame quinoa.

# One-Pan Shrimp and Quinoa Pilau

*This riff on traditional
Indian pilaf gets multiple
layers of texture (shrimp,
peas, peppers and quinoa)
and flavor (curry powder,
lime and cilantro)
without any fussy steps
or ingredients. Serve with
yogurt and/or mango
chutney, as desired.*

| | | |
|---|---|---|
| 2 tsp | vegetable oil | 10 mL |
| 1 | small red bell pepper, chopped | 1 |
| 1 cup | chopped onion | 250 mL |
| 1¼ cups | quinoa, rinsed | 300 mL |
| 1½ tbsp | mild curry powder | 22 mL |
| 1 tsp | ground cumin | 5 mL |
| 2½ cups | ready-to-use reduced-sodium chicken or vegetable broth (GF, if needed) | 625 mL |
| 12 oz | medium shrimp, peeled and deveined | 375 g |
| 1 cup | frozen petite peas | 250 mL |
| ¾ cup | packed fresh cilantro leaves, chopped | 175 mL |
| 2 tbsp | freshly squeezed lime juice | 30 mL |
| | Fine sea salt and freshly cracked black pepper | |

1. In a large, deep skillet, heat oil over medium-high heat. Add red pepper and onion; cook, stirring, for 6 to 8 minutes or until softened. Add quinoa, curry powder and cumin; cook, stirring, for 1 minute.
2. Stir in broth and bring to a boil. Reduce heat to low, cover and simmer for 12 to 15 minutes or until liquid is absorbed. Remove from heat and stir in shrimp and peas; cover and let stand for 5 minutes or until shrimp are pink, firm and opaque. Fluff quinoa with a fork, then gently stir in cilantro and lime juice. Season to taste with salt and pepper.

# Quinoa Paella with Shrimp and Chicken Sausage

*Paella aficionados will flip for this faster (and even healthier) rendition, seasoned with smoked paprika and oregano. The quinoa is an innovation, replacing the traditional rice, but the shrimp and sausage are mainstays; peppers and peas are de rigueur extras.*

| | | |
|---|---|---|
| 2 tsp | olive oil | 10 mL |
| 1 | small red bell pepper, cut into 1/2-inch (1 cm) pieces | 1 |
| 1 cup | chopped onion | 250 mL |
| 3 | links cooked chicken sausages (about 10 oz/300 g total), diced | 3 |
| 2 | cloves garlic, minced | 2 |
| 1 tsp | sweet smoked paprika | 5 mL |
| 1 tsp | dried oregano | 5 mL |
| 1 cup | quinoa, rinsed | 250 mL |
| 2 cups | ready-to-use reduced-sodium chicken or vegetable broth (GF, if needed) | 500 mL |
| 12 oz | medium shrimp, peeled and deveined | 375 g |
| 3/4 cup | frozen petite peas | 175 mL |
| 1/2 cup | packed fresh flat-leaf (Italian) parsley leaves, chopped | 125 mL |
| 1 tbsp | sherry vinegar or white wine vinegar | 15 mL |
| | Fine sea salt and freshly cracked black pepper | |

1. In a large, deep skillet, heat oil over medium-high heat. Add red pepper and onion; cook, stirring, for 6 to 8 minutes or until softened. Add sausages, garlic, paprika and oregano; cook, stirring, for 2 minutes.

2. Stir in quinoa and broth; bring to a boil. Reduce heat to low, cover and simmer for 12 to 15 minutes or until liquid is absorbed. Remove from heat and stir in shrimp and peas; cover and let stand for 5 minutes or until shrimp are pink, firm and opaque. Fluff quinoa with a fork, then gently stir in parsley and vinegar. Season to taste with salt and pepper.

# Balsamic-Glazed Chicken over Quinoa

*Here, red onions move
from the bench to the
starting lineup, joining
roasted chicken for a
dinner with great style.*

- **Preheat oven to 500°F (260°C)**
- **Large rimmed baking sheet, lined with foil and sprayed with nonstick cooking spray (preferably olive oil)**

| | | |
|---|---|---|
| 1½ lbs | red onions, cut into narrow wedges | 750 g |
| 2 tsp | olive oil | 10 mL |
| | Fine sea salt and freshly cracked black pepper | |
| 1½ tbsp | unsalted butter | 22 mL |
| 2 tbsp | liquid honey or pure maple syrup | 30 mL |
| ¼ cup | balsamic vinegar | 60 mL |
| 2 cups | diced or shredded roasted chicken or turkey breast | 500 mL |
| 3 cups | hot cooked quinoa (see page 10) | 750 mL |
| 2 tbsp | chopped fresh flat-leaf (Italian) parsley | 30 mL |

1. In a large bowl, combine red onions and oil, tossing to coat. Sprinkle with salt and pepper. Spread in a single layer on prepared baking sheet. Roast in preheated oven for 40 to 45 minutes, turning two or three times, until onions are browned and tender.

2. In a large, deep skillet, melt butter over medium-high heat. Stir in honey. Remove pan from heat and stir in vinegar. Return to medium heat and bring to a simmer. Add roasted onions and chicken; simmer for 1 to 2 minutes or until warmed through. Season to taste with salt and pepper.

3. Divide quinoa among four shallow bowls and top with chicken mixture. Sprinkle with parsley.

# Mediterranean Quinoa-Stuffed Chicken Breasts

<table>
<tr><td>Makes<br>4 servings</td></tr>
</table>

*The strength of everyday Mediterranean cooking depends largely on a combination of familiar, soulful flavors that culinary fashion can rarely improve. With the exception of quinoa in the filling, these stuffed chicken breasts are a perfect illustration.*

## Tip

Make sure to use fine sea salt in the water you use to cook the quinoa. Conventional table salt contains chemicals and additives, whereas sea salt contains an abundance of naturally occurring trace minerals.

• **Large ovenproof skillet**

| | | |
|---|---|---|
| ¼ cup | white, red or black quinoa, rinsed | 60 mL |
| 2 | cloves garlic, minced | 2 |
| 2 tbsp | chopped fresh flat-leaf (Italian) parsley | 30 mL |
| 1 tsp | dried oregano | 5 mL |
| 3 tbsp | chopped drained oil-packed sun-dried tomatoes | 45 mL |
| 2 tbsp | chopped pitted brine-cured black olives (such as kalamata) | 30 mL |
| 2 tbsp | crumbled feta cheese | 30 mL |
| 2 tbsp | olive oil, divided | 30 mL |
| | Fine sea salt and freshly cracked black pepper | |
| 4 | boneless skinless chicken breasts (each about 6 oz/175 g) | 4 |

1. In a small saucepan of boiling salted water, cook quinoa for 9 minutes. Drain and rinse under cold water until cool. Transfer to a medium bowl and add garlic, parsley, oregano, tomatoes, olives, feta and half the oil, gently stirring to combine. Season to taste with salt and pepper.

2. Preheat oven to 400°F (200°C).

3. Place a chicken breast between two sheets of plastic wrap. Using a kitchen mallet or rolling pin, pound to ¼-inch (0.5 cm) thickness. Repeat with the remaining breasts.

4. Spread quinoa mixture over chicken breasts, dividing evenly. Starting at a long side, roll up like a jelly roll and secure with toothpicks. Sprinkle chicken with salt and pepper.

5. In ovenproof skillet, heat the remaining oil over medium-high heat. Add chicken and cook for 5 to 6 minutes or until browned on the bottom. Turn chicken over (browned side up). Place skillet in oven and bake for 4 to 6 minutes or until chicken is no longer pink inside.

# Almond and Quinoa Chicken Fingers

*Picky children and grown-up gourmets alike will love these chicken fingers. A quick buttermilk brine is the secret to keeping the chicken moist and tender. Don't be alarmed by the amount of salt — it allows you to brine the chicken quickly. Just enough of the salt penetrates the chicken, seasoning it to perfection.*

- **Preheat oven to 350°F (180°C)**
- **Food processor**
- **Large rimmed baking sheet, lined with foil, wire rack set on top**

| | | |
|---|---|---|
| 2 tbsp | coarse sea salt | 30 mL |
| ½ tsp | freshly cracked black pepper | 2 mL |
| 2 cups | buttermilk | 500 mL |
| 1 tbsp | liquid honey | 15 mL |
| 1 tbsp | Dijon mustard | 15 mL |
| 1½ lbs | boneless skinless chicken breasts | 750 g |
| 1¼ cups | quinoa, rinsed | 300 mL |
| 1 cup | lightly salted roasted almonds | 250 mL |
| ¼ cup | freshly grated Parmesan cheese | 60 mL |
| 2 | large eggs | 2 |
| | Nonstick cooking spray (preferably olive oil) | |

1. In a medium non-reactive bowl, whisk together salt, pepper, buttermilk, honey and mustard.
2. Place a chicken breast between two sheets of plastic wrap. Using a kitchen mallet or rolling pin, pound to ¼-inch (0.5 cm) thickness. Repeat with the remaining breasts. Transfer to buttermilk mixture and let stand at room temperature for 30 minutes.
3. Meanwhile, in food processor, combine quinoa and almonds; pulse until finely ground. Transfer to a shallow dish and stir in cheese. In another shallow dish, beat eggs.
4. Remove chicken from buttermilk mixture, shaking off excess, and cut chicken into 3- by ¾-inch (7.5 by 2 cm) wide strips. Dip chicken strips in egg, shaking off excess, then in quinoa mixture, pressing to adhere and shaking off excess. Place on rack on prepared baking sheet and lightly spray with cooking spray. Discard any excess quinoa mixture and egg.
5. Bake in preheated oven for 18 to 22 minutes, turning once halfway through, until coating is golden brown and chicken is no longer pink inside.

# Chicken Quinoa with Chard and Apricots

*A shot of vinegar enlivens the grassy flavor of the chard and quinoa and the concentrated sweetness of dried apricots — a perfect complement to simple chicken breasts. Serve garnished with plain Greek yogurt and/or toasted pine nuts or sliced almonds, as desired.*

| | | |
|---|---|---|
| 1 | large bunch Swiss chard (any variety) | 1 |
| 1 lb | boneless skinless chicken breasts, cut into bite-size pieces | 500 g |
| | Fine sea salt and freshly cracked black pepper | |
| 2 tsp | olive oil | 10 mL |
| 2 | cloves garlic, minced | 2 |
| 1 cup | quinoa, rinsed | 250 mL |
| 1 tsp | ground coriander | 5 mL |
| 2 cups | ready-to-use reduced-sodium chicken or vegetable broth (GF, if needed) | 500 mL |
| ¾ cup | chopped dried apricots | 175 mL |
| 2 tsp | white wine vinegar or sherry vinegar | 10 mL |

1. Trim off tough stems from Swiss chard and discard. Trim tender stems and ribs from leaves and chop stems and ribs. Thinly slice leaves crosswise (to measure about 5 cups/1.25 L). Set chopped stems and sliced leaves aside separately.

2. Sprinkle chicken with salt and pepper. In a large, deep skillet, heat oil over medium-high heat. Add chicken and cook, stirring often, for 4 to 5 minutes or until browned on all sides and no longer pink inside. Using a slotted spoon, transfer chicken to a plate.

3. In the same skillet, combine garlic, quinoa, coriander and broth; bring to a boil over medium-high heat. Stir in apricots and Swiss chard stems; reduce heat to low, cover and simmer for 10 minutes.

4. Return chicken and any accumulated juices to the pan, along with Swiss chard leaves. Simmer, uncovered, stirring occasionally, for 2 to 5 minutes or until liquid is absorbed. Remove from heat, sprinkle with vinegar, cover and let stand for 5 minutes. Fluff with a fork, then season to taste with salt and pepper.

# Chicken, Vegetable and Quinoa Limone

*Quinoa adds a stick-to-the ribs earthiness to this chicken dish, while lemon, peas, mushrooms and asparagus render it just right for spring.*

## Tip

When selecting mushrooms, choose those with a fresh, smooth appearance, free from major blemishes and with a dry surface. Once home, keep mushrooms refrigerated; they're best when used within a few days after purchase. When ready to use, gently wipe mushrooms with a damp cloth or soft brush to remove dirt particles. Alternatively, rinse mushrooms quickly with cold water, then immediately pat dry with paper towels.

| | | |
|---|---|---:|
| 1 tbsp | olive oil | 15 mL |
| 1 cup | finely chopped onion | 250 mL |
| 8 oz | cremini or button mushrooms, sliced | 250 g |
| 1 cup | quinoa, rinsed | 250 mL |
| 2 tsp | dried thyme | 10 mL |
| 2 tsp | finely grated lemon zest | 10 mL |
| 2 cups | ready-to-use reduced-sodium chicken or vegetable broth (GF, if needed) | 500 mL |
| 1 lb | asparagus, trimmed and cut into $\frac{1}{2}$-inch (1 cm) pieces | 500 g |
| 2 cups | diced cooked chicken breast | 500 mL |
| $\frac{2}{3}$ cup | frozen petite peas, thawed | 150 mL |
| 1 tbsp | freshly squeezed lemon juice | 15 mL |
| $\frac{1}{4}$ cup | packed fresh mint leaves, chopped | 60 mL |
| | Fine sea salt and freshly cracked black pepper | |

1. In a large, deep skillet, heat oil over medium heat. Add onion and cook, stirring, for 1 minute. Add mushrooms and cook, stirring, for 5 to 6 minutes or until softened.

2. Stir in quinoa, thyme, lemon zest and broth; bring to a boil. Reduce heat to low, cover and simmer for 10 minutes. Stir in asparagus, cover and simmer for 4 to 5 minutes or until liquid is absorbed and quinoa and asparagus are tender. Remove from heat and stir in chicken, peas and lemon juice. Cover and let stand for 2 minutes to warm through. Stir in mint. Season to taste with salt and pepper.

## Variation

An equal amount of fresh parsley or cilantro leaves may be used in place of the mint.

# Chicken and Quinoa Biryani

*The preparation for
this version of chicken
biryani — a favorite
Punjabi chicken dish from
northern India — may
not be strictly traditional,
but the resulting flavor
is. Raisins are a key
ingredient, offsetting the
spice and heat of the dish
with a delicate sweetness.*

## Tip

An equal amount of fresh
mint can be used in place
of the cilantro.

| | | |
|---|---|---|
| 2 tsp | vegetable oil | 10 mL |
| 1 cup | chopped onion | 250 mL |
| 3 | cloves garlic, minced | 3 |
| 2 tbsp | minced gingerroot | 30 mL |
| 2 tsp | garam masala | 10 mL |
| 2 tsp | ground cumin | 10 mL |
| ¾ tsp | fine sea salt | 3 mL |
| ⅛ tsp | cayenne pepper | 0.5 mL |
| 1 lb | boneless skinless chicken breasts, cut into 1-inch (2.5 cm) cubes | 500 g |
| 1 | can (14 to 15 oz/398 to 425 mL) diced tomatoes, with juice | 1 |
| 1 cup | quinoa, rinsed | 250 mL |
| ⅓ cup | golden raisins | 75 mL |
| 1¾ cups | ready-to-use reduced-sodium chicken broth (GF, if needed) | 425 mL |
| ¼ cup | packed fresh cilantro leaves, chopped | 60 mL |
| 2 tbsp | freshly squeezed lime juice | 30 mL |
| ½ cup | chopped lightly salted roasted cashews or pistachios | 125 mL |

1. In a large, deep skillet, heat oil over medium-high heat. Add onion and cook, stirring, for 5 to 6 minutes or until softened. Add garlic, ginger, garam masala, cumin, salt and cayenne; cook, stirring, for 1 minute. Add chicken and cook, stirring, for 3 to 5 minutes or until browned on all sides.

2. Stir in tomatoes with juice, quinoa, raisins and broth; bring to a boil. Reduce heat to low, cover and simmer, stirring occasionally, for 12 to 15 minutes or until quinoa is tender and chicken is no longer pink inside. Stir in cilantro and lime juice. Serve sprinkled with cashews.

# Broccoli, Chicken and Quinoa Stir-Fry

*This wonderful variation on fried rice is tied together by the hoisin sauce, which adds savory sweetness and hints of five-spice seasoning.*

## Tip

Make sure the quinoa is well chilled before adding it to the stir-fry. This ensures that the grains do not clump together.

| | | |
|---|---|---:|
| 2 tbsp | toasted sesame oil, divided | 30 mL |
| 3 | cloves garlic, minced | 3 |
| 1 | red bell pepper, thinly sliced | 1 |
| 3 cups | small broccoli florets | 750 mL |
| ¾ cup | ready-to-use reduced-sodium chicken or vegetable broth (GF, if needed), divided | 175 mL |
| 1 lb | boneless skinless chicken breasts, cut into thin strips | 500 g |
| | Fine sea salt and freshly ground black pepper | |
| ½ cup | chopped green onions | 125 mL |
| 2 cups | cooked quinoa (see page 10), chilled | 500 mL |
| ⅓ cup | hoisin sauce (GF, if needed) | 75 mL |
| 2 tbsp | freshly squeezed lime juice | 30 mL |

1. In a large, deep skillet, heat half the oil over medium-high heat. Add garlic and cook, stirring, for 30 seconds. Add red pepper, broccoli and ¼ cup (60 mL) of the broth; cover and cook for about 3 minutes or until vegetables are tender-crisp. Transfer vegetable mixture to a bowl.
2. Sprinkle chicken with salt and pepper. In the same skillet, heat the remaining oil over medium-high heat. Add chicken and green onions; cook, stirring, for 3 to 4 minutes or until chicken is browned on all sides and no longer pink inside.
3. Return vegetable mixture to the pan, along with quinoa, hoisin sauce, lime juice and the remaining broth. Cook, stirring, for 2 minutes.

## Variation

Use pork tenderloin, cut into thin strips, in place of the chicken.

# Sausage Quinoa with Apples and Fennel

*Multiple textures and flavors — meaty sausages, nutty quinoa, crisp-sweet apples and faintly licorice fennel — add up to a sophisticated, yet comforting weeknight repast.*

| | | |
|---|---|---|
| 1 tbsp | olive oil, divided | 15 mL |
| 12 oz | cooked chicken sausages (about 5 links), thinly sliced | 375 g |
| 2 | tart-sweet apples (such as Braeburn or Gala), peeled and chopped | 2 |
| 2 cups | chopped fennel bulb (about 1 large bulb), fronds reserved | 500 mL |
| 2 | cloves garlic, minced | 2 |
| 1 cup | quinoa, rinsed | 250 mL |
| 2 cups | ready-to-use reduced-sodium chicken or vegetable broth (GF, if needed) | 500 mL |
| | Fine sea salt and freshly cracked black pepper | |
| ½ cup | chopped toasted pecans | 125 mL |

1. In a large, deep skillet, heat half the oil over medium-high heat. Add sausages and cook, stirring, for 3 to 4 minutes or until browned on both sides. Using a slotted spoon, transfer sausages to a plate.

2. In the same skillet, heat the remaining oil over medium-high heat. Add apples, fennel bulb and garlic; cook, stirring, for 5 to 6 minutes or until softened.

3. Stir in quinoa and broth; bring to a boil. Reduce heat to low, cover and simmer for 12 to 15 minutes or until liquid is absorbed. Remove from heat and return sausages and any accumulated juices to the pan. Cover and let stand for 5 minutes.

4. Meanwhile, chop enough of the reserved fennel fronds to measure 2 tbsp (30 mL). Fluff quinoa with a fork, then season to taste with salt and pepper. Serve sprinkled with fennel fronds and pecans.

# Broccoli Rabe and Sausage Quinoa

*The combination of robust sausage and fresh, faintly bittersweet broccoli rabe is tried and true. The warmth and comfort of the dish are further heightened by the addition of quinoa.*

## Tip

This technique produces a tender-crisp broccoli rabe. If you prefer a more tender texture, blanch the chopped broccoli rabe in a pot of boiling water for 2 minutes or until bright green, then drain and add to the skillet.

| | | |
|---|---|---|
| 1 lb | broccoli rabe | 500 g |
| 1 tbsp | olive oil | 15 mL |
| 12 oz | cooked chicken sausages (about 5 links), thinly sliced | 375 g |
| 3 | cloves garlic, thinly sliced | 3 |
| ½ tsp | hot pepper flakes | 2 mL |
| 2½ cups | hot cooked quinoa (see page 10) | 625 mL |
| ¼ cup | dried currants or raisins | 60 mL |
| 2 tsp | finely grated lemon zest | 10 mL |
| 2 tbsp | freshly squeezed lemon juice | 30 mL |

1. Cut broccoli rabe crosswise into 1-inch (2.5 cm) thick slices. Rinse well and drain, leaving water clinging to it.

2. In a large, deep skillet, heat oil over medium-high heat. Add sausages and cook, stirring, for 3 to 4 minutes or until browned on both sides. Using a slotted spoon, transfer sausages to a plate lined with paper towels.

3. In the same skillet, combine broccoli rabe, garlic and hot pepper flakes; cook over medium-high heat, stirring, for 6 to 10 minutes or until broccoli rabe is tender. Return sausages to the pan, along with quinoa, currants, lemon zest and lemon juice. Reduce heat to medium and cook, stirring, for 1 minute to blend the flavors.

# Cajun Dirty Quinoa

*Rice may be the belle
of the ball in New
Orleans, but quinoa
has an attraction all its
own. Here, it takes on
the signature flavors
of Cajun "dirty rice":
onion, bell pepper, spices
and sausage (albeit
lighter chicken sausage)
in quintessential Big
Easy style.*

| 1 cup | quinoa, rinsed | 250 mL |
| 1 | bay leaf | 1 |
| 2 cups | ready-to-use reduced-sodium chicken or vegetable broth (GF, if needed) | 500 mL |
| 1 tbsp | olive oil | 15 mL |
| 1 | green bell pepper, chopped | 1 |
| 1½ cups | chopped onions | 375 mL |
| ¾ cup | chopped celery | 175 mL |
| 12 oz | cooked chicken sausages (about 5 links), diced | 375 g |
| 1 tbsp | salt-free Cajun spice blend | 15 mL |
| | Fine sea salt and freshly cracked black pepper | |

1. In a medium saucepan, combine quinoa, bay leaf and broth. Bring to a boil over medium-high heat. Reduce heat to low, cover and simmer for 12 to 15 minutes or until liquid is absorbed. Remove from heat and let stand, covered, for 5 minutes. Discard bay leaf and fluff quinoa with a fork.

2. Meanwhile, in a large, deep skillet, heat oil over medium-high heat. Add green pepper, onions and celery; cook, stirring, for 6 to 8 minutes or until softened. Add sausages and Cajun spice blend; cook, stirring, for 2 minutes. Add quinoa and cook, stirring, for 1 minute to blend the flavors. Season to taste with salt and pepper.

# Turkey, Sun-Dried Tomato and Escarole Quinoa

*Turkey and sun-dried tomatoes make this quinoa dish deliciously robust. The bittersweet edge of escarole ties the dish together and eliminates the need to make a salad on the side.*

| | | |
|---|---|---|
| 2 tsp | olive oil | 10 mL |
| 2 cups | thinly sliced red onions | 500 mL |
| 8 cups | roughly chopped escarole (about 1 large head) | 2 L |
| 1½ cups | diced or shredded cooked turkey breast | 375 mL |
| 3 cups | hot cooked quinoa (see page 10) | 750 mL |
| ¼ cup | thinly sliced drained oil-packed sun-dried tomatoes | 60 mL |
| ¼ cup | dry white wine | 60 mL |
| | Fine sea salt and freshly cracked black pepper | |
| 3 tbsp | freshly grated Romano or Parmesan cheese | 45 mL |

1. In a large, deep skillet, heat oil over medium-high heat. Add red onions and cook, stirring, for 6 to 8 minutes or until softened. Add escarole and turkey; cook, stirring, for 2 minutes or until escarole is mostly wilted.
2. Stir in quinoa, sun-dried tomatoes and wine; cook, stirring, for 2 minutes. Season to taste with salt and pepper. Serve sprinkled with cheese.

## Variations

An equal amount of packed tender watercress sprigs or arugula may be used in place of the escarole.

Substitute diced or shredded cooked chicken breast for the turkey.

# Turkey Quinoa Sloppy Joes

*Tired of the same old sloppy Joes? My version has a healthy twist: quinoa and ground turkey. These may be the best sloppy Joes you've ever tasted.*

## Tip

Whenever possible, use whole-grain or multigrain hamburger buns.

| | | |
|---|---|---:|
| ½ cup | quinoa, rinsed | 125 mL |
| 1 tbsp | vegetable oil | 15 mL |
| 1 | small green bell pepper, chopped | 1 |
| 1½ cups | chopped onions | 375 mL |
| ½ cup | chopped celery | 125 mL |
| 2 | cloves garlic, minced | 2 |
| 12 oz | lean ground turkey | 375 g |
| 1 | can (15 oz/425 mL) tomato sauce | 1 |
| ¼ cup | ketchup | 60 mL |
| 1 tbsp | Worcestershire sauce | 15 mL |
| | Fine sea salt and freshly ground black pepper | |
| 6 | hamburger buns (GF, if needed), split and toasted | 6 |

1. In a medium saucepan of boiling salted water, cook quinoa for 9 minutes. Drain.
2. Meanwhile, in a large, deep skillet, heat oil over medium-high heat. Add green pepper, onions, celery and garlic; cook, stirring, for 6 to 8 minutes or until softened. Add turkey and cook, breaking it up with a spoon, for 3 to 5 minutes or until no longer pink.
3. Stir in quinoa, tomato sauce, ketchup and Worcestershire sauce; bring to a boil. Reduce heat and simmer for 6 to 8 minutes, stirring occasionally, until thickened. Season to taste with salt and pepper.
4. Top bottom halves of buns with turkey mixture, dividing evenly. Cover with top halves, pressing down gently.

## Variation

Substitute extra-lean ground beef or pork for the turkey.

# Curried Turkey Quinoa Wraps

*You may never eat an ordinary turkey sandwich again after you've tasted this extraordinary one. Curry loves contrasts of sweet (chutney, apricots) and fresh (lemon, mesclun), and roasted turkey is up for anything.*

## Tip

Whenever possible, use whole-grain or multigrain tortillas.

| | | |
|---|---|---|
| 1 tsp | mild curry powder | 5 mL |
| 1/3 cup | plain Greek yogurt | 75 mL |
| 1 tbsp | freshly squeezed lemon juice | 15 mL |
| | Fine sea salt and freshly cracked black pepper | |
| 2 | 8-inch (20 cm) quinoa tortillas or other GF tortillas (see tip, at left) | 2 |
| 2 cups | packed mesclun or baby spinach | 500 mL |
| 1 cup | chopped roasted turkey or chicken | 250 mL |
| 3/4 cup | cooked quinoa (see page 10), cooled | 175 mL |
| 1/4 cup | chopped dried apricots | 60 mL |

1. In a small bowl, whisk together curry powder, yogurt and lemon juice. Season to taste with salt and pepper.
2. Spread tortillas with yogurt mixture. Top with mesclun, turkey, quinoa and apricots, dividing evenly. Roll up like burritos, enclosing filling, or like jelly rolls (ends open).

## Variation

The ingredients in this recipe are very flexible. For example, other spices or dried herbs, such as ground cumin, dried thyme or ground coriander, may be used in place of the curry powder; other chopped cooked meats, such as ham or roast beef, may be used in place of the turkey; and other dried fruits, such as cranberries or golden raisins, may be used in place of the apricots.

# Chipotle Pork with Quinoa Sweet Potato Hash

*On cool autumn nights, smoky-spiced roasted pork with a quinoa-sweet potato hash alongside is about as comforting as food gets.*

## Tip

If you can't find chipotle chile powder, you can use an equal amount of hot smoked paprika.

- **Preheat oven to 400°F (200°C)**
- **Large ovenproof skillet**

| | | |
|---|---|---|
| 1 lb | pork tenderloin, trimmed | 500 g |
| | Fine sea salt | |
| 1¼ tsp | chipotle chile powder, divided | 6 mL |
| 4 tsp | olive oil, divided | 20 mL |
| 1 | sweet potato (about 8 oz/250 g), peeled and coarsely shredded | 1 |
| 1¼ cups | cooked quinoa (see page 10), cooled | 300 mL |
| 1 cup | chopped green onions | 250 mL |
| ¼ cup | dried cherries or cranberries, chopped | 60 mL |
| 1 tbsp | pure maple syrup | 15 mL |

1. Sprinkle pork with salt and 1 tsp (5 mL) of the chipotle chile powder. In ovenproof skillet, heat half the oil over medium-high heat. Add pork and cook, turning several times, for 3 to 4 minutes or until browned all over.

2. Transfer skillet to preheated oven and roast for 12 to 14 minutes or until an instant-read thermometer inserted in the thickest part of the tenderloin registers 145°F (63°C) for medium-rare, or until desired doneness. Let rest for at least 5 minutes before slicing.

3. Meanwhile, in a large, deep skillet, heat the remaining oil over medium-high heat. Add sweet potato and cook, stirring, for 6 minutes. Add quinoa, green onions and cherries; cook, stirring, for 2 to 4 minutes or until sweet potato is tender. Add maple syrup and the remaining chile powder; cook, stirring, for 1 minute to blend the flavors. Serve with pork.

# Cuban Pork and Beans with Cilantro Quinoa

*Here, classic Cuban
ingredients get a delicious
boost from nutty quinoa.
A last-minute addition of
fresh cilantro adds even
more flavor.*

| | | |
|---|---|---|
| 1 cup | quinoa, rinsed | 250 mL |
| 1 tsp | finely grated orange zest | 5 mL |
| 1¼ cups | orange juice, divided | 300 mL |
| 1 cup | ready-to-use reduced-sodium vegetable or chicken broth (GF, if needed) | 250 mL |
| 2 tsp | olive oil | 10 mL |
| 1 lb | pork tenderloin, trimmed and cut into 1-inch (2.5 cm) cubes | 500 g |
| 2½ tsp | ground cumin | 12 mL |
| 1½ tsp | dried oregano | 7 mL |
| 1 | can (14 to 19 oz/398 to 540 mL) black beans, drained and rinsed | 1 |
| 1 | can (14 to 15 oz/398 to 425 mL) chili-ready diced tomatoes, with juice | 1 |
| | Fine sea salt and freshly cracked black pepper | |
| ½ cup | packed fresh cilantro leaves, chopped | 125 mL |

1. In a medium saucepan, combine quinoa, orange zest, 1 cup (250 mL) of the orange juice and broth. Bring to a boil over medium-high heat. Reduce heat to low, cover and simmer for 12 to 15 minutes or until liquid is absorbed. Remove from heat and let stand, covered, for 5 minutes. Fluff with a fork.

2. Meanwhile, in a large skillet, heat oil over medium-high heat. Add pork, cumin and oregano; cook, stirring, for 4 minutes or until pork is browned on all sides.

3. Stir in beans, tomatoes with juice and the remaining orange juice; bring to a boil. Reduce heat and simmer, stirring occasionally, for 5 to 7 minutes or until sauce is slightly thickened and just a hint of pink remains inside pork. Season to taste with salt and pepper.

4. Just before serving, add cilantro to quinoa, gently stirring to combine. Divide quinoa among four shallow bowls and top with pork mixture.

# Pork Spiedini with Emerald Quinoa

*Your subconscious will register "summer" when you taste this Italian-inspired trio of rosemary-seasoned grilled pork, delicately sweet summer squash and a lemony, grassy, gloriously green quinoa.*

## Tip

If you prefer, an equal amount of boneless skinless chicken breasts can be used in place of the pork.

- **Preheat barbecue grill to medium-high**
- **Blender or food processor**
- **Six 10-inch (25 cm) metal skewers, or wooden skewers soaked in warm water for 30 minutes**

### Emerald Quinoa

| | | |
|---|---|---|
| 1 | clove garlic | 1 |
| 1½ cups | packed fresh flat-leaf (Italian) parsley leaves | 375 mL |
| 2 tbsp | drained capers | 30 mL |
| 1 tsp | finely grated lemon zest | 5 mL |
| 2 tbsp | freshly squeezed lemon juice | 30 mL |
| 2 tbsp | water | 30 mL |
| 2 tbsp | extra virgin olive oil | 30 mL |
| 3 cups | hot cooked quinoa (see page 10) | 750 mL |

### Spiedini

| | | |
|---|---|---|
| 2 tsp | chopped fresh rosemary | 10 mL |
| ½ tsp | fine sea salt | 2 mL |
| ¼ tsp | freshly ground black pepper | 1 mL |
| 1 tbsp | extra virgin olive oil | 15 mL |
| 1 tsp | red wine vinegar | 5 mL |
| 1 lb | pork tenderloin, trimmed and cut into 1-inch (2.5 cm) cubes | 500 g |
| 4 | small summer squash (such as zucchini or yellow crookneck), cut crosswise into 1-inch (2.5 cm) slices | 4 |

1. *Quinoa:* In blender, combine garlic, parsley, capers, lemon zest, lemon juice, water and oil; purée until smooth. Transfer to a large bowl and stir in quinoa; cover and keep warm.

2. *Spiedini:* In a small bowl, whisk together rosemary, salt, pepper, oil and vinegar. Thread pork and squash onto skewers. Generously brush with vinaigrette. Grill on preheated barbecue for 3 to 5 minutes per side or until just a hint of pink remains inside pork. Serve with quinoa mixture.

# Bulgogi Pork with Quinoa Kimchi Slaw

*Often called Korean barbecue in North America,* bulgogi *translates as "fire meat," a reference to the way the meat is grilled over hot coals or an open fire. Beef is the typical meat of choice for bulgogi, but in this rendition I use the distinctive marinade — tamari, sesame oil, fruit juice and ginger — on pork because it requires far less marinating time. A quinoa coleslaw riff on kimchi makes a fantastic and refreshing side dish.*

## Tip

Choose unseasoned rice vinegar over seasoned rice vinegar; the latter has added sugar and salt.

### Kimchi Slaw

| | | |
|---|---|---|
| 3 tbsp | unseasoned rice vinegar | 45 mL |
| 2 tbsp | tamari or soy sauce (GF, if needed) | 30 mL |
| 1 tbsp | Asian chili-garlic sauce | 15 mL |
| 2 tsp | sesame oil | 10 mL |
| 2 cups | shredded purple cabbage | 500 mL |
| 1½ cups | cooked quinoa (see page 10), cooled | 375 mL |
| ½ cup | shredded carrot | 125 mL |
| ½ cup | chopped green onions | 125 mL |

### Sesame Soy Pork

| | | |
|---|---|---|
| 1 tbsp | natural cane sugar or packed brown sugar | 15 mL |
| 2 tsp | ground ginger | 10 mL |
| ¼ cup | tamari or soy sauce (GF, if needed) | 60 mL |
| ¼ cup | unsweetened apple juice | 60 mL |
| 2 tbsp | Asian chili-garlic sauce | 30 mL |
| 2 tbsp | sesame oil | 30 mL |
| 1 lb | pork tenderloin, trimmed and cut crosswise into very thin slices | 500 g |
| 2 tbsp | toasted sesame seeds (optional) | 30 mL |

1. *Slaw:* In a large bowl, whisk together vinegar, tamari, chili-garlic sauce and oil. Add cabbage, quinoa, carrot and green onions, gently tossing to combine. Cover and refrigerate until ready to serve.

2. *Pork:* In a medium bowl, whisk together sugar, ginger, tamari, apple juice, chili-garlic sauce and oil. Add pork and toss to coat. Cover and refrigerate for 15 minutes.

3. Remove half the pork slices from marinade, shaking off excess. In a large, deep skillet, cook pork over medium-high heat, stirring, for 2 to 4 minutes or until browned on all sides and just a hint of pink remains inside. Transfer to a plate. Repeat with the remaining pork, discarding marinade. Return all pork to skillet and cook, stirring, until heated through.

4. Serve pork with slaw. Garnish with sesame seeds, if desired.

# Hoisin Pork and Quinoa Lettuce Wraps

*Sturdy, mild butter lettuce leaves provide the wrapping for a flavorful mix of spicy hoisin pork, crisp fresh vegetables and delicate quinoa. Elegance comes easily with these wraps.*

## Tip

To save time, you can use precut matchstick carrots in place of the coarsely shredded carrots.

| | | |
|---|---|---|
| 2 tsp | vegetable oil | 10 mL |
| 1 lb | extra-lean ground pork | 500 g |
| 5 | cloves garlic, minced | 5 |
| 2 tbsp | minced gingerroot | 30 mL |
| 1/4 cup | hoisin sauce (GF, if needed) | 60 mL |
| 1/4 cup | water | 60 mL |
| 12 | butter lettuce leaves | 12 |
| 1 1/2 cups | cooked quinoa (see page 10), cooled | 375 mL |
| 1 cup | coarsely shredded carrots | 250 mL |
| 1 cup | bean sprouts | 250 mL |
| 1/2 cup | packed fresh mint or cilantro leaves | 125 mL |

1. In a large, deep skillet, heat oil over medium-high heat. Add pork and cook, breaking it up with a spoon, for 5 to 6 minutes or until no longer pink. Add garlic and ginger; cook, stirring, for 30 seconds.

2. Stir in hoisin sauce and water; reduce heat and simmer, stirring occasionally, for 6 to 8 minutes or until thickened.

3. Place lettuce leaves on a work surface, underside of leaves facing up. Spoon quinoa down the center of each leaf, then top with pork mixture, carrots, bean sprouts and mint. Tuck in ends, then tightly roll leaf around filling.

# Ham, Quinoa and Edamame Succotash

**Makes 4 servings**

*Edamame abandons its Asian roots in this fresh, pretty main dish, to delicious effect.*

## Tip

An equal amount of thawed frozen baby lima beans may be used in place of the edamame.

| | | |
|---|---|---|
| ¾ cup | white or black quinoa, rinsed | 175 mL |
| 2 cups | ready-to-use reduced-sodium vegetable or chicken broth (GF, if needed), divided | 500 mL |
| 2 tsp | vegetable oil | 10 mL |
| 1¼ cups | fresh or thawed frozen corn kernels | 300 mL |
| 1 cup | frozen shelled edamame | 250 mL |
| ½ cup | chopped red bell pepper | 125 mL |
| ½ cup | chopped green onions, white and green parts separated | 125 mL |
| 1½ tsp | dried thyme | 7 mL |
| 1⅓ cups | diced cooked lean ham | 325 mL |
| 1 tbsp | freshly squeezed lemon juice | 15 mL |
| | Fine sea salt and freshly cracked black pepper | |

1. In a medium saucepan, combine quinoa and 1½ cups (375 mL) of the broth. Bring to a boil over medium-high heat. Reduce heat to low, cover and simmer for 12 to 15 minutes or until liquid is absorbed. Remove from heat and let stand, covered, for 5 minutes. Fluff with a fork.

2. Meanwhile, in a large, deep skillet, heat oil over medium heat. Add corn, edamame, red pepper, white part of green onions and thyme; cook, stirring, for 3 minutes. Add the remaining broth, cover, leaving lid ajar, and boil gently for 7 to 10 minutes or until edamame is tender. Stir in quinoa, ham, green part of green onions and lemon juice. Season to taste with salt and pepper.

# Ham, Goat Cheese and Quinoa Casserole

*The tried and true casserole moves up in the world when made with quinoa, a smattering of salty ham and sweet apricots, and a sprinkle of goat cheese. You'll return to this recipe again and again, as it can be assembled in advance and delivers serious flavor.*

## Tip

The casserole can be assembled through step 2 up to 24 hours in advance. Cover and refrigerate until ready to bake. Increase the baking time to 20 to 30 minutes.

- **Preheat oven to 400°F (200°C)**
- **8-cup (2 L) glass baking dish, sprayed with nonstick cooking spray**

| | | |
|---|---|---|
| 1¼ cups | quinoa, rinsed | 300 mL |
| 1½ tsp | dried thyme | 7 mL |
| 3 cups | ready-to-use reduced-sodium vegetable or chicken broth (GF, if needed) | 750 mL |
| 6 oz | mild soft goat cheese, crumbled (about 1½ cups/375 mL), divided | 175 g |
| 1½ cups | diced lean cooked ham | 375 mL |
| 1 cup | thinly sliced green onions | 250 mL |
| ½ cup | chopped dried apricots | 125 mL |

1. In a medium saucepan, combine quinoa, thyme and broth. Bring to a boil over medium-high heat. Reduce heat to low, cover and simmer for 10 minutes (broth will not be entirely absorbed). Remove from heat and stir in half the cheese, ham, green onions and apricots.

2. Spread quinoa mixture in prepared baking dish. Sprinkle with the remaining cheese.

3. Bake in preheated oven for 14 to 18 minutes or until top is golden brown. Let cool for 10 minutes before serving.

## Variation

The ingredients for this casserole are quite flexible. Swap other soft, creamy cheeses for the goat cheese, other cooked meats (or beans, lentils or canned tuna) for the ham, and other dried fruits for the apricots.

# Prosciutto and Collard Green Quinoa

**Makes
4 servings**

*Slicing collard greens into
super-thin strips allows
them to cook quickly
while maintaining a bit
of crunch and a glorious
emerald hue. Salty-sweet
prosciutto complements
the greens' grassy flavor.*

| | | |
|---|---|---|
| 1 lb | collard greens | 500 g |
| 1 tbsp | sherry vinegar or white wine vinegar | 15 mL |
| 1 tbsp | liquid honey | 15 mL |
| 1 tbsp | olive oil | 15 mL |
| 3 oz | thinly sliced prosciutto, chopped | 90 g |
| 4 | cloves garlic, minced | 4 |
| 1/4 tsp | hot pepper flakes | 0.5 mL |
| 3 cups | hot cooked quinoa (see page 10) | 750 mL |
| | Fine sea salt | |

1. Stack half the collard greens. Using a very sharp knife, cut away the stems and tough portion of center ribs. Repeat with the remaining collard greens. Discard stems and ribs. Rinse and spin-dry leaves.

2. Stack half the collard leaves and roll them up crosswise into a tight cylinder. Cut the cylinder crosswise into 1/4-inch (0.5 cm) thick slices. Repeat with the remaining leaves. Toss the collard ribbons to uncoil them. Set aside.

3. In a small bowl, whisk together vinegar and honey.

4. In a large skillet, heat oil over medium-high heat. Add prosciutto and cook, stirring, for 2 to 3 minutes or until crisp. Add collard ribbons, garlic and hot pepper flakes; cook, tossing, for about 1 minute or until collard ribbons are coated with oil and just wilted. Add quinoa and cook, tossing, for about 1 minute to blend the flavors. Season to taste with salt. Serve drizzled with vinegar mixture.

# Spicy Kale Quinoa with Pan-Fried Salami

*Spicy salami and red onions add memorable flavors to this hearty kale dish, and quinoa lends both flavor and substance. As a whole, it illustrates that if you start with fresh ingredients, it takes minimal work to produce a stellar meal.*

## Tip

Unlike other greens, kale stems are so tough they are virtually inedible. Hence, they, along with the tougher part of the center rib, must be removed before cooking. To do so, lay a leaf upside down on a cutting board and use a paring knife to cut a V shape along both sides of the rib, cutting it and the stem free from the leaf.

| | | |
|---|---|---|
| 1 lb | kale, tough stems and center ribs removed, leaves very thinly sliced crosswise (about 8 cups/2 L) | 500 g |
| 1½ tbsp | olive oil | 22 mL |
| 4 oz | spicy or regular salami, cut into ¼-inch (0.5 cm) dice | 125 g |
| 2 cups | thinly sliced red onions | 500 mL |
| 2 | cloves garlic, minced | 2 |
| ¼ tsp | hot pepper flakes | 1 mL |
| 3 cups | hot cooked quinoa (see page 10) | 750 mL |
| 2 tsp | sherry vinegar or white wine vinegar | 10 mL |
| | Fine sea salt and freshly cracked black pepper | |

1. In a large pot of boiling salted water, cook kale for about 10 minutes or until just tender. Drain, reserving ¼ cup (60 mL) cooking water.

2. Meanwhile, in a large, deep skillet, heat oil over medium-high heat. Add salami and cook, stirring, for about 5 minutes or until crisp. Using a slotted spoon, transfer salami to a plate.

3. In the same skillet, cook red onions, stirring, for 6 to 8 minutes or until softened. Add garlic and hot pepper flakes; cook, stirring, for 1 minute. Add kale, quinoa and the reserved cooking water; reduce heat to medium and cook, stirring, for 2 minutes or until heated through. Remove from heat and stir in salami and vinegar. Season to taste with salt and black pepper.

# Bacon, Brussels Sprouts and Blue Cheese Quinoa

*When the warm days of summer are waning, welcome fall with this terrific weeknight dish. Bacon and blue cheese flatter quinoa and Brussels sprouts alike.*

## Tip

The Brussels sprouts can be sliced with a kitchen knife, a mandoline or a food processor fitted with a slicing disk.

| | | |
|---|---|---|
| 2 | slices bacon, chopped | 2 |
| 2 | cloves garlic, minced | 2 |
| 12 oz | Brussels sprouts, trimmed and very thinly sliced crosswise | 375 g |
| ½ tsp | fine sea salt | 2 mL |
| ¼ tsp | freshly cracked black pepper | 1 mL |
| 3 cups | hot cooked quinoa (see page 10) | 750 mL |
| 2 tsp | finely grated lemon zest | 10 mL |
| 2 tbsp | freshly squeezed lemon juice | 30 mL |
| ½ cup | crumbled blue cheese | 125 mL |
| ¼ cup | finely chopped toasted walnuts | 60 mL |

1. In a large, deep skillet, cook bacon over medium-high heat, stirring, until crisp. Using a slotted spoon, transfer bacon to a plate lined with paper towels. Drain off all but 2 tsp (10 mL) fat from the pan.

2. Add garlic to the fat remaining in the skillet and cook, stirring, for 30 seconds. Add Brussels sprouts, salt and pepper; cook, stirring, for 3 to 4 minutes or until sprouts are tender and lightly browned. Stir in quinoa, lemon zest and lemon juice; cook, tossing, for 1 minute. Serve sprinkled with bacon, blue cheese and walnuts.

# Sausage and Cherry Tomato Quinoa

*This gorgeous dinner delivers a lot of satisfaction for very little work.*

| 12 oz | Italian pork or turkey sausage (bulk or casings removed) | 375 g |
|---|---|---|
| 2 tsp | olive oil | 10 mL |
| 2 cups | cherry or grape tomatoes | 500 mL |
| 2½ cups | hot cooked quinoa (see page 10) | 625 mL |
| ¼ cup | dry white wine | 60 mL |
| | Fine sea salt and freshly cracked black pepper | |
| ⅓ cup | freshly grated Parmesan cheese | 75 mL |
| 2 tbsp | finely chopped fresh flat-leaf (Italian) parsley | 30 mL |

1. In a large, deep skillet, cook sausage over medium-high heat, breaking it up with a spoon, for 5 to 6 minutes or until no longer pink. Using a slotted spoon, transfer sausage to a plate lined with paper towels. Drain off any fat and wipe out skillet.

2. In the same skillet, heat oil over medium-high heat. Add tomatoes and cook, stirring, for 4 to 5 minutes or until skins begin to split. Reduce heat to medium-low and return sausage to the pan, along with quinoa and wine. Cook, gently tossing to combine, for 2 to 3 minutes or until warmed through. Season to taste with salt and pepper. Serve sprinkled with cheese and parsley.

# Swiss Chard Stuffed with Quinoa and Sausage

*Here, earthy, grassy Swiss chard leaves are folded around a hearty filling of sausage and quinoa, then simmered until fork-tender. Leftovers are wonderful, but unlikely.*

## Tips

Any variety of Swiss chard leaves may be used in this recipe.

Make sure to use fine sea salt in the water you use to cook the quinoa. Conventional table salt contains chemicals and additives, whereas sea salt contains an abundance of naturally occurring trace minerals.

| | | |
|---|---|---|
| ²⁄₃ cup | quinoa, rinsed | 150 mL |
| 12 oz | Italian pork or turkey sausage (bulk or casings removed) | 375 g |
| 2 | cloves garlic, minced | 2 |
| ¾ cup | finely chopped onion | 175 mL |
| 1 tbsp | dried Italian seasoning | 15 mL |
| 1 | large egg, beaten | 1 |
| 8 | large Swiss chard leaves, tough stems removed | 8 |
| 1½ cups | ready-to-use reduced-sodium chicken or vegetable broth (GF, if needed) | 375 mL |
| 2 cups | marinara sauce | 500 mL |
| ⅓ cup | freshly grated Parmesan cheese | 75 mL |

1. In a medium saucepan of boiling salted water, cook quinoa for 9 minutes. Drain and rinse under cold water until cool.

2. In a large bowl, combine quinoa, sausage, garlic, onion, Italian seasoning and egg. Form into eight 3-inch (7.5 cm) oblong portions.

3. Place Swiss chard leaves on a work surface, underside of leaves facing up. Place a portion of sausage mixture in the center of each leaf. Tuck in ends, then tightly roll leaf around filling.

4. Place rolls, seam side down, in a large, deep skillet. Pour in broth, cover and bring to a boil over high heat. Reduce heat and simmer, stirring occasionally, for 8 to 10 minutes or until no longer pink inside. Discard broth.

5. Meanwhile, in a medium saucepan, warm marinara sauce over medium heat, stirring often.

6. Serve rolls topped with marinara sauce and sprinkled with cheese.

# Grilled Steak with Arugula and Parmesan Quinoa

*This dish embodies what's wonderful about grilling: in a short amount of time, a few simple ingredients — lean beef, quinoa, arugula and cheese — are easily transformed into a fabulous, fuss-free dinner that's sure to please all.*

- **Preheat barbecue grill to medium-high**

| | | |
|---|---|---|
| ¾ cup | quinoa, rinsed | 175 mL |
| 1½ cups | ready-to-use reduced-sodium beef or vegetable broth (GF, if needed) | 375 mL |
| 12 oz | boneless beef top loin (strip loin) or top sirloin steak, trimmed | 375 g |
| | Nonstick cooking spray | |
| | Fine sea salt and freshly cracked black pepper | |
| 1 tbsp | extra virgin olive oil | 15 mL |
| 1 tsp | freshly squeezed lemon juice | 5 mL |
| 1 tsp | balsamic vinegar | 5 mL |
| 3 cups | packed arugula, roughly chopped | 750 mL |
| ¼ cup | freshly grated Parmesan cheese | 60 mL |

1. In a medium saucepan, combine quinoa and broth. Bring to a boil over medium-high heat. Reduce heat to low, cover and simmer for 12 to 15 minutes or until liquid is absorbed. Remove from heat and let stand, covered, for 5 minutes. Fluff with a fork.

2. Meanwhile, pat steak dry with paper towels. Lightly spray with cooking spray. Sprinkle with salt and generously season with pepper. Grill on preheated barbecue, turning once, for 5 to 6 minutes per side for medium-rare, or to desired doneness. Transfer to a cutting board and let rest for 5 minutes.

3. In a small bowl, whisk together oil, lemon juice and vinegar. Season to taste with salt and pepper.

4. To the quinoa, add arugula and cheese, gently tossing to combine. Divide quinoa mixture among four dinner plates. Thinly slice steak and arrange on top of arugula. Drizzle with dressing.

# Tangerine Beef with Almond Quinoa

*Forget about fancy steps and time-intensive marinating — this tangerine-scented stir-fry is staggeringly simple. Thin slices of flank steak are quickly cooked, then cloaked in a citrus-sweet, faintly spicy sauce. A bed of almond quinoa helps to soak up all the delectable sauce.*

## Tips

If you can't find tangerines, use orange zest and juice instead.

To toast sliced almonds, place up to ½ cup (125 mL) almonds in a medium skillet set over medium heat. Cook, shaking the skillet, for 2 to 3 minutes or until almonds are golden brown and fragrant. Let cool completely before use.

| | | |
|---|---|---|
| 1 lb | beef flank steak, trimmed and cut across the grain into thin strips | 500 g |
| | Fine sea salt and freshly ground black pepper | |
| 2 tsp | vegetable oil, divided | 10 mL |
| 1 tbsp | minced gingerroot | 15 mL |
| ¼ tsp | hot pepper flakes | 1 mL |
| 1 tsp | finely grated tangerine zest | 5 mL |
| ⅓ cup | freshly squeezed tangerine juice | 75 mL |
| 3 tbsp | orange marmalade | 45 mL |
| 3 tbsp | tamari or soy sauce (GF, if needed) | 45 mL |
| 1 tbsp | rice or cider vinegar | 15 mL |
| ½ cup | sliced almonds, toasted (see tip, at left) | 125 mL |
| 2½ cups | hot cooked quinoa (see page 10) | 625 mL |
| ½ cup | thinly sliced green onions | 125 mL |

1. Sprinkle beef with salt and pepper. In a large, deep skillet, heat half the oil over medium-high heat. Add half the beef and cook, stirring, for 3 minutes. Using a slotted spoon, transfer beef to a plate. Repeat with the remaining oil and beef.

2. Return all beef to the skillet. Stir in ginger, hot pepper flakes, tangerine zest, tangerine juice, marmalade, tamari and vinegar; bring to a boil, stirring constantly. Boil, stirring, for 1 minute or until sauce is slightly thickened. Remove from heat.

3. Stir almonds into hot quinoa. Divide quinoa mixture among four dinner plates and top with beef mixture. Sprinkle with green onions.

# Skillet Quinoa Moussaka

**Makes 4 servings**

*Moussaka is Greece's answer for an abundance of eggplant. Here, the favorite casserole is reinvented in a quick-to-the-table dish loaded with all of the traditional flavors of the original.*

| | | |
|---|---|---|
| 2 tsp | olive oil | 10 mL |
| 1 | large eggplant (about 1 lb/500 g), peeled and cut into ½-inch (1 cm) cubes | 1 |
| 1¼ cups | chopped onions | 300 mL |
| 12 oz | extra-lean ground beef | 375 g |
| 2 | cloves garlic, minced | 2 |
| ½ tsp | fine sea salt | 2 mL |
| 1 | can (28 oz/796 mL) crushed tomatoes | 1 |
| 2 tsp | dried oregano | 10 mL |
| ½ tsp | ground cinnamon | 2 mL |
| 2 cups | hot cooked quinoa (see page 10) | 500 mL |
| ½ cup | packed fresh flat-leaf (Italian) parsley leaves, chopped | 125 mL |
| ½ cup | crumbled feta cheese | 125 mL |

1. In a Dutch oven or a large saucepan, heat oil over medium-high heat. Add eggplant and onions; cook, stirring, for 6 to 8 minutes or until softened. Transfer to a bowl.

2. In the same skillet, combine beef, garlic and salt; cook, breaking up beef with a spoon, for 6 to 9 minutes or until beef is no longer pink. Drain off any fat.

3. Stir in eggplant mixture, tomatoes, oregano and cinnamon; bring to a boil. Reduce heat and simmer, stirring occasionally, for 20 to 25 minutes or until sauce is thickened and eggplant is very tender. Add quinoa and simmer, stirring occasionally, for 2 minutes. Stir in parsley. Serve sprinkled with cheese.

# Beef and Quinoa Picadillo

*Picadillo — which means
"small bits and pieces" —
is a spicy, sweet and
savory ground meat dish
served throughout Latin
America. It is served
warm, cold, stuffed into
empanadas, rolled into
tortillas or spooned into
lettuce leaves, as in this
recipe. Quinoa makes
a fantastic addition,
absorbing all of the robust
flavors while adding
a unique nutty-earthy
flavor of its own.*

| | | |
|---|---|---|
| 8 oz | extra-lean ground beef | 250 g |
| 2 cups | hot cooked quinoa (see page 10) | 500 mL |
| 1/3 cup | dried currants or chopped raisins | 75 mL |
| 2 tsp | ground cumin | 10 mL |
| 1 tsp | ground cinnamon | 5 mL |
| 1 1/2 cups | salsa | 375 mL |
| 2 | large hard-cooked eggs (see tip, page 292), peeled and chopped | 2 |
| 1/2 cup | packed fresh cilantro leaves, chopped | 125 mL |
| 1/3 cup | chopped pimento-stuffed green olives | 75 mL |
| 1 | small head Boston or butter lettuce, leaves separated | 1 |

1. In a large, deep skillet, cook beef over medium-high heat, breaking it up with a spoon, for 5 to 6 minutes or until no longer pink. Drain off any fat. Add quinoa, currants, cumin, cinnamon and salsa; reduce heat and simmer, stirring occasionally, for 5 minutes. Remove from heat and stir in eggs, cilantro and olives.

2. Place lettuce leaves on a work surface, underside of leaves facing up. Spoon quinoa mixture down the center of each leaf. Tuck in ends, then tightly roll leaf around filling.

# Barbecue Quinoa Meatloaf Minis

*The umami flavor of beef, the binding qualities of quinoa and the sweet-tangy taste of barbecue sauce combine to make these miniature meatloaves wonderfully delicious and appealing to one and all. And they cook in a fraction of the time of traditional meatloaf!*

## Tip

Make sure to use fine sea salt in the water you use to cook the quinoa. Conventional table salt contains chemicals and additives, whereas sea salt contains an abundance of naturally occurring trace minerals.

- **Preheat oven to 350°F (180°C)**
- **12-cup muffin pan, sprayed with nonstick cooking spray**

| | | |
|---|---|---|
| ½ cup | quinoa, rinsed | 125 mL |
| 2 tsp | olive oil | 10 mL |
| 1 cup | finely chopped onion | 250 mL |
| ⅔ cup | finely shredded carrot | 150 mL |
| 3 | cloves garlic, minced | 3 |
| 1 tbsp | dried Italian seasoning | 15 mL |
| 1½ lbs | extra-lean ground beef | 750 g |
| ¼ tsp | freshly ground black pepper | 1 mL |
| 2 | large eggs, lightly beaten | 2 |
| 1 cup | barbecue sauce, divided | 250 mL |

1. In a medium saucepan of boiling salted water, cook quinoa for 9 minutes. Drain and rinse under cold water until cool.

2. Meanwhile, in a large nonstick skillet, heat oil over medium-high heat. Add onion, carrot, garlic and Italian seasoning; cook, stirring, for 2 minutes. Let cool completely.

3. In a large bowl, combine quinoa, onion mixture, beef, pepper, eggs and half the barbecue sauce. Divide meat mixture equally among prepared muffin cups. Spoon 2 tsp (10 mL) of the remaining barbecue sauce over each.

4. Bake in preheated oven for 22 to 25 minutes or until an instant-read thermometer inserted in the center of a meatloaf registers 160°F (71°C). Let stand for 5 minutes. Serve warm.

# Spiced Moroccan Meatballs with Feta

**Makes 4 servings**

*Quinoa makes these spicy meatballs light; a quick tomato sauce and a crumble of feta cheese make them irresistible.*

- • **Preheat oven to 400°F (200°C)**
- • **Large rimmed baking sheet, sprayed with nonstick cooking spray (preferably olive oil)**

| | | |
|---|---|---|
| 1 lb | extra-lean ground beef | 500 g |
| 1⅓ cups | cooked quinoa (see page 10), cooled | 325 mL |
| 1 cup | packed fresh cilantro leaves, chopped | 250 mL |
| 2 tsp | ground cumin, divided | 10 mL |
| ½ tsp | fine sea salt | 2 mL |
| ¼ tsp | cayenne pepper, divided | 1 mL |
| 1 | large egg, lightly beaten | 1 |
| 2 cups | marinara sauce | 500 mL |
| ¾ tsp | ground cinnamon | 3 mL |
| ½ cup | crumbled feta cheese | 125 mL |

1. In a large bowl, combine beef, quinoa, half the cilantro, 1½ tsp (7 mL) of the cumin, salt, half the cayenne and egg. Form into twenty 1½-inch (4 cm) meatballs and arrange on prepared baking sheet.

2. Bake in preheated oven for 14 to 18 minutes or until no longer pink inside.

3. Meanwhile, in a large, deep skillet, combine marinara sauce, cinnamon, the remaining cumin and the remaining cayenne. Cook over medium heat, stirring occasionally, for 5 to 6 minutes or until warmed though and slightly thickened. Add meatballs, spooning sauce over top. Reduce heat to low and cook for 3 to 4 minutes to blend the flavors. Serve sprinkled with cheese and the remaining cilantro.

# Beef and Quinoa Power Burgers

**Makes
4 servings**

*There are burgers and
then there are burgers.
This is definitely one of
the latter. This superfood
variation takes the classic
beef burger in an entirely
new direction.*

## Tips

Be careful to mix the beef
mixture as little as possible;
over-mixing can make the
burgers tough.

Whenever possible, use
whole-grain or multigrain
hamburger buns.

| | | |
|---|---|---|
| ⅔ cup | quinoa, rinsed | 150 mL |
| 1 cup | water | 250 mL |
| ⅓ cup | barbecue sauce | 75 mL |
| 1 lb | extra-lean ground beef | 500 g |
| ½ cup | finely chopped green onions | 125 mL |
| 2 tsp | ground cumin | 10 mL |
| ½ tsp | fine sea salt | 2 mL |
| ¼ tsp | freshly cracked black pepper | 1 mL |
| 2 tsp | olive oil | 10 mL |
| 4 | hamburger buns (GF, if needed), split and toasted | 4 |

### Suggested Accompaniments

Thinly sliced cheese (such as sharp Cheddar
or Gruyère) or crumbled goat cheese

Large tomato slices

Baby spinach, arugula or tender watercress
sprigs

Additional barbecue sauce

**1.** In a medium saucepan, combine quinoa, water and
barbecue sauce. Bring to a boil over medium-high
heat. Reduce heat to low, cover and simmer for 12 to
15 minutes or until liquid is absorbed. Remove from
heat and let cool to room temperature.

**2.** In a large bowl, combine quinoa, beef, green onions,
cumin, salt and pepper. Form into four ¾-inch (2 cm)
thick patties.

**3.** In a large, deep skillet, heat oil over medium-high heat.
Add patties and cook for 4 minutes. Turn and cook for
4 to 5 minutes or until no longer pink inside.

**4.** Transfer patties to toasted buns. Top with any of the
suggested accompaniments, as desired.

## Variation

Substitute lean ground turkey or extra-lean ground
pork for the beef.

# Roast Beef and Crimson Quinoa Wraps

*Two common sandwich fillings, roast beef and hummus, make room for some newfangled newcomers — beets, quinoa, feta cheese and watercress — resulting in a sassy take on the ho-hum wrap.*

## Tip

Whenever possible, use whole-grain or multigrain tortillas.

| | | |
|---|---|---|
| 1 cup | cooked quinoa (see page 10), cooled | 250 mL |
| ½ cup | finely shredded peeled beet (about 1 small) | 125 mL |
| ⅓ cup | crumbled feta cheese | 75 mL |
| 1 tbsp | freshly squeezed lemon juice | 15 mL |
| 2 tsp | extra virgin olive oil | 10 mL |
| | Fine sea salt and freshly cracked black pepper | |
| 2 | 8-inch (20 cm) quinoa tortillas or other GF tortillas (see tip, at left) | 2 |
| ¼ cup | hummus | 60 mL |
| 4 | thin slices deli roast beef | 4 |
| 1½ cups | packed arugula or tender watercress sprigs | 375 mL |

1. In a small bowl, combine quinoa, beet, cheese, lemon juice and oil. Season to taste with salt and pepper.
2. Spread tortillas with hummus. Top with quinoa mixture, roast beef and arugula, dividing evenly. Roll up like burritos, enclosing filling, or like jelly rolls (ends open).

# Middle Eastern Lamb, Greens and Quinoa

*Ground lamb and Middle Eastern spices add deep flavor to a simple dish of chickpeas and chard; quinoa absorbs the flavorful juices.*

| | | |
|---|---|---|
| 1 | large bunch red Swiss chard | 1 |
| 8 oz | lean or extra-lean ground lamb | 250 g |
| 4 | cloves garlic, minced | 4 |
| 2 tbsp | minced gingerroot | 30 mL |
| 1½ tsp | ground cumin | 7 mL |
| 1 tsp | ground coriander | 5 mL |
| ¼ tsp | cayenne pepper | 1 mL |
| ½ cup | ready-to-use reduced-sodium chicken or vegetable broth (GF, if needed) | 125 mL |
| 1 | can (14 to 19 oz/398 to 540 mL) chickpeas, drained and rinsed | 1 |
| 2 tsp | finely grated lemon zest | 10 mL |
| 2 tbsp | freshly squeezed lemon juice | 30 mL |
| | Fine sea salt and freshly cracked black pepper | |
| 3 cups | hot cooked quinoa (see page 10) | 750 mL |
| ¾ cup | plain yogurt | 175 mL |

1. Trim off tough stems from Swiss chard and discard. Trim tender stems and ribs from leaves and finely chop stems and ribs. Thinly slice leaves crosswise (to measure about 5 cups/1.25 L).
2. In a large, deep skillet, cook lamb, garlic, ginger, cumin, coriander and cayenne over medium-high heat, breaking lamb up with a spoon, for 5 to 6 minutes or until lamb is no longer pink.
3. Stir in Swiss chard and broth; cook, stirring, for 3 to 4 minutes or until Swiss chard is just wilted. Stir in chickpeas, lemon zest and lemon juice; cook, tossing, for 2 to 3 minutes to warm through and blend the flavors. Season to taste with salt and black pepper.
4. Divide quinoa among four dinner plates and top with lamb mixture. Drizzle with yogurt.

## Variation

Substitute lean ground turkey or extra-lean ground beef for the lamb.

# Turkish Lamb and Quinoa Kebabs

*Have leftover quinoa? Add it to Turkish-spiced lamb kebabs. Combining grains and ground meat is a common practice in Turkish and Middle Eastern cooking, and quinoa works deliciously, adding a nutty flavor and texture that complements the richness of the lamb.*

## Tips

The kebabs can be broiled instead of grilled. Preheat the broiler to high and place the kebabs on a broiler tray sprayed with nonstick cooking spray. Broil for 6 to 10 minutes, turning once halfway through, until no longer pink inside.

Whenever possible, use whole-grain or multigrain pitas or tortillas.

- **Preheat barbecue grill to medium-high**
- **Eight 10-inch (25 cm) metal skewers, or wooden skewers soaked in warm water for 30 minutes**

| | | |
|---|---|---|
| 1 lb | lean or extra-lean ground lamb | 500 g |
| 1 cup | cooked quinoa (see page 10), cooled | 250 mL |
| ¾ cup | packed fresh flat-leaf (Italian) parsley leaves, chopped | 175 mL |
| ¼ cup | finely chopped green onions | 60 mL |
| 1 tbsp | sweet smoked paprika | 15 mL |
| 1 tsp | dried oregano | 5 mL |
| ½ tsp | fine sea salt | 2 mL |
| ¼ tsp | cayenne pepper | 1 mL |
| 1 | large egg, lightly beaten | 1 |

### Suggested Accompaniments

Warm pitas or tortillas (GF, if needed)

Plain Greek yogurt

Diced tomatoes

1. In a large bowl, combine lamb, quinoa, parsley, green onions, paprika, oregano, salt, cayenne and egg. Divide mixture into 8 portions. Form each portion around a skewer, shaping the meat into a 6- by 1-inch (15 by 2.5 cm) cylinder around the skewer.

2. Grill kebabs on preheated barbecue, turning once or twice, for 6 to 10 minutes or until no longer pink inside.

## Variation

Substitute lean ground turkey or extra-lean ground beef for the lamb.

# Breads

# Basic Quinoa Muffins

*Simple is so often best. Bite into one of these tender, nutty muffins and you'll agree. A short list of good-for-you ingredients — quinoa flour, coconut oil, yogurt — and a few optional accents (perhaps some spice, a handful of dried fruit or toasted nuts) yields wondrous results.*

## Storage Tip

Store the cooled muffins in an airtight container in the refrigerator for up to 3 days. Or wrap them in plastic wrap, then foil, completely enclosing them, and freeze for up to 6 months. Let thaw at room temperature for 2 hours before serving.

- **Preheat oven to 350°F (180°C)**
- **12-cup muffin pan, 10 cups sprayed with nonstick cooking spray**

| | | |
|---|---|---|
| 1½ cups | quinoa flour | 375 mL |
| 1½ tbsp | cornstarch or arrowroot | 22 mL |
| 1½ tsp | baking powder (GF, if needed) | 7 mL |
| ¾ tsp | fine sea salt | 3 mL |
| ¼ tsp | baking soda | 1 mL |
| 2 | large eggs | 2 |
| ¾ cup | plain yogurt or buttermilk | 175 mL |
| ⅓ cup | unrefined virgin coconut oil, warmed, or unsalted butter, melted | 75 mL |
| ⅓ cup | liquid honey, pure maple syrup, brown rice syrup or agave nectar | 75 mL |
| 1 tsp | vanilla extract (GF, if needed) | 5 mL |

1. In a large bowl, whisk together quinoa flour, cornstarch, baking powder, salt and baking soda.
2. In a medium bowl, whisk together eggs, yogurt, oil, honey and vanilla until well blended.
3. Add the egg mixture to the flour mixture and stir until just blended.
4. Divide batter equally among prepared muffin cups.
5. Bake in preheated oven for 20 to 25 minutes or until tops are golden brown and a toothpick inserted in the center comes out clean. Let cool in pan on a wire rack for 3 minutes, then transfer to the rack to cool.

## Variations

*Spiced Muffins:* Add 1 tsp (5 mL) ground cinnamon, ½ tsp (2 mL) ground cardamom or nutmeg and ½ tsp (2 mL) ground allspice to the flour mixture.

*Double Ginger Muffins:* Add 2 tsp (10 mL) ground ginger to the flour mixture. Gently fold in ¼ cup (60 mL) finely chopped crystallized ginger at the end of step 3.

*Dried Fruit Muffins:* Replace the vanilla with ½ tsp (2 mL) almond extract. Gently fold in ½ cup (125 mL) dried fruit (such as raisins, cranberries, chopped apricots or blueberries) at the end of step 3.

*Quinoa Crunch Muffins:* In a small bowl, combine 2 tbsp (30 mL) rinsed quinoa, 1½ tbsp (22 mL) turbinado sugar and ½ tsp (2 mL) ground cinnamon. Sprinkle over muffin tops before baking.

*Toasted Nut Muffins:* Gently fold in 1 cup (250 mL) chopped toasted nuts (such as pecans, walnuts or almonds) at the end of step 3.

# Bowl of Oatmeal Muffins

**Makes
12 muffins**

*I love a bowl of warm oatmeal (preferably with ample amounts of brown sugar), but when I'm on the run, I like to have a batch of these quinoa-enriched oat muffins ready to pack into my bag.*

## Tip

Plain soy yogurt or rice yogurt may be used in place of the yogurt.

## Storage Tip

Store the cooled muffins in an airtight container in the refrigerator for up to 3 days. Or wrap them in plastic wrap, then foil, completely enclosing them, and freeze for up to 6 months. Let thaw at room temperature for 2 hours before serving.

- **Preheat oven to 400°F (200°C)**
- **12-cup muffin pan, sprayed with nonstick cooking spray**

| | | |
|---|---|---|
| 1 cup | quinoa flour | 250 mL |
| 2 tsp | baking powder (GF, if needed) | 10 mL |
| ¾ tsp | fine sea salt | 3 mL |
| ½ tsp | ground cinnamon | 2 mL |
| ½ tsp | baking soda | 2 mL |
| 1⅓ cups | quick-cooking rolled oats (certified GF, if needed) | 325 mL |
| 2 | large eggs | 2 |
| 1 cup | plain yogurt | 250 mL |
| ½ cup | liquid honey, pure maple syrup or brown rice syrup | 125 mL |
| ¼ cup | unsalted butter, melted, or vegetable oil | 60 mL |
| 1 tsp | vanilla extract (GF, if needed) | 5 mL |
| 1 cup | dried fruit (such as raisins, cranberries or cherries) | 250 mL |

1. In a large bowl, whisk together quinoa flour, baking powder, salt, cinnamon and baking soda. Stir in oats.
2. In a medium bowl, whisk together eggs, yogurt, honey, butter and vanilla until well blended.
3. Add the egg mixture to the flour mixture and stir until just combined. Gently fold in dried fruit.
4. Divide batter equally among prepared muffin cups.
5. Bake in preheated oven for 20 to 25 minutes or until tops are golden and a toothpick inserted in the center comes out clean. Let cool in pan on a wire rack for 3 minutes, then transfer to the rack to cool.

# Quinoa Muesli Muffins

*Serve these hearty
muffins, based on the
traditional Scandinavian
cereal, alongside a cup
of yogurt or skim latte
to start the day off with
both good health and
great taste.*

## Tips

For the dried fruit, try
raisins, cranberries or
blueberries, or chopped
apricots, apples, figs
or cherries.

You can use almonds or
hazelnuts — or seeds,
such as green pumpkin
seeds (pepitas) or
sunflower seeds — in
place of the pecans.

## Storage Tip

Store the cooled muffins
in an airtight container
in the refrigerator for up
to 3 days. Or wrap them
in plastic wrap, then foil,
completely enclosing
them, and freeze for up
to 6 months. Let thaw
at room temperature for
2 hours before serving.

- **Preheat oven to 375°F (190°C)**
- **12-cup muffin pan, lined with paper liners**

### Muesli

| | | |
|---|---|---|
| ½ cup | quinoa flakes or large-flake (old-fashioned) rolled oats (certified GF, if needed) | 125 mL |
| ½ cup | dried fruit (see tip, at left)) | 125 mL |
| ½ cup | chopped toasted pecans or walnuts | 125 mL |
| ⅓ cup | ground flax seeds (flaxseed meal) | 75 mL |

### Muffins

| | | |
|---|---|---|
| 1⅓ cups | quinoa flour | 325 mL |
| ½ cup | quinoa flakes or large-flake (old-fashioned) rolled oats (certified GF, if needed) | 125 mL |
| 1 tsp | baking soda | 5 mL |
| ½ tsp | fine sea salt | 2 mL |
| ¼ tsp | ground cinnamon | 1 mL |
| 2 | large eggs | 2 |
| ⅔ cup | unsweetened applesauce | 150 mL |
| ⅓ cup | vegetable oil | 75 mL |
| ⅓ cup | liquid honey, brown rice syrup or pure maple syrup | 75 mL |
| 1 tsp | vanilla extract (GF, if needed) | 5 mL |
| 1 cup | finely chopped ripe bananas | 250 mL |

1. *Muesli:* In a medium bowl, combine quinoa flakes, dried fruit, pecans and flax seeds. Set aside.
2. *Muffins:* In a medium bowl, whisk together quinoa flour, quinoa flakes, baking soda, salt and cinnamon.
3. In a large bowl, whisk together eggs, applesauce, oil, honey and vanilla until well blended. Stir in bananas.
4. Add the flour mixture to the egg mixture and stir until just blended. Stir in ¾ cup (175 mL) of the muesli.
5. Divide batter equally among prepared muffin cups. Sprinkle with the remaining muesli and press lightly into batter.
6. Bake in preheated oven for 20 to 23 minutes or until tops are golden and a toothpick inserted in the center comes out clean. Let cool in pan on a wire rack for 5 minutes, then transfer to the rack to cool.

# Four-Grain Fruit Muffins

**Makes
12 muffins**

*These hearty multigrain muffins are at once homestyle and modern. They are great for toasting, spreading with marmalade or eating as is.*

## Tip

Measure the oil in a glass measuring cup, then measure the honey in the same cup; the residue from the oil will allow the honey to slide right out without sticking.

## Storage Tip

Store the cooled muffins in an airtight container in the refrigerator for up to 3 days. Or wrap them in plastic wrap, then foil, completely enclosing them, and freeze for up to 6 months. Let thaw at room temperature for 2 hours before serving.

- **Preheat oven to 400°F (200°C)**
- **Food processor**
- **12-cup muffin pan, sprayed with nonstick cooking spray**

| | | |
|---|---|---|
| 1¼ cups | quick-cooking rolled oats (certified GF, if needed) | 300 mL |
| 1 cup | quinoa flour | 250 mL |
| ¼ cup | yellow cornmeal (GF, if needed) | 60 mL |
| ¼ cup | ground flax seeds (flaxseed meal) | 60 mL |
| 1 tsp | baking powder (GF, if needed) | 5 mL |
| 1 tsp | baking soda | 5 mL |
| ¾ tsp | fine sea salt | 3 mL |
| 2 | large eggs | 2 |
| ¼ cup | vegetable oil | 60 mL |
| ½ cup | liquid honey, pure maple syrup or brown rice syrup | 125 mL |
| 1 tsp | almond extract (GF, if needed) | 5 mL |
| 1½ cups | buttermilk | 375 mL |
| 1½ cups | berries or chopped fruit | 375 mL |

1. In food processor, pulse oats five or six times or until oats resemble coarse meal.
2. In a large bowl, whisk together oats, quinoa flour, cornmeal, flax seeds, baking powder, baking soda and salt.
3. In a medium bowl, whisk together eggs, oil, honey and almond extract until well blended. Whisk in buttermilk until blended.
4. Add the egg mixture to the oat mixture and stir until just blended. Gently fold in berries.
5. Divide batter equally among prepared muffin cups.
6. Bake in preheated oven for 18 to 23 minutes or until tops are golden and a toothpick inserted in the center comes out clean. Let cool in pan on a wire rack for 5 minutes, then transfer to the rack to cool.

# Apple Walnut Muffins

*Apples add moistness
and natural sweetness to
these delicious, healthful
muffins. A sprinkling of
toasted walnuts in the
batter adds a delectable,
complementary crunch.*

## Tip

For the apples, try
Braeburn, Gala or Golden
Delicious.

## Storage Tip

Store the cooled muffins
in an airtight container
in the refrigerator for up
to 3 days. Or wrap them
in plastic wrap, then foil,
completely enclosing
them, and freeze for up
to 6 months. Let thaw
at room temperature for
2 hours before serving.

- **Preheat oven to 400°F (200°C)**
- **12-cup muffin pan, sprayed with nonstick cooking spray**

| | | |
|---|---|---|
| 2 cups | quinoa flour | 500 mL |
| 2 tbsp | cornstarch or arrowroot | 30 mL |
| 1 tbsp | baking powder (GF, if needed) | 15 mL |
| ½ tsp | fine sea salt | 2 mL |
| ½ tsp | ground cinnamon | 2 mL |
| ½ cup | natural cane sugar or packed light brown sugar | 125 mL |
| 2 | large eggs | 2 |
| ¾ cup | buttermilk | 175 mL |
| ¼ cup | toasted walnut oil or vegetable oil | 60 mL |
| 1½ cups | chopped tart-sweet apples (unpeeled) | 375 mL |
| ½ cup | toasted chopped walnuts | 125 mL |

1. In a large bowl, whisk together quinoa flour, cornstarch, baking powder, salt and cinnamon.
2. In a medium bowl, whisk together sugar, eggs, buttermilk and oil until well blended.
3. Add the egg mixture to the flour mixture and stir until just blended. Gently fold in apples and walnuts.
4. Divide batter equally among prepared muffin cups.
5. Bake in preheated oven for 18 to 23 minutes or until tops are golden and a toothpick inserted in the center comes out clean. Let cool in pan on a wire rack for 3 minutes, then transfer to the rack to cool.

## Variation

*Pear Pecan Muffins:* Replace the cinnamon with ground nutmeg, the apples with chopped pears (unpeeled) and the walnuts with toasted chopped pecans.

# Blueberry Muffins

*Quinoa flour lends a subtle, nutty flavor to these honey-sweetened blueberry muffins.*

## Tip

If using frozen blueberries, opt for wild blueberries. Do not thaw the berries for more than 5 minutes, or they will bleed into the batter.

## Storage Tip

Store the cooled muffins in an airtight container in the refrigerator for up to 3 days. Or wrap them in plastic wrap, then foil, completely enclosing them, and freeze for up to 6 months. Let thaw at room temperature for 2 hours before serving.

- **Preheat oven to 400°F (200°C)**
- **12-cup muffin pan, sprayed with nonstick cooking spray**

| | | |
|---|---|---|
| 2 cups | quinoa flour | 500 mL |
| 2 tbsp | cornstarch or arrowroot | 30 mL |
| 2½ tsp | baking powder (GF, if needed) | 12 mL |
| ½ tsp | ground cinnamon | 2 mL |
| ½ tsp | baking soda | 2 mL |
| ½ tsp | fine sea salt | 2 mL |
| 2 | large eggs | 2 |
| 1 cup | buttermilk | 250 mL |
| ⅓ cup | unsalted butter, melted, or unrefined virgin coconut oil, warmed | 75 mL |
| ½ cup | liquid honey or pure maple syrup | 125 mL |
| 1 tsp | vanilla extract (GF, if needed) | 5 mL |
| 1⅓ cups | fresh or frozen blueberries | 325 mL |

1. In a large bowl, whisk together quinoa flour, cornstarch, baking powder, cinnamon, baking soda and salt.
2. In a medium bowl, whisk together eggs, buttermilk, butter, honey and vanilla until well blended.
3. Add the egg mixture to the flour mixture and stir just until blended. Gently fold in blueberries.
4. Divide batter equally among prepared muffin cups.
5. Bake in preheated oven for 18 to 23 minutes or until tops are golden brown and a toothpick inserted in the center comes out clean. Let cool in pan on a wire rack for 3 minutes, then transfer to the rack to cool.

# Orange Poppy Seed Muffins

*You know those big, buttery poppy seed muffins in the coffeehouse case? The ones that tempt you every time you order a skim latte? Well, it's a good thing you held out, because my version is the one you really want. These freeze particularly well, so you can savor just a few at a time.*

## Tip

Be sure to get your poppy seeds from a good source. They need to be fresh, as they can go rancid very quickly.

## Storage Tip

Store the cooled muffins in an airtight container in the refrigerator for up to 3 days. Or wrap them in plastic wrap, then foil, completely enclosing them, and freeze for up to 6 months. Let thaw at room temperature for 2 hours before serving.

- **Preheat oven to 375°F (190°C)**
- **12-cup muffin pan, 10 cups sprayed with nonstick cooking spray**

| | | |
|---|---|---:|
| 1½ cups | quinoa flour | 375 mL |
| 2 tbsp | poppy seeds | 30 mL |
| 1½ tbsp | cornstarch or arrowroot | 22 mL |
| 1½ tsp | baking powder (GF, if needed) | 7 mL |
| ½ tsp | fine sea salt | 2 mL |
| ¼ tsp | baking soda | 1 mL |
| 2 | large eggs | 2 |
| ¾ cup | plain yogurt | 175 mL |
| ¼ cup | unrefined virgin coconut oil, warmed, or unsalted butter, melted | 60 mL |
| ½ cup | liquid honey, brown rice syrup or agave nectar | 125 mL |
| 2 tsp | finely grated orange or tangerine zest | 10 mL |

1. In a large bowl, whisk together quinoa flour, poppy seeds, cornstarch, baking powder, salt and baking soda.
2. In a medium bowl, whisk together eggs, yogurt, oil, honey and orange zest until well blended.
3. Add the egg mixture to the flour mixture and stir until just blended.
4. Divide batter equally among prepared muffin cups.
5. Bake in preheated oven for 20 to 24 minutes or until tops are golden and a toothpick inserted in the center comes out clean. Let cool in pan on a wire rack for 3 minutes, then transfer to the rack to cool.

## Variations

*Glazed Orange Muffins:* In a small saucepan, melt ⅓ cup (75 mL) orange marmalade over low heat. Spoon over warm muffins as soon as they have been removed from the pan.

*Almond Poppy Seed Muffins:* Replace the orange zest with 1 tsp (5 mL) almond extract.

# Banana and Toasted Quinoa Muffins

*By the end of the school or work week, most bananas are past their prime — but they're perfect for these moist double quinoa muffins. Toasting the quinoa enhances its nutty flavor and crunch.*

## Tip

Plain soy yogurt or rice yogurt may be used in place of the yogurt.

## Storage Tip

Store the cooled muffins in an airtight container in the refrigerator for up to 3 days. Or wrap them in plastic wrap, then foil, completely enclosing them, and freeze for up to 6 months. Let thaw at room temperature for 2 hours before serving.

- **12-cup muffin pan, sprayed with nonstick cooking spray**

| | | |
|---|---|---|
| 1/2 cup | quinoa, rinsed | 125 mL |
| 2 cups | quinoa flour | 500 mL |
| 1/4 cup | ground flax seeds (flaxseed meal) | 60 mL |
| 2 1/2 tsp | ground cinnamon | 12 mL |
| 1 tsp | baking soda | 5 mL |
| 1 tsp | fine sea salt | 5 mL |
| 2 | large eggs | 2 |
| 1 1/2 cups | mashed ripe bananas | 375 mL |
| 3/4 cup | plain yogurt | 175 mL |
| 1/2 cup | liquid honey or agave nectar | 125 mL |
| 3 tbsp | vegetable oil | 45 mL |
| 2 tsp | vanilla extract (GF, if needed) | 10 mL |

1. Heat a large skillet over medium-high heat. Toast quinoa, stirring occasionally, for 3 to 4 minutes or until golden brown and just beginning to pop. Transfer to a large bowl and let cool completely.
2. Preheat oven to 350°F (180°C).
3. Whisk quinoa flour, flax seeds, cinnamon, baking soda and salt into cooled quinoa.
4. In a medium bowl, whisk together eggs, bananas, yogurt, honey, oil and vanilla until well blended.
5. Add the egg mixture to the flour mixture and stir until just blended.
6. Divide batter equally among prepared muffin cups.
7. Bake for 23 to 28 minutes or until tops are golden and a toothpick inserted in the center comes out clean. Let cool in pan on a wire rack for 3 minutes, then transfer to the rack to cool.

# Morning Glory Muffins

**Makes 12 muffins**

*These morning glory muffins are chock full of goodness and great taste. A quartet of flavorful ingredients — shredded carrots, crushed pineapple, flaked coconut and dried cranberries — add gentle sweetness and keep the muffins moist, allowing the added sugar and fat to be kept to a minimum.*

## Tips

For the ideal texture, thoroughly drain the pineapple and pat it dry with paper towels; otherwise, the muffins will be somewhat gummy.

These muffins taste best when the carrots are shredded using the large holes of a box grater. That way, the carrots maintain their texture while baking.

## Storage Tip

Store the cooled muffins in an airtight container in the refrigerator for up to 3 days. Or wrap them in plastic wrap, then foil, completely enclosing them, and freeze for up to 6 months. Let thaw at room temperature for 2 hours before serving.

- **Preheat oven to 375°F (190°C)**
- **12-cup muffin pan, sprayed with nonstick cooking spray**

| | | |
|---|---|---|
| 1½ cups | quinoa flour | 375 mL |
| ¾ cup | quick-cooking rolled oats (certified GF, if needed) | 175 mL |
| 2 tsp | baking soda | 10 mL |
| 1 tsp | ground cinnamon | 5 mL |
| ½ tsp | fine sea salt | 2 mL |
| ½ cup | natural cane sugar or packed light brown sugar | 125 mL |
| 3 | large eggs | 3 |
| ¼ cup | unrefined virgin coconut oil, warmed, or vegetable oil | 60 mL |
| 1 tsp | vanilla extract (GF, if needed) | 5 mL |
| 1 | can (8 oz/227 mL) crushed pineapple, drained (see tip, at left) | 1 |
| 2 cups | coarsely shredded carrots (see tip, at left) | 500 mL |
| ⅔ cup | unsweetened flaked coconut | 150 mL |
| ½ cup | dried cranberries or raisins | 125 mL |
| ½ cup | chopped toasted walnuts or pecans | 125 mL |

1. In a large bowl, whisk together quinoa flour, oats, baking soda, cinnamon and salt.
2. In a medium bowl, whisk together sugar, eggs, oil and vanilla until blended.
3. Add the egg mixture to the flour mixture and stir until just blended. Gently fold in pineapple, carrots, coconut, cranberries and walnuts.
4. Divide batter equally among prepared muffin cups.
5. Bake in preheated oven for 25 to 30 minutes or until tops are golden and a toothpick inserted in the center comes out with just a few crumbs attached. Let cool in pan on a wire rack for 5 minutes, then transfer to the rack to cool.

# Double Quinoa Raisin Muffins

**Makes 12 muffins**

*Perfect for anyone looking to amp up the whole grains in their diet, these moist muffins are subtly scented with cinnamon and accented with plump raisins.*

## Tip

Measure the butter in a glass measuring cup, then measure the honey in the same cup; the residue from the butter will allow the honey to slide right out without sticking.

## Storage Tip

Store the cooled muffins in an airtight container in the refrigerator for up to 3 days. Or wrap them in plastic wrap, then foil, completely enclosing them, and freeze for up to 6 months. Let thaw at room temperature for 2 hours before serving.

- **Preheat oven to 400°F (200°C)**
- **12-cup muffin pan, lined with paper liners**

| | | |
|---|---|---|
| 2 cups | quinoa flour | 500 mL |
| 2 tbsp | cornstarch or arrowroot | 30 mL |
| 2½ tsp | baking powder (GF, if needed) | 12 mL |
| 1 tsp | ground cinnamon | 5 mL |
| ½ tsp | baking soda | 2 mL |
| ½ tsp | fine sea salt | 2 mL |
| 2 | large eggs | 2 |
| 1 cup | buttermilk | 250 mL |
| ¼ cup | unsalted butter, melted | 60 mL |
| ½ cup | liquid honey, pure maple syrup or brown rice syrup | 125 mL |
| 1½ tsp | vanilla extract (GF, if needed) | 7 mL |
| 2 cups | cooked quinoa (see page 10), cooled | 500 mL |
| ⅔ cup | raisins | 150 mL |

1. In a large bowl, whisk together quinoa flour, cornstarch, baking powder, cinnamon, baking soda and salt.
2. In a medium bowl, whisk together eggs, buttermilk, butter, honey and vanilla until well blended.
3. Add the egg mixture to the flour mixture and stir until just blended. Gently fold in quinoa and raisins.
4. Divide batter equally among prepared muffin cups.
5. Bake in preheated oven for 18 to 23 minutes or until tops are golden and a toothpick inserted in the center comes out clean. Let cool in pan on a wire rack for 5 minutes, then transfer to the rack to cool.

# Flax Quinoa Date Muffins

*Flax is rich in nutrients that protect against heart disease and cancer. It has a very mild taste and, when used in quick breads, contributes great moisture. Dates and molasses contribute deep, natural, caramel-like sweetness.*

## Storage Tip

Store the cooled muffins in an airtight container in the refrigerator for up to 3 days. Or wrap them in plastic wrap, then foil, completely enclosing them, and freeze for up to 6 months. Let thaw at room temperature for 2 hours before serving.

- **Preheat oven to 350°F (180°C)**
- **12-cup muffin pan, sprayed with nonstick cooking spray**

| | | |
|---|---|---|
| 1½ cups | quinoa flour | 375 mL |
| ¾ cup | ground flax seeds (flaxseed meal) | 175 mL |
| 1 tsp | ground cinnamon | 5 mL |
| 1 tsp | baking soda | 5 mL |
| ½ tsp | fine sea salt | 2 mL |
| 2 | large eggs | 2 |
| 1 cup | plain yogurt | 250 mL |
| ⅓ cup | dark (cooking) molasses | 75 mL |
| 1 tsp | vanilla extract (GF, if needed) | 5 mL |
| 1 cup | pitted dates, chopped | 250 mL |

1. In a large bowl, whisk together quinoa flour, flax seeds, cinnamon, baking soda and salt.
2. In a medium bowl, whisk together eggs, yogurt, molasses and vanilla until well blended.
3. Add the egg mixture to the flour mixture and stir until just blended. Gently fold in dates.
4. Divide batter equally among prepared muffin cups.
5. Bake in preheated oven for 22 to 27 minutes or until tops are light golden brown and a toothpick inserted in the center comes out clean. Let cool in pan on a wire rack for 3 minutes, then transfer to the rack to cool.

# Health Nut Muffins

*These not-so-humble, but oh-so-healthy muffins pack a range of flavors and textures that add up to irresistible.*

## Storage Tip

Store the cooled muffins in an airtight container in the refrigerator for up to 3 days. Or wrap them in plastic wrap, then foil, completely enclosing them, and freeze for up to 6 months. Let thaw at room temperature for 2 hours before serving.

- **Preheat oven to 350°F (180°C)**
- **12-cup muffin pan, sprayed with nonstick cooking spray**

| | | |
|---|---|---|
| 1½ cups | quinoa flour | 375 mL |
| ¾ cup | quick-cooking rolled oats (certified GF, if needed) | 175 mL |
| ¼ cup | ground flax seeds (flaxseed meal) | 60 mL |
| 2 tsp | baking powder (GF, if needed) | 10 mL |
| ½ tsp | baking soda | 2 mL |
| ½ tsp | fine sea salt | 2 mL |
| 2 | large eggs | 2 |
| ¾ cup | buttermilk | 175 mL |
| ¼ cup | vegetable oil | 60 mL |
| ⅔ cup | liquid honey, brown rice syrup or pure maple syrup | 150 mL |
| ⅔ cup | dried cherries or blueberries | 150 mL |
| ½ cup | chopped toasted walnuts or pecans | 125 mL |
| ½ cup | lightly salted roasted sunflower seeds | 125 mL |

1. In a large bowl, whisk together quinoa flour, oats, flax seeds, baking powder, baking soda and salt.
2. In a medium bowl, whisk together eggs, buttermilk, oil and honey until well blended.
3. Add the egg mixture to the flour mixture and stir until just blended. Gently fold in cherries, walnuts and sunflower seeds.
4. Divide batter equally among prepared muffin cups.
5. Bake in preheated oven for 18 to 22 minutes or until tops are golden and a toothpick inserted in the center comes out clean. Let cool in pan on a wire rack for 3 minutes, then transfer to the rack to cool.

# Almond Butter Muffins

*Alternative nut butters
used to be sold only at
health food stores, but
now they are widely
available at supermarkets
and superstores. Here,
almond butter enriches
quinoa flour, creating
hearty muffins that will
sustain you through the
most rigorous morning
without a thought
of lunch.*

## Tips

Any variety of natural nut
or seed butter (such as
peanut, cashew, sunflower
seed or sesame seed) may
be used in place of the
almond butter.

For the dried fruit, try
raisins, cranberries,
chopped cherries or
chopped apricots, or a
combination.

## Storage Tip

Store the cooled muffins
in an airtight container
in the refrigerator for up
to 3 days. Or wrap them
in plastic wrap, then foil,
completely enclosing
them, and freeze for up
to 6 months. Let thaw
at room temperature for
2 hours before serving.

- **Preheat oven to 400°F (200°C)**
- **12-cup muffin pan, sprayed with nonstick cooking spray**

| | | |
|---|---|---:|
| 1¾ cups | quinoa flour | 425 mL |
| 1 tbsp | baking powder (GF, if needed) | 15 mL |
| ½ tsp | fine sea salt | 2 mL |
| 2 | large eggs | 2 |
| ½ cup | unsweetened natural almond butter, well stirred | 125 mL |
| ¼ cup | vegetable oil or unrefined virgin coconut oil, warmed | 60 mL |
| ¼ cup | liquid honey or brown rice syrup | 60 mL |
| 1 tsp | vanilla extract (GF, if needed) | 5 mL |
| 1¼ cups | milk or plain non-dairy milk (such as soy, almond, rice or hemp) | 300 mL |
| ½ cup | dried fruit | 125 mL |

1. In a large bowl, whisk together quinoa flour, baking powder and salt.
2. In a medium bowl, whisk together eggs, almond butter, oil, honey and vanilla until well blended. Whisk in milk until blended.
3. Add the egg mixture to the flour mixture and stir until just blended. Gently fold in dried fruit.
4. Divide batter equally among prepared muffin cups.
5. Bake in preheated oven for 18 to 22 minutes or until tops are golden and a toothpick inserted in the center comes out clean. Let cool in pan on a wire rack for 5 minutes, then transfer to the rack to cool.

# Dark Chocolate Muffins

*Healthy and decadent all in one, these will soon become your most requested muffins. Moist and chocolatey, they are absolutely delicious and a snap to make.*

## Storage Tip

Store the cooled muffins in an airtight container in the refrigerator for up to 3 days. Or wrap them in plastic wrap, then foil, completely enclosing them, and freeze for up to 6 months. Let thaw at room temperature for 2 hours before serving.

- Preheat oven to 350°F (180°C)
- 12-cup muffin pan, sprayed with nonstick cooking spray

| | | |
|---|---|---|
| 1½ cups | quinoa flour | 375 mL |
| ½ cup | unsweetened cocoa powder (not Dutch process) | 125 mL |
| 1½ tsp | baking powder (GF, if needed) | 7 mL |
| ½ tsp | baking soda | 2 mL |
| ¼ tsp | fine sea salt | 1 mL |
| 2 | large eggs | 2 |
| 1 cup | buttermilk | 250 mL |
| ¼ cup | vegetable oil | 60 mL |
| ½ cup | agave nectar or liquid honey | 125 mL |
| 1 tsp | vanilla extract (GF, if needed) | 5 mL |

1. In a large bowl, whisk together quinoa flour, cocoa powder, baking powder, baking soda and salt.
2. In a medium bowl, whisk together eggs, buttermilk, oil, agave nectar and vanilla until well blended.
3. Add the egg mixture to the flour mixture and stir until just blended.
4. Divide batter equally among prepared muffin cups.
5. Bake in preheated oven for 18 to 22 minutes or until a toothpick inserted in the center comes out clean. Let cool in pan on a wire rack for 3 minutes, then transfer to the rack to cool.

## Variations

Gently fold in ½ cup (125 mL) miniature semisweet chocolate chips (GF, if needed) at the end of step 3.

*Carob-Quinoa Muffins:* Use unsweetened carob powder in place of the cocoa powder. If desired, gently fold in ½ cup (125 mL) carob chips, chopped, at the end of step 3.

# Honey Ricotta Muffins

*Nutty from quinoa flour
and fragrant from orange
zest and mace, these
tender muffins are plain
and simple without being
the least bit boring. They
melt in your mouth and
are as delicious a day or
two after baking as they
are warm.*

## Storage Tip

Store the cooled muffins
in an airtight container
in the refrigerator for up
to 3 days. Or wrap them
in plastic wrap, then foil,
completely enclosing
them, and freeze for up
to 6 months. Let thaw
at room temperature for
2 hours before serving.

- **Preheat oven to 400°F (200°C)**
- **12-cup muffin pan, sprayed with nonstick cooking spray**

| | | |
|---|---|---|
| 2 cups | quinoa flour | 500 mL |
| 2½ tsp | baking powder (GF, if needed) | 12 mL |
| ½ tsp | fine sea salt | 2 mL |
| ¼ tsp | baking soda | 1 mL |
| ¼ tsp | ground mace or nutmeg | 1 mL |
| 1 | large egg | 1 |
| 1 cup | ricotta cheese (reduced-fat or regular) | 250 mL |
| ½ cup | plain yogurt | 125 mL |
| ¼ cup | olive or vegetable oil | 60 mL |
| ⅓ cup | liquid honey | 75 mL |
| 1 tbsp | finely grated orange zest | 15 mL |

1. In a large bowl, whisk together quinoa flour, baking powder, salt, baking soda and mace.
2. In a medium bowl, whisk together egg, cheese, yogurt, oil, honey and orange zest until well blended.
3. Add the egg mixture to the flour mixture and stir until just blended.
4. Divide batter equally among prepared muffin cups.
5. Bake in preheated oven for 15 to 20 minutes or until tops are golden and a toothpick inserted in the center comes out clean. Let cool in pan on a wire rack for 3 minutes, then transfer to the rack to cool.

# Old-Fashioned Molasses Muffins

*I like to bake these dark muffins, redolent with rich spices and notes of caramel from the molasses, throughout the winter months — they're perfect with a cup of tea on chilly mornings.*

## Storage Tip

Store the cooled muffins in an airtight container in the refrigerator for up to 3 days. Or wrap them in plastic wrap, then foil, completely enclosing them, and freeze for up to 6 months. Let thaw at room temperature for 2 hours before serving.

- **Preheat oven to 400°F (200°C)**
- **12-cup muffin pan, sprayed with nonstick cooking spray**

| | | |
|---|---|---|
| 1½ cups | quinoa flour | 375 mL |
| ¾ cup | quick-cooking rolled oats (certified GF, if needed) | 175 mL |
| 2¼ tsp | baking powder (GF, if needed) | 11 mL |
| ¾ tsp | ground cinnamon | 3 mL |
| ½ tsp | baking soda | 2 mL |
| ½ tsp | fine sea salt | 2 mL |
| 2 | large eggs | 2 |
| ¼ cup | unsalted butter, melted | 60 mL |
| ⅓ cup | dark (cooking) molasses | 75 mL |
| 1⅓ cups | buttermilk | 325 mL |

1. In a large bowl, whisk together quinoa flour, oats, baking powder, cinnamon, baking soda and salt.
2. In a medium bowl, whisk together eggs, butter and molasses until well blended. Whisk in buttermilk until blended.
3. Add the egg mixture to the flour mixture and stir until just blended.
4. Divide batter equally among prepared muffin cups.
5. Bake in preheated oven for 21 to 26 minutes or until tops are golden and a toothpick inserted in the center comes out clean. Let cool in pan on a wire rack for 5 minutes, then transfer to the rack to cool.

# Salsa Muffins

*Salsa is great with chips, but it is also a fantastic pantry staple. Think about it: tomatoes, peppers, onions, spice and heat — it's a quick foundation for chili, soup, omelets and casseroles. I love what it does to these quinoa-corn muffins, too. I especially like these made with chipotle salsa, but any thick tomato salsa will do.*

## Storage Tip

Store the cooled muffins in an airtight container in the refrigerator for up to 3 days. Or wrap them in plastic wrap, then foil, completely enclosing them, and freeze for up to 6 months. Let thaw at room temperature for 2 hours before serving.

- **Preheat oven to 400°F (200°C)**
- **12-cup muffin pan, sprayed with nonstick cooking spray**

| | | |
|---|---|---|
| 1 cup | quinoa flour | 250 mL |
| 1 cup | yellow cornmeal (GF, if needed) | 250 mL |
| 1 tbsp | cornstarch or arrowroot | 15 mL |
| 1 tbsp | baking powder (GF, if needed) | 15 mL |
| 2 tsp | ground cumin | 10 mL |
| ½ tsp | fine sea salt | 2 mL |
| 2 | large eggs | 2 |
| ⅔ cup | milk or plain non-dairy milk (such as soy, almond, rice or hemp) | 150 mL |
| ¼ cup | vegetable oil | 60 mL |
| ¾ cup | chunky tomato salsa | 175 mL |

1. In a large bowl, whisk together quinoa flour, cornmeal, cornstarch, baking powder, cumin and salt.
2. In a medium bowl, whisk together eggs, milk and oil until well blended. Stir in salsa until blended.
3. Add the egg mixture to the flour mixture and stir until just blended.
4. Divide batter equally among prepared muffin cups.
5. Bake in preheated oven for 23 to 28 minutes or until tops are golden and a toothpick inserted in the center comes out clean. Let cool in pan on a wire rack for 5 minutes, then transfer to the rack to cool slightly. Serve warm or let cool completely.

# Mushroom Walnut Muffins

**Makes 9 muffins**

*Cottage cheese may sound like an unusual ingredient for muffins, but it has transformative properties: it makes quick breads almost soufflé-like in texture, imparting both lightness and a tender crumb. You can add any combination of extras you like, but I love them with mushrooms and walnuts.*

## Tip

For best results, do not use nonfat cottage cheese.

## Storage Tip

Store the cooled muffins in an airtight container in the refrigerator for up to 3 days.

• **12-cup muffin pan, 9 cups greased**

| | | |
|---|---|---|
| 1 tsp | olive oil | 5 mL |
| 8 oz | cremini or button mushrooms, coarsely chopped | 250 g |
| 1 cup | quinoa flour | 250 mL |
| 1 tsp | baking powder | 5 mL |
| ¼ tsp | fine sea salt | 1 mL |
| ¼ tsp | freshly ground black pepper | 1 mL |
| 4 | large eggs, lightly beaten | 4 |
| ⅔ cup | small-curd cottage cheese | 150 mL |
| 2 tbsp | freshly grated Parmesan cheese | 30 mL |
| ½ cup | chopped toasted walnuts | 125 mL |

1. In a large skillet, heat oil over medium-high heat. Add mushrooms and cook, stirring, for 4 to 5 minutes or until starting to brown and liquid has evaporated. Remove from heat and let cool.
2. Preheat oven to 375°F (190°C).
3. In a large bowl, whisk together quinoa flour, baking powder, salt and pepper. Stir in eggs, cottage cheese and Parmesan until just blended. Fold in sautéed mushrooms and walnuts.
4. Divide batter equally among prepared muffin cups.
5. Bake for 23 to 25 minutes or until tops are golden and a toothpick inserted in the center comes out clean. Let cool in pan on a wire rack for 5 minutes, then transfer to the rack to cool slightly. Serve warm or let cool to room temperature.

# Roasted Pepper Feta Muffins

**Makes
12 muffins**

*These are outstanding muffins, substantial yet tender. I love them alongside a bowl of soup or a salad — they're ideal for mopping up every last bit of soup in the bowl or dressing on the plate.*

## Storage Tip

Store the cooled muffins in an airtight container in the refrigerator for up to 3 days. Or wrap them in plastic wrap, then foil, completely enclosing them, and freeze for up to 6 months. Let thaw at room temperature for 2 hours before serving.

- **Preheat oven to 375°F (190°C)**
- **12-cup muffin pan, sprayed with nonstick cooking spray**

| | | |
|---|---|---|
| 1½ cups | quinoa flour | 375 mL |
| ½ cup | yellow cornmeal (preferably stone-ground; GF, if needed) | 125 mL |
| 2 tsp | baking powder (GF, if needed) | 10 mL |
| 1 tsp | dried oregano | 5 mL |
| ½ tsp | baking soda | 2 mL |
| ½ tsp | fine sea salt | 2 mL |
| 2 | large eggs | 2 |
| 1 cup | buttermilk | 250 mL |
| ¼ cup | olive oil | 60 mL |
| ¾ cup | crumbled feta cheese | 175 mL |
| ½ cup | chopped drained roasted red bell peppers, patted dry | 125 mL |

1. In a large bowl, whisk together quinoa flour, cornmeal, baking powder, oregano, baking soda and salt.
2. In a medium bowl, whisk together eggs, buttermilk and oil until well blended.
3. Add the egg mixture to the flour mixture and stir until just blended. Gently fold in cheese and roasted peppers.
4. Divide batter equally among prepared muffin cups.
5. Bake in preheated oven for 18 to 22 minutes or until tops are golden and a toothpick inserted in the center comes out clean. Let cool in pan on a wire rack for 5 minutes, then transfer to the rack to cool slightly. Serve warm or let cool completely.

# Scallion Cheese Muffins

*Green onions, also called scallions, are commonly paired with cheese, but something really great happens when you team them up with the earthy, nutty flavor of quinoa.*

## Storage Tip

Store the cooled muffins in an airtight container in the refrigerator for up to 3 days. Or wrap them in plastic wrap, then foil, completely enclosing them, and freeze for up to 6 months. Let thaw at room temperature for 2 hours before serving.

- **Preheat oven to 375°F (190°C)**
- **12-cup muffin pan, sprayed with nonstick cooking spray**

| | | |
|---|---|---|
| 2 cups | quinoa flour | 500 mL |
| 2½ tsp | baking powder (GF, if needed) | 12 mL |
| 1½ tsp | dried oregano | 7 mL |
| ½ tsp | fine sea salt | 2 mL |
| 2 | cloves garlic, minced | 2 |
| 2 | large eggs | 2 |
| ¼ cup | olive oil or vegetable oil | 60 mL |
| 1 cup | cottage cheese | 250 mL |
| ½ cup | milk | 125 mL |
| ½ cup | chopped green onions (scallions) | 125 mL |
| ½ cup | freshly grated Parmesan cheese | 125 mL |

1. In a large bowl, whisk together quinoa flour, baking powder, oregano and salt.
2. In a medium bowl, whisk together garlic, eggs and oil until well blended. Whisk in cottage cheese and milk until blended.
3. Add the egg mixture to the flour mixture and stir until just blended. Gently fold in green onions and Parmesan.
4. Divide batter equally among prepared muffin cups.
5. Bake in preheated oven for 20 to 25 minutes or until a toothpick inserted in the center comes out clean. Let cool in pan on a wire rack for 5 minutes, then transfer to the rack to cool slightly. Serve warm or let cool completely.

# Cinnamon Sugar Doughnuts

*Nothing beats these spiced, buttery doughnuts fresh from the oven — and you get the pleasure of filling your house with their warm, cinnamon scent as they bake.*

## Tips

The donuts may also be prepared in two batches in a 12-count mini doughnut pan. Prepare as directed, baking donuts for 5 to 9 minutes.

If you don't own a donut pan, you can prepare the batter in a regular or mini muffin pan. For a regular muffin pan, spray 6 cups with nonstick cooking spray, fill with batter and bake for 11 to 14 minutes or until a toothpick inserted in the center comes out clean. For a mini muffin pan, spray 12 cups with nonstick cooking spray, fill with batter and bake for 7 to 10 minutes or until a toothpick inserted in the center comes out clean.

- **Preheat oven to 375°F (190°C)**
- **6-count doughnut pan, sprayed with nonstick cooking spray**

| | | |
|---|---|---|
| 1 cup | quinoa flour | 250 mL |
| 1¼ tsp | ground cinnamon, divided | 6 mL |
| 1 tsp | baking powder (GF, if needed) | 5 mL |
| ¼ tsp | fine sea salt | 1 mL |
| ⅛ tsp | ground nutmeg | 0.5 mL |
| ⅔ cup | natural cane sugar or packed light brown sugar, divided | 150 mL |
| 2 | large eggs | 2 |
| ¼ cup | buttermilk | 60 mL |
| 3 tbsp | unsalted butter, melted, or vegetable oil | 45 mL |

1. In a medium bowl, whisk together quinoa flour, 1 tsp (5 mL) of the cinnamon, baking powder, salt and nutmeg.
2. In a small bowl, whisk together ½ cup (125 mL) of the sugar, eggs, buttermilk and butter until well blended.
3. Add the egg mixture to the flour mixture and stir until just blended.
4. Divide half the batter equally among prepared doughnut forms (they should be about half full).
5. Bake in preheated oven for 9 to 12 minutes or until doughnuts are golden and spring back when lightly touched. Let cool in pan on a wire rack for 2 minutes, then transfer to the rack. Repeat with the remaining batter.
6. In a shallow dish, combine the remaining sugar and the remaining cinnamon. Sprinkle over both sides of warm doughnuts. Let cool completely.

# Brown Sugar Quinoa Scones

*In this recipe, simple
pantry ingredients come
together with quinoa flour
in homey scones that are
so delicious, you'll be
fighting over the last one.*

## Storage Tip

Store the cooled scones
in an airtight container at
room temperature for up
to 2 days or in the freezer
for up to 3 months. Let
thaw at room temperature
for 1 to 2 hours
before serving.

- **Preheat oven to 400°F (200°C)**
- **Large rimmed baking sheet, lined with parchment paper**

| | | |
|---|---|---|
| 2 cups | quinoa flour | 500 mL |
| 1/4 cup | packed dark brown sugar or natural cane sugar | 60 mL |
| 1 tbsp | baking powder (GF, if needed) | 15 mL |
| 1/2 tsp | fine sea salt | 2 mL |
| 6 tbsp | cold unsalted butter, cut into small pieces | 90 mL |
| 2 | large eggs | 2 |
| 1/2 cup | milk or plain non-dairy milk (such as soy, almond, rice or hemp) | 125 mL |
| 1 tsp | vanilla extract (GF, if needed) | 5 mL |
| 1 tbsp | milk or plain non-dairy milk (such as soy, almond, rice or hemp) | 15 mL |
| 2 tbsp | turbinado sugar (optional) | 30 mL |

1. In a large bowl, whisk together quinoa flour, brown sugar, baking powder and salt. Using a pastry blender or two knives, cut in butter until crumbly. Refrigerate for 10 minutes.

2. In a small bowl, whisk together eggs, 1/2 cup (125 mL) milk and vanilla until well blended.

3. Add the egg mixture to the flour mixture and stir until just blended.

4. Turn dough out onto a work surface lightly floured with quinoa flour. Knead briefly until dough comes together. Gently pat into a 9-inch (23 cm) circle about 3/4 inch (2 cm) thick. Brush with 1 tbsp (15 mL) milk and sprinkle with turbinado sugar (if using). Cut into 10 wedges and place 2 inches (5 cm) apart on prepared baking sheet.

5. Bake in preheated oven for 15 to 20 minutes or until tops are golden brown and a toothpick inserted in the center comes out clean. Transfer scones to a wire rack and let cool for 5 minutes. Serve warm or let cool completely.

# Scottish Oat Scones

*The Scots have long known that oats are not just for porridge: they add flavor, crunch and character to everything. Here, they work their magic in harmony with quinoa flour in a newfangled take on old-fashioned Scottish oat scones. Serve them with ample amounts of jam or marmalade and a mug of tea.*

## Storage Tip

Store the cooled scones in an airtight container at room temperature for up to 2 days or in the freezer for up to 3 months. Let thaw at room temperature for 1 to 2 hours before serving.

- **Preheat oven to 425°F (220°C)**
- **Large rimmed baking sheet, lined with parchment paper**

| | | |
|---|---|---|
| 1⅓ cups | quinoa flour | 325 mL |
| 1¼ cups | large-flake (old-fashioned) rolled oats (certified GF, if needed) | 300 mL |
| ⅓ cup | natural cane sugar or packed light brown sugar | 75 mL |
| 1 tbsp | baking powder (GF, if needed) | 15 mL |
| 1 tsp | ground cinnamon | 5 mL |
| ½ tsp | baking soda | 2 mL |
| ½ tsp | fine sea salt | 2 mL |
| 6 tbsp | cold unsalted butter, cut into small pieces | 90 mL |
| 2 | large eggs | 2 |
| ¾ cup | buttermilk | 175 mL |

1. In a large bowl, whisk together quinoa flour, oats, sugar, baking powder, cinnamon, baking soda and salt. Using a pastry blender or two knives, cut in butter until crumbly. Refrigerate for 10 minutes.

2. In a medium bowl, whisk together eggs and buttermilk until well blended.

3. Add the egg mixture to the flour mixture and stir until just blended.

4. Turn dough out onto a work surface lightly floured with quinoa flour. Knead briefly until dough comes together. Gently pat into an 8-inch (20 cm) circle about ¾ inch (2 cm) thick. Cut into 8 wedges and place 2 inches (5 cm) apart on prepared baking sheet.

5. Bake in preheated oven for 10 to 13 minutes or until tops are golden brown and a toothpick inserted in the center comes out clean. Let cool on pan on a wire rack for 5 minutes, then transfer to the rack to cool for 5 minutes. Serve warm or let cool completely.

## Variations

Replace the butter with 6 tbsp (90 mL) of unrefined virgin coconut oil.

Gently fold in ½ cup (125 mL) raisins, dried cranberries, chopped dates or chopped dried cherries at the end of step 3.

# Dried Cherry Maple Scones

*Dried cherries and maple syrup infuse a simple scone recipe with the rich flavors of fall.*

## Storage Tip

Store the cooled scones in an airtight container at room temperature for up to 2 days or in the freezer for up to 3 months. Let thaw at room temperature for 1 to 2 hours before serving.

- **Preheat oven to 350°F (180°C)**
- **Large rimmed baking sheet, lined with parchment paper**

| | | |
|---|---|---|
| 1¼ cups | quinoa flour | 300 mL |
| 1 cup | large-flake (old-fashioned) rolled oats (certified GF, if needed) | 250 mL |
| ¼ cup | natural cane sugar or packed light brown sugar | 60 mL |
| 2¼ tsp | baking powder (GF, if needed) | 11 mL |
| ¾ tsp | ground cinnamon | 3 mL |
| ½ tsp | baking soda | 2 mL |
| ½ tsp | fine sea salt | 2 mL |
| 6 tbsp | cold unsalted butter, cut into small pieces | 90 mL |
| 2 | large eggs | 2 |
| ¼ cup | buttermilk | 60 mL |
| 4 tbsp | pure maple syrup, divided | 60 mL |
| 1 tsp | vanilla extract (GF, if needed) | 5 mL |
| ½ cup | dried tart cherries | 125 mL |
| 1 tbsp | turbinado sugar | 15 mL |

1. In a large bowl, whisk together quinoa flour, oats, cane sugar, baking powder, cinnamon, baking soda and salt. Using a pastry blender or two knives, cut in butter until crumbly. Refrigerate for 10 minutes.

2. In a medium bowl, whisk together eggs, buttermilk, 3 tbsp (45 mL) of the maple syrup and vanilla until well blended.

3. Add the egg mixture and dried cherries to the flour mixture and stir until just blended.

4. Turn dough out onto a work surface lightly floured with quinoa flour. Knead briefly until dough comes together. Gently pat into an 8-inch (20 cm) circle about ¾ inch (2 cm) thick. Brush top with the remaining maple syrup and sprinkle with turbinado sugar. Cut into 8 wedges and place 2 inches (5 cm) apart on prepared baking sheet.

5. Bake in preheated oven for 18 to 21 minutes or until tops are golden brown and a toothpick inserted in the center comes out clean. Let cool on pan on a wire rack for 5 minutes, then transfer to the rack to cool for 5 minutes. Serve warm or let cool completely.

# Pumpkin Spice Scones

**Makes
10 scones**

*Quinoa flour underscores
these scones with an
aromatic, nutty nuance,
boosting the autumnal
flavors of pumpkin and
spice. The dough is egg-
free, resulting in a tender
yet sturdy texture that
holds up well to toasting
or a generous schmear
of jam.*

## Storage Tip

Store the cooled scones
in an airtight container at
room temperature for up
to 2 days or in the freezer
for up to 3 months. Let
thaw at room temperature
for 1 to 2 hours
before serving.

- **Preheat oven to 400°F (200°C)**
- **Large rimmed baking sheet, lined with parchment paper**

| | | |
|---|---|---|
| 2 cups | quinoa flour | 500 mL |
| 1 tbsp | baking powder (GF, if needed) | 15 mL |
| 2 tsp | ground cinnamon | 10 mL |
| ½ tsp | ground nutmeg | 2 mL |
| ½ tsp | fine sea salt | 2 mL |
| ⅓ cup | cold unsalted butter or chilled unrefined virgin coconut oil, cut into small pieces | 75 mL |
| ⅓ cup | packed light brown sugar or natural cane sugar | 75 mL |
| 1 cup | pumpkin purée (not pie filling) | 250 mL |
| ⅓ cup | milk or plain non-dairy milk (such as soy, almond, rice or hemp) | 75 mL |
| 1 tsp | vanilla extract (GF, if needed) | 5 mL |
| 1 tbsp | turbinado sugar (optional) | 15 mL |

1. In a large bowl, whisk together quinoa flour, baking powder, cinnamon, nutmeg and salt. Using a pastry blender or two knives, cut in butter until crumbly. Refrigerate for 10 minutes.
2. In a small bowl, whisk together brown sugar, pumpkin, milk and vanilla until well blended.
3. Add the pumpkin mixture to the flour mixture and stir until just blended.
4. Turn dough out onto a work surface lightly floured with quinoa flour. Knead briefly until dough comes together. Gently pat into a 9-inch (23 cm) circle about ¾ inch (2 cm) thick. If desired, sprinkle top with turbinado sugar. Cut into 10 wedges and place 2 inches (5 cm) apart on prepared baking sheet.
5. Bake in preheated oven for 13 to 17 minutes or until a toothpick inserted in the center comes out clean. Transfer scones to a wire rack and let cool for 5 minutes. Serve warm or let cool completely.

# Ginger Cardamom Drop Scones

*Cardamom and ginger play starring roles in Swedish baked goods. Combined with quinoa flour and oats, the duo gives drop scones an irresistible Scandinavian bakery aroma.*

## Storage Tip

Store the cooled scones in an airtight container at room temperature for up to 2 days or in the freezer for up to 3 months. Let thaw at room temperature for 1 to 2 hours before serving.

- **Preheat oven to 400°F (200°C)**
- **Large rimmed baking sheet, lined with parchment paper**

| | | |
|---|---|---|
| 1½ cups | quinoa flour | 375 mL |
| ½ cup | large-flake (old-fashioned) rolled oats (certified GF, if needed) | 125 mL |
| 3 tbsp | natural cane sugar or packed light brown sugar | 45 mL |
| 2 tsp | baking powder (GF, if needed) | 10 mL |
| 1½ tsp | ground ginger | 7 mL |
| ¾ tsp | ground cardamom | 3 mL |
| ½ tsp | fine sea salt | 2 mL |
| 2 | large eggs | 2 |
| 1 cup | buttermilk | 250 mL |
| 3 tbsp | unsalted butter, melted and cooled | 45 mL |
| 1 tsp | vanilla extract (GF, if needed) | 5 mL |
| ¼ cup | finely chopped crystallized ginger | 60 mL |
| 3 tbsp | turbinado sugar (optional) | 45 mL |

1. In a large bowl, whisk together quinoa flour, oats, cane sugar, baking powder, ground ginger, cardamom and salt.

2. In a small bowl, whisk together eggs, buttermilk, butter and vanilla until well blended.

3. Add the egg mixture and crystallized ginger to the flour mixture and stir until just blended.

4. Drop dough by ⅓-cup (75 mL) measures 2 inches (5 cm) apart on prepared baking sheet. Sprinkle tops with turbinado sugar (if using).

5. Bake in preheated oven for 15 to 20 minutes or until tops are golden brown and a toothpick inserted in the center comes out clean. Transfer scones to a wire rack and let cool for 5 minutes. Serve warm or let cool completely.

# Gingerbread Scones with Lemon Drizzle

## Makes 8 scones

*A robust trio of gingerbread spices — ginger, cinnamon and cloves — coalesce with nutty quinoa and a lemon drizzle to give tender scones newfound vibrancy.*

## Tips

For a tropical twist, substitute virgin coconut oil for the butter in the muffins, and lime zest and juice for the lemon zest and juice in the glaze.

If you like, you can add ½ cup (125 mL) dried cranberries or tart dried cherries at the end of step 3.

## Storage Tip

Store the cooled, unglazed scones in an airtight container at room temperature for up to 2 days or in the freezer for up to 3 months. Let thaw at room temperature for 1 to 2 hours before glazing and serving.

- **Preheat oven to 400°F (200°C)**
- **Large rimmed baking sheet, lined with parchment paper**

| | | |
|---|---|---|
| 2 cups | quinoa flour | 500 mL |
| 3 tbsp | natural cane sugar or packed dark brown sugar | 45 mL |
| 2 tbsp | cornstarch or arrowroot | 30 mL |
| 1 tbsp | ground ginger | 15 mL |
| 2 tsp | baking powder (GF, if needed) | 10 mL |
| 1½ tsp | ground cinnamon | 7 mL |
| ½ tsp | ground cloves | 2 mL |
| ½ tsp | baking soda | 2 mL |
| ½ tsp | fine sea salt | 2 mL |
| ¼ cup | cold unsalted butter, cut into small pieces | 60 mL |
| 2 | large eggs | 2 |
| ½ cup | buttermilk or plain yogurt | 125 mL |
| ⅓ cup | dark (cooking) molasses | 75 mL |

### Lemon Glaze

| | | |
|---|---|---|
| 1 cup | confectioners' (icing) sugar | 250 mL |
| ½ tsp | finely grated lemon zest | 2 mL |
| 1 tsp | freshly squeezed lemon juice | 5 mL |

1. In a large bowl, whisk together quinoa flour, sugar, cornstarch, ginger, baking powder, cinnamon, cloves, baking soda and salt. Using a pastry blender or two knives, cut in butter until crumbly. Refrigerate for 10 minutes.

2. In a medium bowl, whisk together eggs, buttermilk and molasses until well blended.

3. Add the egg mixture to the flour mixture and stir until just blended.

4. Turn dough out onto a work surface lightly floured with quinoa flour. Knead briefly until dough comes together. Gently pat into an 8-inch (20 cm) circle about ¾ inch (2 cm) thick. Cut into 8 wedges and place 2 inches (5 cm) apart on prepared baking sheet.

5. Bake in preheated oven for 12 to 15 minutes or until a toothpick inserted in the center comes out clean. Let cool on pan on a wire rack for 5 minutes, then transfer to the rack to cool completely.

6. *Glaze:* In a small bowl, combine confectioners' sugar, lemon zest and lemon juice until smooth. Drizzle over tops of cooled scones.

# Mixed Berry Drop Scones

**Makes
12 scones**

*A little easy preparation, plus a short spell in the oven, yields gorgeous quinoa scones that showcase summer berries in a most delicious way.*

**Tip**

For the berries, try blueberries, cranberries, blackberries and/or raspberries.

**Storage Tip**

Store the cooled scones in an airtight container at room temperature for up to 2 days or in the freezer for up to 3 months. Let thaw at room temperature for 1 to 2 hours before serving.

- **Preheat oven to 400°F (200°C)**
- **Large rimmed baking sheet, lined with parchment paper**

| 2 cups | quinoa flour | 500 mL |
|---|---|---|
| 2 tsp | baking powder (GF, if needed) | 10 mL |
| 1/2 tsp | baking soda | 2 mL |
| 1/2 tsp | fine sea salt | 2 mL |
| 6 tbsp | cold unsalted butter, cut into small pieces | 90 mL |
| 1 1/2 cups | assorted berries (see tip, at left) | 375 mL |
| 2 | large eggs | 2 |
| 1 cup | buttermilk | 250 mL |
| 3 tbsp | liquid honey, pure maple syrup or brown rice syrup | 45 mL |
| 2 tsp | finely grated orange zest or lemon zest | 10 mL |
| 2 tbsp | turbinado sugar (optional) | 30 mL |

1. In a large bowl, whisk together quinoa flour, baking powder, baking soda and salt. Using a pastry blender or two knives, cut in butter until crumbly. Refrigerate for 10 minutes. Toss in berries.

2. In a small bowl, whisk together eggs, buttermilk, honey and orange zest until well blended.

3. Add the egg mixture to the flour mixture and stir until just blended.

4. Drop dough by 1/4-cup (60 mL) measures 2 inches (5 cm) apart on prepared baking sheet. Sprinkle tops with sugar (if using).

5. Bake in preheated oven for 15 to 20 minutes or until tops are golden brown and a toothpick inserted in the center comes out clean. Transfer scones to a wire rack and let cool for 5 minutes. Serve warm or let cool completely.

# Quinoa Buttermilk Biscuits

*Homey and old-fashioned, these comforting biscuits can be on the table in a flash, thanks to a quick method for shaping and cutting out the biscuits (no rolling, rerolling or biscuit cutters involved).*

## Storage Tip

Store the cooled biscuits in an airtight container at room temperature for up to 2 days or in the freezer for up to 3 months. Let thaw at room temperature for 1 to 2 hours before serving.

- **Preheat oven to 400°F (200°C)**
- **Large rimmed baking sheet, lined with parchment paper**

| | | |
|---|---|---|
| 2 cups | quinoa flour | 500 mL |
| 1 tbsp | cornstarch or arrowroot | 15 mL |
| 2¼ tsp | baking powder (GF, if needed) | 11 mL |
| ½ tsp | fine sea salt | 2 mL |
| ¼ tsp | baking soda | 1 mL |
| ⅓ cup | cold unsalted butter, cut into small pieces | 75 mL |
| ¾ cup | buttermilk | 175 mL |
| 3 tbsp | liquid honey or pure maple syrup | 45 mL |
| 1 tbsp | buttermilk | 15 mL |

1. In a large bowl, whisk together quinoa flour, cornstarch, baking powder, salt and baking soda. Using a pastry blender or two knives, cut in butter until crumbly. Refrigerate for 10 minutes.

2. In a small bowl, whisk together ¾ cup (175 mL) buttermilk and honey until well blended.

3. Add the buttermilk mixture to the flour mixture and stir until just blended.

4. Turn dough out onto a work surface lightly floured with quinoa flour. Knead briefly until dough comes together. Gently pat into an 8- by 6-inch (20 by 15 cm) rectangle about ¾ inch (2 cm) thick. Cut into twelve 2-inch (5 cm) squares and place 2 inches (5 cm) apart on prepared baking sheet. Brush with 1 tbsp (15 mL) buttermilk.

5. Bake in preheated oven for 12 to 15 minutes or until golden brown. Transfer biscuits to a wire rack and let cool slightly. Serve warm or let cool completely.

# Cheddar Biscuits

*These are everything cheese biscuits should be: crisp golden brown exteriors, yet pillowy inside, stuffed with a generous amount of Cheddar that bursts forth as they bake.*

## Storage Tip

Store the cooled biscuits in an airtight container at room temperature for up to 2 days or in the freezer for up to 3 months. Let thaw at room temperature for 1 to 2 hours before serving.

- **Preheat oven to 400°F (200°C)**
- **Large rimmed baking sheet, lined with parchment paper**

| | | |
|---|---|---|
| 1½ cups | quinoa flour | 375 mL |
| ½ cup | stone-ground cornmeal (GF, if needed) | 125 mL |
| 2½ tsp | baking powder (GF, if needed) | 12 mL |
| ½ tsp | fine sea salt | 2 mL |
| ⅛ tsp | cayenne pepper | 0.5 mL |
| ⅓ cup | cold unsalted butter, cut into small pieces | 75 mL |
| 1 | large egg | 1 |
| ⅔ cup | buttermilk | 150 mL |
| 1 tbsp | Dijon mustard | 15 mL |
| 4 oz | extra-sharp (extra-old) Cheddar cheese, cut into small pieces | 125 g |
| 1 tbsp | buttermilk | 15 mL |

1. In a large bowl, whisk together quinoa flour, cornmeal, baking powder, salt and cayenne. Using a pastry blender or two knives, cut in butter until crumbly. Refrigerate for 10 minutes.

2. In a small bowl, whisk together egg, ⅔ cup (150 mL) buttermilk and mustard until well blended.

3. Add the buttermilk mixture and cheese to the flour mixture and stir until just blended.

4. Turn dough out onto a work surface lightly floured with quinoa flour. Knead briefly until dough comes together. Gently pat into an 8- by 6-inch (20 by 15 cm) rectangle about ¾ inch (2 cm) thick. Cut into twelve 2-inch (5 cm) squares and place 2 inches (5 cm) apart on prepared baking sheet. Brush with 1 tbsp (15 mL) buttermilk.

5. Bake in preheated oven for 12 to 15 minutes or until golden brown. Transfer biscuits to a wire rack and let cool slightly. Serve warm or let cool completely.

# Seeded Multigrain Biscuits

*These multi-textured multigrain biscuits are as good with scrambled eggs or a bowl of midday soup as they are with a robust supper.*

## Storage Tip

Store the cooled biscuits in an airtight container at room temperature for up to 2 days or in the freezer for up to 3 months. Let thaw at room temperature for 1 to 2 hours before serving.

- **Preheat oven to 400°F (200°C)**
- **Large rimmed baking sheet, lined with parchment paper**

| | | |
|---|---|---|
| 1¾ cups | quinoa flour | 425 mL |
| ½ cup | stone-ground cornmeal (GF, if needed) | 125 mL |
| 1 tbsp | cornstarch or arrowroot | 15 mL |
| 1 tbsp | sesame seeds | 15 mL |
| 1 tbsp | poppy seeds | 15 mL |
| 1 tbsp | fennel seeds | 15 mL |
| 1½ tsp | baking soda | 7 mL |
| ½ tsp | baking powder (GF, if needed) | 2 mL |
| ½ tsp | fine sea salt | 2 mL |
| 6 tbsp | cold unsalted butter, cut into small pieces | 90 mL |
| 1 cup | buttermilk | 250 mL |
| 2 tbsp | liquid honey or brown rice syrup | 30 mL |

1. In a large bowl, whisk together quinoa flour, cornmeal, cornstarch, sesame seeds, poppy seeds, fennel seeds, baking soda, baking powder and salt. Using a pastry blender or two knives, cut in butter until crumbly. Refrigerate for 10 minutes.

2. In a small bowl, whisk together buttermilk and honey until well blended.

3. Add the buttermilk mixture to the flour mixture and stir until just blended.

4. Turn dough out onto a work surface lightly floured with quinoa flour. Knead briefly until dough comes together. Gently pat into an 8-inch (20 cm) square about ½ inch (1 cm) thick. Cut into sixteen 2-inch (5 cm) squares and place 2 inches (5 cm) apart on prepared baking sheet.

5. Bake in preheated oven for 12 to 15 minutes or until golden brown. Transfer biscuits to a wire rack and let cool slightly. Serve warm or let cool completely.

# Parmesan Pepper Drop Biscuits

**Makes
12 biscuits**

*Buttermilk gives these quick, cheesy biscuits their exceptionally light texture; freshly cracked black pepper and Dijon mustard provide the kick. But it's the salty flurry of Parmesan in combination with nutty-sweet quinoa that makes the biscuits extra-special.*

## Storage Tip

Store the cooled biscuits in an airtight container at room temperature for up to 2 days or in the freezer for up to 3 months. Let thaw at room temperature for 1 to 2 hours before serving.

- **Preheat oven to 400°F (200°C)**
- **Large rimmed baking sheet, lined with parchment paper**

| | | |
|---|---|---|
| 1⅓ cups | quinoa flour | 325 mL |
| ⅓ cup | quick-cooking rolled oats (certified GF, if needed) | 75 mL |
| ¼ cup | stone-ground cornmeal (GF, if needed) | 60 mL |
| 2¼ tsp | baking powder (GF, if needed) | 11 mL |
| 1 tsp | freshly cracked black pepper | 5 mL |
| 1 tsp | natural cane sugar or packed light brown sugar | 5 mL |
| ½ tsp | fine sea salt | 2 mL |
| ¼ tsp | baking soda | 1 mL |
| 1 | large egg | 1 |
| 1 cup | buttermilk | 250 mL |
| ¼ cup | unsalted butter, melted and cooled | 60 mL |
| 2 tsp | Dijon mustard | 10 mL |
| ½ cup | freshly grated Parmesan cheese | 125 mL |

1. In a large bowl, whisk together quinoa flour, oats, cornmeal, baking powder, pepper, sugar, salt and baking soda.
2. In a small bowl, whisk together egg, buttermilk, butter and mustard until well blended.
3. Add the buttermilk mixture and cheese to the flour mixture and stir until just blended.
4. Drop dough by ¼-cup (60 mL) measures 2 inches (5 cm) apart on prepared baking sheet.
5. Bake in preheated oven for 12 to 15 minutes or until golden brown. Transfer biscuits to a wire rack and let cool slightly. Serve warm or let cool completely.

# Sweet Potato Biscuits

*Sweet potatoes lend
heartiness and a
natural sweetness to
these biscuits. Team
with savory dishes as
a sidekick, or split and
spread with jam or nut
butter for a healthy
breakfast to go.*

## Tip

Prepare the mashed
sweet potato without milk
and butter. Here's how
to easily cook it in the
microwave: Scrub sweet
potato (about 1 medium
for this recipe) and pierce
a few times with a fork.
Place on a microwave-safe
plate lined with a paper
towel. Microwave on High,
turning halfway through,
for 4 to 5 minutes or until
tender. Let cool. Cut in half,
scoop the flesh into a bowl
and mash with a fork.

## Storage Tip

Store the cooled biscuits
in an airtight container at
room temperature for up
to 2 days or in the freezer
for up to 3 months. Let
thaw at room temperature
for 1 to 2 hours
before serving.

- **Preheat oven to 400°F (200°C)**
- **Large rimmed baking sheet, lined with parchment paper**

| | | |
|---|---|---|
| 2 cups | quinoa flour | 500 mL |
| 1 tbsp | cornstarch or arrowroot | 15 mL |
| 2½ tsp | baking powder (GF, if needed) | 12 mL |
| 1 tsp | dried rubbed sage or ground cinnamon | 5 mL |
| ½ tsp | fine sea salt | 2 mL |
| ⅓ cup | cold unsalted butter, cut into small pieces | 75 mL |
| ¾ cup | mashed cooked sweet potato | 175 mL |
| ⅓ cup | buttermilk | 75 mL |
| 3 tbsp | pure maple syrup or liquid honey | 45 mL |

1. In a large bowl, whisk together quinoa flour, cornstarch, baking powder, sage and salt. Using a pastry blender or two knives, cut in butter until crumbly. Refrigerate for 10 minutes.

2. In a small bowl, whisk together sweet potato, buttermilk and maple syrup until well blended.

3. Add the sweet potato mixture to the flour mixture and stir until just blended.

4. Turn dough out onto a work surface lightly floured with quinoa flour. Knead briefly until dough comes together. Gently pat into an 8- by 6-inch (20 by 15 cm) rectangle about ¾ inch (2 cm) thick. Cut into twelve 2-inch (5 cm) squares and place 2 inches (5 cm) apart on prepared baking sheet.

5. Bake in preheated oven for 13 to 17 minutes or until golden brown. Transfer biscuits to a wire rack and let cool slightly. Serve warm or let cool completely.

# Quinoa Popovers

*Offering tremendous
homestyle appeal, these
light, airy popovers make
a wonderful complement
to almost any meal. No
matter how tempting
the aroma coming from
your oven as they bake,
resist opening the oven
to check them until
about 5 minutes before
they're finished baking;
check too soon, and they
will deflate.*

## Tips

These popovers may
also be made in a 12-cup
muffin pan with 6 cups
buttered. Reduce the
second baking time by
about 5 minutes.

If using a 12-cup popover
pan or muffin pan, butter
every other cup for
even baking.

- **Preheat oven to 450°F (230°C)**
- **Blender or food processor**
- **6-cup nonstick popover pan, generously buttered**

| | | |
|---|---|---:|
| 1 cup | quinoa flour | 250 mL |
| ¼ tsp | fine sea salt | 1 mL |
| 3 | large eggs, at room temperature | 3 |
| 1 cup | milk | 250 mL |
| 1 tbsp | unsalted butter, melted, or olive oil | 15 mL |

**1.** In blender, combine flour, salt, eggs, milk and butter; process until smooth.

**2.** Divide batter equally among prepared muffin cups.

**3.** Bake in preheated oven for 10 minutes. Without opening oven door, reduce heat to 375°F (190°C). Bake for 15 to 20 minutes or until puffed and golden brown. Run a thin knife between the edge of each popover and the cup to loosen. Lift popovers from cups and serve immediately.

## Variations

*Sharp Cheddar Quinoa Popovers:* Add 1 tsp (5 mL) Dijon mustard and a pinch of cayenne pepper in step 1. Sprinkle popovers with ½ cup (125 mL) shredded extra-sharp (extra-old) Cheddar cheese before the final 5 minutes of baking.

*Parmesan Sage Quinoa Popovers:* Add ¼ cup (60 mL) freshly grated Parmesan cheese and 1 tsp (5 mL) rubbed dried sage in step 1. Sprinkle popovers with an additional ¼ cup (60 mL) Parmesan before the final 5 minutes of baking.

# Multigrain Sandwich Bread

This no-nonsense, yeast-free, gluten-free sandwich loaf is guaranteed to please. Its subtle sweetness works beautifully with any number of sandwich fillings, from turkey to cream cheese to roasted vegetables.

## Storage Tip

Store the cooled bread, wrapped in foil or plastic wrap, in the refrigerator for up to 5 days. Alternatively, wrap it in plastic wrap, then foil, completely enclosing bread, and freeze for up to 3 months. Let thaw at room temperature for 4 to 6 hours before serving.

- **8- by 4-inch (20 by 10 cm) metal loaf pan, sprayed with nonstick cooking spray**

| | | |
|---|---|---|
| 1½ cups | multigrain hot cereal (GF, if needed) | 375 mL |
| 2 cups | buttermilk | 500 mL |
| 1⅓ cups | quinoa flour | 325 mL |
| 1 tbsp | cornstarch or arrowroot | 15 mL |
| 2 tsp | baking powder (GF, if needed) | 10 mL |
| 1¼ tsp | baking soda | 6 mL |
| 1¼ tsp | fine sea salt | 6 mL |
| 2 | large eggs | 2 |
| ½ cup | olive or vegetable oil | 125 mL |
| ¼ cup | dark (cooking) molasses or liquid honey | 60 mL |

1. In a large bowl, combine cereal and buttermilk. Let stand for 20 minutes.
2. Preheat oven to 375°F (190°C).
3. In another large bowl, whisk together quinoa flour, cornstarch, baking powder, baking soda and salt.
4. Whisk eggs, oil and molasses into cereal mixture until well blended.
5. Add the egg mixture to the flour mixture and stir until just blended.
6. Spread batter evenly in prepared pan.
7. Bake for 55 to 60 minutes or until a toothpick inserted in the center comes out clean. Let cool in pan on a wire rack for 5 minutes, then transfer to the rack. Serve warm or let cool completely.

# Quinoa Irish Soda Bread

*Dense, hearty and easy to make, this quinoa version of Irish soda bread has an earthy, subtle sweetness that makes a slice as delightful with a bowl of stew as it is slathered with jam. Some soda breads are baked free-form, but this one is best baked in a loaf pan.*

## Storage Tip

Store the cooled bread, wrapped in foil or plastic wrap, in the refrigerator for up to 3 days. Alternatively, wrap it in plastic wrap, then foil, completely enclosing bread, and freeze for up to 3 months. Let thaw at room temperature for 4 to 6 hours before serving.

- **Preheat oven to 350°F (180°C)**
- **8- by 4-inch (20 by 10 cm) metal loaf pan, sprayed with nonstick cooking spray**

| | | |
|---|---|---|
| 2 cups | quinoa flour | 500 mL |
| 1¾ tsp | baking powder (GF, if needed) | 8 mL |
| ½ tsp | fine sea salt | 5 mL |
| ¼ tsp | baking soda | 1 mL |
| 1 cup | buttermilk | 250 mL |
| 1 tbsp | liquid honey | 15 mL |

1. In a medium bowl, whisk together quinoa flour, baking powder, salt and baking soda.
2. In a small bowl, whisk together buttermilk and honey until well blended.
3. Add the buttermilk mixture to the flour mixture and stir until just blended.
4. Spread batter evenly in prepared pan. Using a serrated knife, cut 3 to 4 deep, diagonal slashes across the top.
5. Bake in preheated oven for 35 to 40 minutes or until a toothpick inserted in the center comes out clean. Let cool in pan on a wire rack for 5 minutes, then transfer to the rack. Serve warm or let cool completely.

## Variations

*Caraway Currant Soda Bread:* Gently fold in ½ cup (125 mL) dried currants and 1 tbsp (15 mL) caraway seeds at the end of step 3.

*Sesame Soda Bread:* Gently fold in 2 tbsp (30 mL) toasted sesame seeds at the end of step 3.

*Golden Raisin Soda Bread:* Gently fold in ½ cup (125 mL) golden raisins and 2 tsp (10 mL) finely grated orange zest at the end of step 3.

# Lager Quinoa Bread

*Got beer? Then you've got bread. Beer and quinoa have a natural affinity, so don't be surprised if one slice isn't enough.*

## Storage Tip

Store the cooled bread, wrapped in foil or plastic wrap, in the refrigerator for up to 3 days. Alternatively, wrap it in plastic wrap, then foil, completely enclosing bread, and freeze for up to 3 months. Let thaw at room temperature for 4 to 6 hours before serving.

- **Preheat oven to 375°F (190°C)**
- **9- by 5-inch (23 by 12.5 cm) metal loaf pan, sprayed with nonstick cooking spray**

| | | |
|---|---|---|
| 3 cups | quinoa flour | 750 mL |
| 1 tbsp | baking powder (GF, if needed) | 15 mL |
| 1 tsp | fine sea salt | 5 mL |
| 1 | bottle (12 oz/341 mL) lager beer (GF, if needed), at room temperature | 1 |
| ¼ cup | unsalted butter, melted | 60 mL |
| 3 tbsp | liquid honey | 45 mL |

1. In a large bowl, whisk together quinoa flour, baking powder and salt. Add beer, butter and honey all at once and stir as little as possible until just blended.
2. Spread batter evenly in prepared pan.
3. Bake in preheated oven for 55 to 60 minutes or until top is golden and a toothpick inserted in the center comes out clean. Let cool in pan on a wire rack for 5 minutes, then transfer to the rack. Serve warm or let cool completely.

## Variations

*Cheese Dill Beer Bread:* Add 1 tbsp (15 mL) dried dillweed to the flour mixture. Gently fold in 1¼ cups (300 mL) shredded Gruyère or extra-sharp (extra-old) Cheddar cheese at the end of step 1.

*Guinness Quinoa Bread:* Substitute an equal amount of Guinness or another dark beer for the lager-style beer. Replace the honey with 3 tbsp (45 mL) dark (cooking) molasses.

# White Cheddar Herb Bread

*A sprinkling of herbs and a punch of extra-sharp white Cheddar cheese brings out the earthy nuances of quinoa flour in this inventive bread.*

## Storage Tip

Store the cooled bread, wrapped in foil or plastic wrap, in the refrigerator for up to 5 days. Alternatively, wrap it in plastic wrap, then foil, completely enclosing bread, and freeze for up to 3 months. Let thaw at room temperature for 4 to 6 hours before serving.

- **Preheat oven to 350°F (180°C)**
- **8- by 4-inch (20 by 10 cm) metal loaf pan, sprayed with nonstick cooking spray**

| | | |
|---|---|---|
| 1½ cups | quinoa flour | 375 mL |
| 2 tsp | baking powder (GF, if needed) | 10 mL |
| 1¼ tsp | fine sea salt | 6 mL |
| ¼ tsp | freshly ground black pepper | 1 mL |
| 1¼ cups | shredded extra-sharp (extra-old) white Cheddar cheese | 300 mL |
| 1 | clove garlic, minced | 1 |
| ½ cup | packed fresh flat-leaf (Italian) parsley leaves, chopped | 125 mL |
| 2 tsp | minced fresh thyme | 10 mL |
| 2 tsp | minced fresh sage | 10 mL |
| 1 | egg | 1 |
| ½ cup | milk | 125 mL |
| ¼ cup | olive oil | 60 mL |

1. In a medium bowl, whisk together quinoa flour, baking powder, salt and pepper. Stir in cheese.
2. In a small bowl, whisk together garlic, parsley, thyme, sage, egg, milk and oil until blended.
3. Add the egg mixture to the flour mixture and stir until just blended.
4. Spread batter evenly in prepared pan.
5. Bake in preheated oven for 45 to 50 minutes or until top is golden and a toothpick inserted in the center comes out clean. Let cool in pan on a wire rack for 5 minutes, then transfer to the rack. Serve warm or let cool completely.

# Fresh Herb and Pesto Bread

*Ready-made pesto is a harried cook's best friend, adding an instant punch of basil-garlic flavor to a wide range of dishes. Here, it co-stars with fresh herbs in a fantastic quinoa loaf that delivers the concentrated taste of summer.*

## Storage Tip

Store the cooled bread, wrapped in foil or plastic wrap, in the refrigerator for up to 5 days. Alternatively, wrap it in plastic wrap, then foil, completely enclosing bread, and freeze for up to 3 months. Let thaw at room temperature for 4 to 6 hours before serving.

- **Preheat oven to 350°F (180°C)**
- **8- by 4-inch (20 by 10 cm) metal loaf pan, sprayed with nonstick cooking spray**

| | | |
|---|---|---|
| 2 cups | quinoa flour | 500 mL |
| 2 tsp | baking powder (GF, if needed) | 10 mL |
| ½ tsp | fine sea salt | 2 mL |
| ½ tsp | baking soda | 2 mL |
| 2 | large eggs | 2 |
| 1 cup | buttermilk | 250 mL |
| ⅓ cup | basil pesto | 75 mL |
| ½ cup | packed fresh flat-leaf (Italian) parsley leaves, chopped | 125 mL |
| 3 tbsp | minced fresh chives | 45 mL |

1. In a large bowl, whisk together quinoa flour, baking powder, salt and baking soda.
2. In a medium bowl, whisk together eggs, buttermilk and pesto until well blended. Stir in parsley and chives.
3. Add the egg mixture to the flour mixture and stir until just blended.
4. Spread batter evenly in prepared pan.
5. Bake in preheated oven for 50 to 55 minutes or until top is golden brown and a toothpick inserted in the center comes out clean. Let cool in pan on a wire rack for 10 minutes, then transfer to the rack to cool.

# Rosemary Walnut Bread

*Rosemary does something splendid to quinoa, resulting in an especially delicious quick bread that is terrific on its own or layered into a sandwich. Studded with crunchy walnuts, it is also worth savoring as morning toast with a spread of orange marmalade.*

## Tip

An equal amount of chopped toasted pecans may be used in place of the walnuts.

## Storage Tip

Store the cooled bread, wrapped in foil or plastic wrap, in the refrigerator for up to 5 days. Alternatively, wrap it in plastic wrap, then foil, completely enclosing bread, and freeze for up to 3 months. Let thaw at room temperature for 4 to 6 hours before serving.

- Preheat oven to 350°F (180°C)
- 8- by 4-inch (20 by 10 cm) metal loaf pan, sprayed with nonstick cooking spray

| | | |
|---|---|---|
| 2¼ cups | quinoa flour | 550 mL |
| 1 tbsp | minced fresh rosemary | 15 mL |
| 1½ tsp | baking soda | 7 mL |
| ¾ tsp | fine sea salt | 3 mL |
| 2 | large eggs, beaten | 2 |
| 1 cup | buttermilk | 250 mL |
| ⅓ cup | liquid honey, brown rice syrup or dark (cooking) molasses | 75 mL |
| 2 tbsp | extra virgin olive oil | 30 mL |
| 1 cup | chopped toasted walnuts | 250 mL |

1. In a large bowl, whisk together quinoa flour, rosemary, baking soda and salt.
2. In a medium bowl, whisk together eggs, buttermilk, honey and oil until blended.
3. Add the buttermilk mixture to the flour mixture and stir until just blended. Gently fold in walnuts.
4. Spread batter evenly in prepared pan.
5. Bake in preheated oven for 45 to 55 minutes or until top is golden brown and a toothpick inserted in the center comes out clean. Let cool in pan on a wire rack for 10 minutes, then transfer to the rack to cool.

## Variation

*Toasted Walnut Bread:* Omit the rosemary.

# Caraway Bread

*Caraway seeds have a subtle licorice flavor that gives an Old World nuance to this modern quick bread.*

## Tip

Crushing the caraway seeds greatly enhances their aromatic flavor. The process is a snap: place the seeds in a small sealable plastic bag, seal and pound with a mallet or rolling pin until coarsely crushed.

## Storage Tip

Store the cooled bread, wrapped in foil or plastic wrap, in the refrigerator for up to 5 days. Alternatively, wrap it in plastic wrap, then foil, completely enclosing bread, and freeze for up to 3 months. Let thaw at room temperature for 4 to 6 hours before serving.

- Preheat oven to 350°F (180°C)
- 8- by 4-inch (20 by 10 cm) metal loaf pan, sprayed with nonstick cooking spray

| | | |
|---|---|---|
| 2 cups | quinoa flour | 500 mL |
| 2 tbsp | caraway seeds, crushed (see tip, at left) | 30 mL |
| 1½ tsp | baking powder (GF, if needed) | 7 mL |
| 1 tsp | fine sea salt | 5 mL |
| ½ tsp | baking soda | 2 mL |
| 2 | eggs | 2 |
| ⅔ cup | buttermilk | 150 mL |
| ¼ cup | unsalted butter, melted, or olive oil | 60 mL |
| 3 tbsp | liquid honey | 45 mL |

1. In a large bowl, whisk together quinoa flour, caraway seeds, baking powder, salt and baking soda.
2. In a medium bowl, whisk together eggs, buttermilk, butter and honey until well blended.
3. Add the egg mixture to the flour mixture and stir until just blended.
4. Spread batter evenly in prepared pan.
5. Bake in preheated oven for 50 to 55 minutes or until top is golden brown and a toothpick inserted in the center comes out clean. Let cool in pan on a wire rack for 10 minutes, then transfer to the rack to cool.

# Multi-Seed Bread

With a satisfying mix of seeds throughout — flax, sesame, poppy and caraway — this bread makes the most of contrasting textures and flavors. The subtle, nutty flavor of quinoa flour (also made from seeds) connects all of the components.

## Storage Tip

Store the cooled bread, wrapped in foil or plastic wrap, in the refrigerator for up to 5 days. Alternatively, wrap it in plastic wrap, then foil, completely enclosing bread, and freeze for up to 3 months. Let thaw at room temperature for 4 to 6 hours before serving.

- **Preheat oven to 350°F (180°C)**
- **8- by 4-inch (20 by 10 cm) metal loaf pan, sprayed with nonstick cooking spray**

| | | |
|---|---|---|
| 1¾ cups | quinoa flour | 425 mL |
| ⅓ cup | ground flax seeds (flaxseed meal) | 75 mL |
| 3 tbsp | sesame seeds, divided | 45 mL |
| 1 tbsp | poppy seeds | 15 mL |
| 1 tbsp | caraway seeds, slightly crushed (see tip, page 420) | 15 mL |
| 1 tbsp | baking powder (GF, if needed) | 15 mL |
| 1 tsp | fine sea salt | 5 mL |
| 2 | large eggs | 2 |
| 1 cup | milk or plain non-dairy milk (such as soy, almond, rice or hemp) | 250 mL |
| ¼ cup | olive oil | 60 mL |
| 1 tbsp | dark (cooking) molasses or liquid honey | 15 mL |

1. In a large bowl, whisk together quinoa flour, flax seeds, 2 tbsp (30 mL) of the sesame seeds, poppy seeds, caraway seeds, baking powder and salt.
2. In a medium bowl, whisk together eggs, milk, oil and molasses until well blended.
3. Add the egg mixture to the flour mixture and stir until just blended.
4. Spread batter evenly in prepared pan. Sprinkle with the remaining sesame seeds.
5. Bake in preheated oven for 55 to 60 minutes or until top is golden brown and a toothpick inserted in the center comes out clean. Let cool in pan on a wire rack for 10 minutes, then transfer to the rack to cool.

# Maple and Toasted Quinoa Bread

**Makes 14 slices**

*Maple syrup for natural sweetness, yogurt for calcium and two forms of quinoa for protein — eating well never tasted so good. Stirring nutty, toasted quinoa into the batter adds a delicate crunch and deep flavor to the bread.*

## Tip

Liquid honey, agave nectar or brown rice syrup may be used in place of the maple syrup.

## Storage Tip

Store the cooled bread, wrapped in foil or plastic wrap, in the refrigerator for up to 5 days. Alternatively, wrap it in plastic wrap, then foil, completely enclosing bread, and freeze for up to 3 months. Let thaw at room temperature for 4 to 6 hours before serving.

- **8- by 4-inch (20 by 10 cm) metal loaf pan, sprayed with nonstick cooking spray**

| | | |
|---|---|---:|
| ½ cup | quinoa, rinsed | 125 mL |
| 2 cups | quinoa flour | 500 mL |
| 2 tbsp | cornstarch or arrowroot | 30 mL |
| 1½ tsp | baking powder (GF, if needed) | 7 mL |
| 1 tsp | baking soda | 5 mL |
| ¾ tsp | fine sea salt | 3 mL |
| 2 | large eggs | 2 |
| 1 cup | plain yogurt | 250 mL |
| ⅓ cup | unrefined virgin coconut oil, warmed, or vegetable oil | 75 mL |
| ½ cup | pure maple syrup | 125 mL |
| 2 tbsp | turbinado sugar | 30 mL |

1. Heat a large skillet over medium-high heat. Toast quinoa, stirring occasionally, for 3 to 4 minutes or until golden brown and just beginning to pop. Transfer to a plate and let cool completely.
2. Preheat oven to 350°F (180°C).
3. In a large bowl, whisk together quinoa, quinoa flour, cornstarch, baking powder, baking soda and salt.
4. In a medium bowl, whisk together eggs, yogurt, oil and maple syrup until well blended.
5. Add the egg mixture to the flour mixture and stir until just blended.
6. Spread batter evenly in prepared pan. Sprinkle top with sugar.
7. Bake for 50 to 55 minutes or until top is golden and a toothpick inserted in the center comes out clean. Let cool in pan on a wire rack for 5 minutes, then transfer to the rack. Serve warm or let cool completely.

# Chocolate Ricotta Bread

**Makes 14 slices**

*Ricotta cheese is an excellent option for baked goods such as this very chocolatey quinoa bread, imparting richness while offering high levels of calcium and protein.*

## Storage Tip

Store the cooled bread, wrapped in foil or plastic wrap, in the refrigerator for up to 5 days. Alternatively, wrap it in plastic wrap, then foil, completely enclosing bread, and freeze for up to 3 months. Let thaw at room temperature for 4 to 6 hours before serving.

- Preheat oven to 350°F (180°C)
- 8- by 4-inch (20 by 10 cm) metal loaf pan, sprayed with nonstick cooking spray

| | | |
|---|---|---|
| 2 cups | quinoa flour | 500 mL |
| ½ cup | unsweetened cocoa powder (not Dutch process) | 125 mL |
| 2 tsp | baking powder (GF, if needed) | 10 mL |
| ¾ tsp | fine sea salt | 3 mL |
| ¾ cup | natural cane sugar or packed light brown sugar | 175 mL |
| 2 | large eggs | 2 |
| 1 cup | ricotta cheese (reduced-fat or regular) | 250 mL |
| ¼ cup | unrefined virgin coconut oil, warmed, or vegetable oil | 60 mL |
| 1 tsp | almond extract (GF, if needed) | 5 mL |
| 1½ cups | milk or plain non-dairy milk (such as soy, almond, rice or hemp) | 375 mL |
| ½ cup | miniature semisweet chocolate chips (GF, if needed) | 125 mL |

1. In a large bowl, whisk together quinoa flour, cocoa powder, baking powder and salt.
2. In a medium bowl, whisk together sugar, eggs, cheese, oil and almond extract until well blended. Whisk in milk until blended.
3. Add the egg mixture to the flour mixture and stir until just blended. Gently fold in chocolate chips.
4. Spread batter evenly in prepared pan.
5. Bake in preheated oven for 50 to 55 minutes or until a toothpick inserted in the center comes out clean. Let cool in pan on a wire rack for 5 minutes, then transfer to the rack. Serve warm or let cool completely.

## Variation

*Carob Ricotta Bread:* Substitute unsweetened carob powder for the cocoa powder and carob chips, chopped, for the chocolate chips.

# Cinnamon Applesauce Bread

*Ground cinnamon gives this applesauce bread its signature zing. Nutty quinoa flour draws out and enhances the flavor of the applesauce and added cranberries.*

## Storage Tip

Store the cooled bread, wrapped in foil or plastic wrap, in the refrigerator for up to 5 days. Alternatively, wrap it in plastic wrap, then foil, completely enclosing bread, and freeze for up to 3 months. Let thaw at room temperature for 4 to 6 hours before serving.

- **Preheat oven to 350°F (180°C)**
- **8- by 4-inch (20 by 10 cm) metal loaf pan, sprayed with nonstick cooking spray**

| | | |
|---|---|---|
| 1½ cups | quinoa flour | 375 mL |
| 1½ tbsp | cornstarch or arrowroot | 22 mL |
| 2 tsp | ground cinnamon | 10 mL |
| ¾ tsp | baking soda | 3 mL |
| ½ tsp | fine sea salt | 2 mL |
| ⅔ cup | natural cane sugar or packed light brown sugar | 150 mL |
| 2 | large eggs | 2 |
| ¼ cup | unsalted butter, melted, or vegetable oil | 60 mL |
| 1¼ cups | unsweetened applesauce | 300 mL |
| ½ cup | dried cranberries or raisins (optional) | 125 mL |

1. In a large bowl, whisk together quinoa flour, cornstarch, cinnamon, baking soda and salt.
2. In a medium bowl, whisk together sugar, eggs and butter until well blended. Whisk in applesauce until blended.
3. Add the egg mixture to the flour mixture and stir until just blended. Gently fold in cranberries (if using).
4. Spread batter evenly in prepared pan.
5. Bake in preheated oven for 50 to 55 minutes or until golden and a toothpick inserted in the center comes out clean. Let cool in pan on a wire rack for 10 minutes, then transfer to the rack to cool.

# Cranberry Orange Bread

*Oranges, with their clean, citrusy spark, are an excellent foil for both the earthy quinoa flour and the tart-sweet cranberries in this simple quick bread.*

## Storage Tip

Store the cooled bread, wrapped in foil or plastic wrap, in the refrigerator for up to 5 days. Alternatively, wrap it in plastic wrap, then foil, completely enclosing bread, and freeze for up to 3 months. Let thaw at room temperature for 4 to 6 hours before serving.

- **Preheat oven to 350°F (180°C)**
- **8- by 4-inch (20 by 10 cm) metal loaf pan, sprayed with nonstick cooking spray**

| | | |
|---|---|---|
| 1¼ cups | quinoa flour | 300 mL |
| ¼ cup | quick-cooking rolled oats (certified GF, if needed) | 60 mL |
| 1 tbsp | cornstarch or arrowroot | 15 mL |
| 1½ tsp | baking powder (GF, if needed) | 7 mL |
| 1 tsp | ground nutmeg | 5 mL |
| ½ tsp | baking soda | 2 mL |
| ½ tsp | fine sea salt | 2 mL |
| ⅔ cup | natural cane sugar or packed light brown sugar | 150 mL |
| 1 | large egg | 1 |
| 2 tsp | finely grated orange zest | 10 mL |
| ½ cup | freshly squeezed orange juice | 125 mL |
| ⅓ cup | olive or vegetable oil | 75 mL |
| 1 cup | dried cranberries | 250 mL |
| 1 cup | chopped toasted pecans | 250 mL |

1. In a large bowl, whisk together quinoa flour, oats, cornstarch, baking powder, nutmeg, baking soda and salt.
2. In a medium bowl, whisk together sugar, egg, orange zest, orange juice and oil until blended.
3. Add the egg to the flour mixture and stir until just blended. Gently fold in cranberries and pecans.
4. Spread batter evenly in prepared pan.
5. Bake in preheated oven for 50 to 55 minutes or until a toothpick inserted in the center comes out clean. Let cool in pan on a wire rack for 10 minutes, then transfer to the rack to cool.

# Fresh Ginger Lemon Bread

*Here comes the sun: graced with ample amounts of ginger and lemon, this golden bread is always a cheery sight.*

## Storage Tip

Store the cooled bread, wrapped in foil or plastic wrap, in the refrigerator for up to 5 days. Alternatively, wrap it in plastic wrap, then foil, completely enclosing bread, and freeze for up to 3 months. Let thaw at room temperature for 4 to 6 hours before serving.

- **8- by 4-inch (20 by 10 cm) metal loaf pan, sprayed with nonstick cooking spray**

| | | |
|---|---|---|
| ²⁄₃ cup | natural cane sugar or packed light brown sugar, divided | 150 mL |
| ¹⁄₃ cup | chopped gingerroot | 75 mL |
| 1 tbsp | finely grated lemon zest | 15 mL |
| 6 tbsp | freshly squeezed lemon juice, divided | 90 mL |
| 1 cup | buttermilk | 250 mL |
| 2 cups | quinoa flour | 500 mL |
| 2 tbsp | cornstarch or arrowroot | 30 mL |
| 1½ tsp | baking powder (GF, if needed) | 7 mL |
| ¾ tsp | baking soda | 3 mL |
| ½ tsp | fine sea salt | 2 mL |
| 2 | large eggs | 2 |
| ¼ cup | unsalted butter, melted | 60 mL |
| 2 tbsp | liquid honey | 30 mL |

1. In a small saucepan, combine half the cane sugar, ginger, lemon zest and 4 tbsp (60 mL) of the lemon juice. Cook over medium-high heat, stirring constantly, for 4 to 5 minutes or until sugar is dissolved. Scrape into a medium bowl and whisk in buttermilk. Let cool completely.
2. Preheat oven to 350°F (180°C).
3. In a large bowl, whisk together quinoa flour, cornstarch, baking powder, baking soda and salt.
4. Whisk the remaining sugar, eggs and butter into buttermilk mixture until well blended.
5. Add the egg mixture to the flour mixture and stir until just blended.
6. Spread batter evenly in prepared pan.
7. Bake for 50 to 55 minutes or until golden and a toothpick inserted in the center comes out clean. Let cool in pan on a wire rack for 10 minutes, then transfer to the rack.
8. In a small cup, combine honey and the remaining lemon juice. Brush over top and sides of warm bread. Let cool completely.

# Banana Quinoa Bread

*This otherwise humble bread is a delicious example of true comfort food. It's the perfect use for bananas that are past their prime.*

## Storage Tip

Store the cooled bread, wrapped in foil or plastic wrap, in the refrigerator for up to 5 days. Alternatively, wrap it in plastic wrap, then foil, completely enclosing bread, and freeze for up to 3 months. Let thaw at room temperature for 4 to 6 hours before serving.

- **Preheat oven to 350°F (180°C)**
- **8- by 4-inch (20 by 10 cm) metal loaf pan, sprayed with nonstick cooking spray**

| | | |
|---|---|---|
| 1⅓ cups | quinoa flour | 325 mL |
| 2 tsp | baking powder (GF, if needed) | 10 mL |
| ½ tsp | fine sea salt | 2 mL |
| ½ tsp | ground cinnamon | 2 mL |
| ½ tsp | ground nutmeg | 2 mL |
| ½ cup | natural cane sugar or packed brown sugar | 125 mL |
| 1 | large egg | 1 |
| 1 cup | mashed ripe bananas | 250 mL |
| 1 cup | plain yogurt | 250 mL |
| ¼ cup | unrefined virgin coconut oil, warmed, or unsalted butter, melted | 60 mL |
| ½ cup | chopped toasted walnuts or pecans (optional) | 125 mL |

1. In a large bowl, whisk together quinoa flour, baking powder, salt, cinnamon and nutmeg.
2. In a medium bowl, whisk together sugar, egg, bananas, yogurt and oil until blended.
3. Add the egg mixture to the flour mixture and stir until just blended. Gently fold in walnuts (if using).
4. Spread batter evenly in prepared pan.
5. Bake in preheated oven for 50 to 55 minutes or until a toothpick inserted in the center comes out clean. Let cool in pan on a wire rack for 10 minutes, then transfer to the rack to cool.

# Peanut Butter and Banana Bread

*The indulgent flavor combination of peanut butter and banana (reportedly Elvis Presley's favorite) is actually an exemplary duo of superfoods. Add in quinoa flour, flax seeds and yogurt, and you have yourself an incredibly nutritious and delicious bread.*

## Tip

Other unsweetened natural nut or seed butters (such as cashew, almond or sunflower seed) may be used in place of the peanut butter.

## Storage Tip

Store the cooled bread, wrapped in foil or plastic wrap, in the refrigerator for up to 5 days. Alternatively, wrap it in plastic wrap, then foil, completely enclosing bread, and freeze for up to 3 months. Let thaw at room temperature for 4 to 6 hours before serving.

- **Preheat oven to 350°F (180°C)**
- **8- by 4-inch (20 by 10 cm) metal loaf pan, sprayed with nonstick cooking spray**

| | | |
|---|---|---|
| 1½ cups | quinoa flour | 375 mL |
| ¼ cup | ground flax seeds (flaxseed meal) | 60 mL |
| 1 tsp | baking soda | 5 mL |
| ½ tsp | fine sea salt | 2 mL |
| ½ tsp | ground cinnamon | 2 mL |
| ⅔ cup | natural cane sugar or packed light brown sugar | 150 mL |
| 2 | large eggs | 2 |
| 1½ cups | mashed ripe bananas | 375 mL |
| ⅔ cup | plain yogurt | 150 mL |
| ⅓ cup | unsweetened natural peanut butter | 75 mL |
| 3 tbsp | unrefined virgin coconut oil, warmed, or vegetable oil | 45 mL |
| ⅓ cup | lightly salted roasted peanuts, chopped | 75 mL |

**Glaze**

| | | |
|---|---|---|
| 1 tbsp | unsweetened natural peanut butter | 15 mL |
| 1 tbsp | liquid honey or pure maple syrup | 15 mL |

1. In a large bowl, whisk together quinoa flour, flax seeds, baking soda, salt and cinnamon.
2. In a medium bowl, whisk together sugar, eggs, bananas, yogurt, peanut butter and oil until blended.
3. Add the egg mixture to the flour mixture and stir until just blended. Gently fold in peanuts.
4. Spread batter evenly in prepared pan.
5. Bake in preheated oven for 60 to 65 minutes or until a toothpick inserted in the center comes out clean. Let cool in pan on a wire rack for 10 minutes, then transfer to the rack.
6. *Glaze:* In a small bowl, combine 1 tbsp (15 mL) peanut butter and honey until smooth. Spoon and spread over top of warm bread. Let cool completely.

# Cinnamon Raisin Bread

*Tender, moist and studded with raisins, this cinnamon-spiced bread is a perfect way to welcome any morning, but especially a chilly one.*

## Tip

Other dried fruits, such as cranberries, chopped dates or chopped apricots, may be used in place of the raisins.

## Storage Tip

Store the cooled bread, wrapped in foil or plastic wrap, in the refrigerator for up to 4 days. Alternatively, wrap it in plastic wrap, then foil, completely enclosing bread, and freeze for up to 3 months. Let thaw at room temperature for 4 to 6 hours before serving.

- **Preheat oven to 350°F (180°C)**
- **8- by 4-inch (20 by 10 cm) metal loaf pan, sprayed with nonstick cooking spray**

| | | |
|---|---|---|
| 1⅔ cups | quinoa flour | 400 mL |
| ¾ cup | quick-cooking rolled oats (certified GF, if needed) | 175 mL |
| ¼ cup | ground flax seeds (flaxseed meal) | 60 mL |
| 2¼ tsp | baking powder (GF, if needed) | 11 mL |
| ½ tsp | baking soda | 2 mL |
| ½ tsp | fine sea salt | 2 mL |
| ⅔ cup | natural cane sugar or packed light brown sugar | 150 mL |
| 2 | large eggs | 2 |
| 1 cup | buttermilk | 250 mL |
| ¼ cup | vegetable oil or unsalted butter, melted | 60 mL |
| 1 tsp | vanilla extract (GF, if needed) | 5 mL |
| 1 cup | raisins | 250 mL |
| ½ cup | chopped toasted pecans or walnuts (optional) | 125 mL |

1. In a large bowl, whisk together quinoa flour, oats, flax seeds, baking powder, baking soda and salt.
2. In a medium bowl, whisk together sugar, eggs, buttermilk, oil and vanilla until well blended.
3. Add the egg mixture to the flour mixture and stir until just blended. Gently fold in raisins and pecans (if using).
4. Spread batter evenly in prepared pan.
5. Bake in preheated oven for 55 to 60 minutes or until golden and a toothpick inserted in the center comes out clean. Let cool in pan on a wire rack for 10 minutes, then transfer to the rack to cool.

# Quinoa Date Bread

**Makes 12 slices**

*Ingredients of Sephardic cooking — dates, cardamom and honey — bring a mosaic of Mediterranean scents to this delicious bread. You can use any variety of dates, but I prefer Medjool dates for their caramel-and-molasses flavor and pronounced sweetness.*

## Tip

Measure the oil in a glass measuring cup, then measure the honey in the same cup; the residue from the oil will allow the honey to slide right out without sticking.

## Storage Tip

Store the cooled bread, wrapped in foil or plastic wrap, in the refrigerator for up to 5 days. Alternatively, wrap it in plastic wrap, then foil, completely enclosing bread, and freeze for up to 3 months. Let thaw at room temperature for 4 to 6 hours before serving.

- **Preheat oven to 350°F (180°C)**
- **8- by 4-inch (20 by 10 cm) metal loaf pan, sprayed with nonstick cooking spray**

| | | |
|---|---|---|
| ¾ cup | milk | 175 mL |
| 1 cup | chopped pitted dates (preferably Medjool) | 250 mL |
| 2 cups | quinoa flour | 500 mL |
| 2 tbsp | cornstarch or arrowroot | 30 mL |
| 2½ tsp | baking powder (GF, if needed) | 12 mL |
| 1 tsp | ground cardamom or cinnamon | 5 mL |
| ½ tsp | fine sea salt | 2 mL |
| ¼ tsp | baking soda | 1 mL |
| 2 | large eggs | 2 |
| ⅓ cup | vegetable oil | 75 mL |
| ⅔ cup | liquid honey or brown rice syrup | 150 mL |
| 1 tsp | vanilla extract (GF, if needed) | 5 mL |
| 1 cup | chopped toasted pecans or walnuts (optional) | 250 mL |

1. In a small saucepan, combine dates and milk. Bring to a simmer over low heat. Remove from heat, cover and let stand for 10 minutes.
2. In a large bowl, whisk together quinoa flour, cornstarch, baking powder, cardamom, salt and baking soda.
3. In a medium bowl, whisk together eggs, oil, honey and vanilla until well blended. Stir in date mixture until blended.
4. Add the egg mixture to the flour mixture and stir until just blended. Gently fold in pecans (if using).
5. Spread batter evenly in prepared pan.
6. Bake in preheated oven for 55 to 60 minutes or until a toothpick inserted in the center comes out clean. Let cool in pan on a wire rack for 10 minutes, then transfer to the rack to cool.

# Apricot Almond Bread

*Vivid apricots and sweet almonds in a honey-sweetened multigrain loaf? Oh yes, please.*

## Storage Tip

Store the cooled bread, wrapped in foil or plastic wrap, in the refrigerator for up to 5 days. Alternatively, wrap it in plastic wrap, then foil, completely enclosing bread, and freeze for up to 3 months. Let thaw at room temperature for 4 to 6 hours before serving.

- **Preheat oven to 350°F (180°C)**
- **8- by 4-inch (20 by 10 cm) metal loaf pan, sprayed with nonstick cooking spray**

| | | |
|---|---|---|
| 1⅓ cups | quick-cooking rolled oats (certified GF, if needed) | 325 mL |
| 1 cup | quinoa flour | 250 mL |
| 1 tbsp | cornstarch or arrowroot | 15 mL |
| 2¼ tsp | baking powder (GF, if needed) | 11 mL |
| 1 tsp | ground cardamom or nutmeg | 5 mL |
| ½ tsp | fine sea salt | 2 mL |
| ¼ tsp | baking soda | 1 mL |
| 2 | large eggs | 2 |
| 1 cup | plain yogurt | 250 mL |
| ¼ cup | unrefined virgin coconut oil, warmed, or vegetable oil | 60 mL |
| ½ cup | liquid honey or brown rice syrup | 125 mL |
| 1 tsp | almond extract (GF, if needed) | 2 mL |
| 1 cup | finely chopped dried apricots | 250 mL |
| ½ cup | slivered almonds | 125 mL |

1. In a large bowl, whisk together oats, quinoa flour, cornstarch, baking powder, cardamom, salt and baking soda.
2. In a medium bowl, whisk together eggs, yogurt, oil, honey and almond extract until well blended.
3. Add the egg mixture to the flour mixture and stir until just blended. Gently fold in apricots.
4. Spread batter evenly in prepared pan. Sprinkle with almonds.
5. Bake in preheated oven for 50 to 55 minutes or until top is golden and a toothpick inserted in the center comes out clean. Let cool in pan on a wire rack for 5 minutes, then transfer to the rack. Serve warm or let cool completely.

# Pumpkin Quinoa Bread

*Embrace the flavors of fall with this moist, delicious bread. Pumpkin not only lends richness and color, but, like quinoa, is one of the healthiest ingredients you can keep in your pantry.*

## Storage Tip

Store the cooled bread, wrapped in foil or plastic wrap, in the refrigerator for up to 3 days. Alternatively, wrap it in plastic wrap, then foil, completely enclosing bread, and freeze for up to 3 months. Let thaw at room temperature for 4 to 6 hours before serving.

- **Preheat oven to 350°F (180°C)**
- **8- by 4-inch (20 by 10 cm) metal loaf pan, sprayed with nonstick cooking spray**

| | | |
|---|---|---:|
| 1¾ cups | quinoa flour | 425 mL |
| 1 tbsp | pumpkin pie spice | 15 mL |
| 2 tsp | baking powder (GF, if needed) | 10 mL |
| ¼ tsp | baking soda | 1 mL |
| ¼ tsp | fine sea salt | 1 mL |
| ⅔ cup | natural cane sugar or packed light brown sugar | 150 mL |
| 1 | large egg | 1 |
| 1¼ cups | pumpkin purée (not pie filling) | 300 mL |
| ½ cup | plain yogurt or buttermilk | 125 mL |
| ⅓ cup | vegetable oil or unsalted butter, melted | 75 mL |
| 1 tsp | vanilla extract (GF, if needed) | 5 mL |
| 1 cup | chopped toasted walnuts (optional) | 250 mL |

1. In a large bowl, whisk together quinoa flour, pumpkin pie spice, baking powder, baking soda and salt.
2. In a medium bowl, whisk together sugar, egg, pumpkin, yogurt, oil and vanilla until well blended.
3. Add the egg mixture to the flour mixture and stir until just blended. Gently fold in walnuts (if using).
4. Spread batter evenly in prepared pan.
5. Bake in preheated oven for about 1 hour or until golden and a toothpick inserted in the center comes out clean. Let cool in pan on a wire rack for 10 minutes, then transfer to the rack to cool.

# Sun-Dried Tomato and Spinach Bread

*Savory-sweet sun-dried tomatoes, earthy spinach and creamy ricotta take center stage in this Mediterranean bread. A slice is almost a meal unto itself.*

## Storage Tip

Store the cooled bread, wrapped in foil or plastic wrap, in the refrigerator for up to 3 days. Alternatively, wrap it in plastic wrap, then foil, completely enclosing bread, and freeze for up to 3 months. Let thaw at room temperature for 4 to 6 hours before serving.

- **Preheat oven to 350°F (180°C)**
- **9- by 5-inch (23 by 12.5 cm) metal loaf pan, sprayed with nonstick cooking spray**

| | | |
|---|---|---|
| 2 cups | quinoa flour | 500 mL |
| 1 cup | quick-cooking rolled oats (certified GF, if needed) | 250 mL |
| 1 tbsp | baking powder (GF, if needed) | 15 mL |
| 2 tsp | dried basil | 10 mL |
| 1 tsp | fine sea salt | 5 mL |
| 1 | large egg | 1 |
| ¼ cup | olive or vegetable oil | 60 mL |
| 1 cup | milk | 250 mL |
| ¾ cup | ricotta cheese (reduced-fat or regular) | 175 mL |
| 1 | package (10 oz/300 g) frozen chopped spinach, thawed and squeezed dry | 1 |
| ⅓ cup | chopped drained oil-packed sun-dried tomatoes | 75 mL |

1. In a large bowl, whisk together quinoa flour, oats, baking powder, basil and salt.
2. In a medium bowl, whisk together egg and oil until well blended. Whisk in milk and cheese until blended. Gently fold in spinach and tomatoes.
3. Add the egg mixture to the flour mixture and stir until just blended.
4. Spread batter evenly in prepared pan.
5. Bake in preheated oven for 60 to 65 minutes or until top is golden and a toothpick inserted in the center comes out clean. Let cool in pan on a wire rack for 5 minutes, then transfer to the rack. Serve warm or let cool completely.

# Mediterranean Quinoa Bread

*The ripe, salty flavor of brine-cured olives and the gentle sweetness of sun-dried tomatoes combine in this deeply satisfying, Mediterranean-inspired bread. Serve with a green salad for an instant lunch or light dinner.*

## Tip

Fresh flat-leaf (Italian) parsley leaves may be used in place of the basil. Alternatively, use 2 tsp (10 mL) dried basil in place of the fresh.

## Storage Tip

Store the cooled bread, wrapped in foil or plastic wrap, in the refrigerator for up to 3 days. Alternatively, wrap it in plastic wrap, then foil, completely enclosing bread, and freeze for up to 3 months. Let thaw at room temperature for 4 to 6 hours before serving.

- **Preheat oven to 350°F (180°C)**
- **8- by 4-inch (20 by 10 cm) metal loaf pan, sprayed with nonstick cooking spray**

| | | |
|---|---|---|
| 2 cups | quinoa flour | 500 mL |
| 2 tsp | baking powder (GF, if needed) | 10 mL |
| ¾ tsp | fine sea salt | 3 mL |
| ½ tsp | baking soda | 2 mL |
| 2 | large eggs | 2 |
| 1 cup | buttermilk | 250 mL |
| ¼ cup | olive oil | 60 mL |
| ½ cup | packed fresh basil, chopped | 125 mL |
| ⅓ cup | chopped drained oil-packed sun-dried tomatoes | 75 mL |
| ⅓ cup | crumbled feta cheese | 75 mL |
| ¼ cup | chopped pitted brine-cured black olives (such as kalamata) | 60 mL |

1. In a large bowl, whisk together quinoa flour, baking powder, salt and baking soda.
2. In a medium bowl, whisk together eggs, buttermilk and oil until smooth.
3. Add the egg mixture to the flour mixture and stir until just blended. Gently fold in basil, tomatoes, cheese and olives.
4. Spread batter evenly in prepared pan.
5. Bake in preheated oven for 50 to 55 minutes or until top is golden and a toothpick inserted in the center comes out clean. Let cool in pan on a wire rack for 5 minutes, then transfer to the rack. Serve warm or let cool completely.

# Zucchini Quinoa Bread

*Most zucchini recipes taste far more like cake than quick bread; not so here. This quinoa-based version steers clear of being overly sweet. Toasty walnuts add great crunch while also enhancing the nutty flavor of the quinoa flour.*

## Tip

For maximum health benefits, leave the zucchini unpeeled. Zucchini provides large amounts of folate and potassium, and the dark green peel contains beta carotene. It also adds pretty specks of emerald throughout the bread.

## Storage Tip

Store the cooled bread, wrapped in foil or plastic wrap, in the refrigerator for up to 5 days. Alternatively, wrap it in plastic wrap, then foil, completely enclosing bread, and freeze for up to 3 months. Let thaw at room temperature for 4 to 6 hours before serving.

- Preheat oven to 325°F (160°C)
- 8- by 4-inch (20 by 10 cm) metal loaf pan, sprayed with nonstick cooking spray

| | | |
|---|---|---|
| 2 cups | quinoa flour | 500 mL |
| 2 tbsp | cornstarch or arrowroot | 30 mL |
| 1 tsp | ground cinnamon | 5 mL |
| ½ tsp | baking powder (GF, if needed) | 2 mL |
| ½ tsp | baking soda | 2 mL |
| ½ tsp | fine sea salt | 2 mL |
| ¾ cup | natural cane sugar or packed light brown sugar | 175 mL |
| 2 | large eggs | 2 |
| ¾ cup | plain yogurt | 175 mL |
| ⅓ cup | vegetable oil or unrefined virgin coconut oil, warmed | 75 mL |
| 1 tsp | vanilla extract (GF, if needed) | 5 mL |
| 1 cup | shredded zucchini | 250 mL |
| 1 cup | chopped toasted walnuts or pecans (optional) | 250 mL |

1. In a large bowl, whisk together quinoa flour, cornstarch, cinnamon, baking powder, baking soda and salt.
2. In a medium bowl, whisk together sugar, eggs, yogurt, oil and vanilla until well blended.
3. Add the egg mixture to the flour mixture and stir until just blended. Gently fold in zucchini and walnuts (if using).
4. Spread batter evenly in prepared pan.
5. Bake in preheated oven for about 70 minutes or until golden and a toothpick inserted in the center comes out clean. Let cool in pan on a wire rack for 10 minutes, then transfer to the rack to cool.

# Leek and Gruyère Bread

*Pan-fried leeks, tarragon and Gruyère melt into each other and make a rich, but not heavy bread. Pair it with soup for a quietly spectacular weeknight repast.*

## Tip

After cutting leeks lengthwise, rinse them well under running water and rub out any sand and grit before slicing.

- **8- by 4-inch (20 by 10 cm) metal loaf pan, sprayed with nonstick cooking spray**

| | | |
|---|---|---|
| 4 tbsp | olive oil, divided | 60 mL |
| 2 | medium-large leeks (white and light green parts only), cut in half lengthwise, then sliced crosswise | 2 |
| 2 cups | quinoa flour | 500 mL |
| 1 tbsp | baking powder (GF, if needed) | 15 mL |
| 1½ tsp | dried tarragon | 7 mL |
| ½ tsp | fine sea salt | 2 mL |
| 2 | large eggs | 2 |
| 1 cup | milk | 250 mL |
| 2 tsp | Dijon mustard | 10 mL |
| 4 oz | Gruyère or Swiss cheese, cut into small cubes | 125 g |

1. In a large nonstick skillet, heat 1 tbsp (15 mL) of the oil over medium heat. Add leeks and cook, stirring, for 7 to 10 minutes or until softened. Remove from heat and let cool completely.
2. Preheat oven to 350°F (180°C).
3. In a large bowl, whisk together quinoa flour, baking powder, tarragon and salt.
4. In a medium bowl, whisk together eggs, milk, mustard and the remaining oil until well blended.
5. Add the egg mixture to the flour mixture and stir until just blended. Gently fold in leeks and cheese.
6. Spread batter evenly in prepared pan.
7. Bake for 50 to 55 minutes or until top is golden brown and a toothpick inserted in the center comes out clean. Let cool in pan on a wire rack for 10 minutes, then transfer to the rack to cool.

# Scallion Sesame Bread

*Quinoa already has a toasty flavor that hints of sesame, so imagine how delicious this bread is when toasted sesame oil is added to the batter. Chopped scallions add plenty of verdant verve, and a sprinkle of sesame seeds tops the loaf off with flavor and crunch.*

## Storage Tip

Store the cooled bread, wrapped in foil or plastic wrap, in the refrigerator for up to 3 days. Alternatively, wrap it in plastic wrap, then foil, completely enclosing bread, and freeze for up to 3 months. Let thaw at room temperature for 4 to 6 hours before serving.

- Preheat oven to 350°F (180°C)
- 8- by 4-inch (20 by 10 cm) metal loaf pan, sprayed with nonstick cooking spray

| | | |
|---|---|---|
| 2 cups | quinoa flour | 500 mL |
| 2 tbsp | cornstarch or arrowroot | 30 mL |
| 2¼ tsp | baking powder (GF, if needed) | 11 mL |
| 1 tsp | baking soda | 5 mL |
| ½ tsp | fine sea salt | 2 mL |
| 2 | large eggs | 2 |
| 1¼ cups | buttermilk | 300 mL |
| 3 tbsp | vegetable oil | 45 mL |
| 2 tbsp | toasted sesame oil | 30 mL |
| 1 cup | chopped green onions (scallions) | 250 mL |
| 3 tbsp | sesame seeds | 45 mL |

1. In a large bowl, whisk together quinoa flour, cornstarch, baking powder, baking soda and salt.
2. In a medium bowl, whisk together eggs, buttermilk, vegetable oil and sesame oil until well blended.
3. Add the egg mixture to the flour mixture and stir until just blended. Gently fold in green onions.
4. Spread batter evenly in prepared pan. Sprinkle with sesame seeds.
5. Bake in preheated oven for 50 to 55 minutes or until top is golden brown and a toothpick inserted in the center comes out clean. Let cool in pan on a wire rack for 10 minutes, then transfer to the rack. Serve warm or let cool completely.

# Skillet Quinoa Cornbread

*Quinoa and corn —
two prized New World
crops — make perfect
(and delicious) sense
in this golden, crusty
cornbread.*

## Tip

If you don't have a cast-iron skillet, use a 9-inch (23 cm) metal baking pan instead. Do not preheat the pan; simply spray it with nonstick cooking spray or rub it with oil. The bread will not be as crusty as when baked in the skillet.

## Storage Tip

Store the cooled bread, wrapped in foil or plastic wrap, in the refrigerator for up to 3 days. Alternatively, wrap it in plastic wrap, then foil, completely enclosing bread, and freeze for up to 3 months. Let thaw at room temperature for 4 to 6 hours before serving.

- **Preheat oven to 400°F (200°C)**
- **9-inch (23 cm) cast-iron skillet, oiled**

| | | |
|---|---|---|
| 1½ cups | quinoa flour | 375 mL |
| 1¼ cups | cornmeal (preferably stone-ground; GF, if needed) | 300 mL |
| 2 tsp | baking powder (GF, if needed) | 10 mL |
| ½ tsp | fine sea salt | 2 mL |
| ½ tsp | baking soda | 2 mL |
| 1 | large egg | 1 |
| ⅓ cup | vegetable oil or unsalted butter, melted | 75 mL |
| 2 tbsp | liquid honey or pure maple syrup | 30 mL |
| 1½ cups | buttermilk | 375 mL |

1. Place prepared skillet in preheated oven for 10 minutes while you prepare the batter.
2. In a large bowl, whisk together quinoa flour, cornmeal, baking powder, salt and baking soda.
3. In a medium bowl, whisk together egg, oil and honey until well blended. Whisk in buttermilk until blended.
4. Add the egg mixture to the flour mixture and stir until just blended.
5. Carefully spread batter evenly in hot skillet.
6. Bake for 22 to 25 minutes or until golden and a toothpick inserted in the center comes out clean. Let cool in skillet on a wire rack for 10 minutes, then transfer to the rack. Serve warm or let cool completely.

## Variations

*Mexican Cornbread:* Reduce the buttermilk to 1 cup (250 mL) and omit the honey. Add 1½ tsp (7 mL) ground cumin to the flour mixture. Add ¾ cup (175 mL) thick, chunky salsa with the buttermilk. Gently fold in 1 cup (250 mL) fresh or thawed frozen corn kernels at the end of step 4.

*Jalapeño Cumin Cornbread:* Add 2 tsp (10 mL) ground cumin to the flour mixture. Gently fold in 1½ tbsp (22 mL) minced jalapeño pepper at the end of step 4. Depending on the level of heat you like, you can omit or include some or all of the jalapeño seeds.

# Rosemary Quinoa Focaccia

*With quinoa flour and baking powder in place of wheat flour and yeast, this focaccia is anything but traditional. Nevertheless, it is irresistible. Like the original, the dough is finished with the delicate crunch of coarse sea salt and is puckered to allow small pockets of flavorful olive oil to remain once the loaf is baked.*

## Storage Tip

Store the cooled focaccia, wrapped in foil or plastic wrap, in the refrigerator for up to 1 day.

- Preheat oven to 425°F (220°C)
- 13- by 9-inch (33 by 23 cm) glass or metal baking pan, oiled (preferably olive oil)

| | | |
|---|---|---|
| 2 cups | quinoa flour | 500 mL |
| 1 tbsp | baking powder (GF, if needed) | 15 mL |
| ½ tsp | fine sea salt | 2 mL |
| 1 cup | water | 250 mL |
| 3 tbsp | olive oil, divided | 45 mL |
| 1 tbsp | chopped fresh rosemary | 15 mL |
| 1½ tsp | coarse sea salt | 7 mL |

1. In a large bowl, whisk together quinoa flour, baking powder and fine sea salt. Using a wooden spoon, stir in water and 1 tbsp (15 mL) of the oil until blended.

2. Turn dough out onto a work surface lightly floured with quinoa flour. Knead for 1 minute.

3. Transfer dough to prepared pan and pat into a ½-inch (1 cm) thick rectangle (it will not cover entire bottom of pan). Poke indentations all over top of bread with your fingertips. Brush or drizzle dough with the remaining oil and sprinkle with rosemary and coarse sea salt.

4. Bake in preheated oven for 20 to 25 minutes or until golden brown. Let cool in pan on a wire rack for 5 minutes, then transfer to the rack to cool. Serve warm or let cool completely.

# Middle Eastern Flatbread

My version of the Middle Eastern spice blend za'atar flavors this simple flatbread.

## Tip

If you prefer, you can omit the za'atar topping and simply sprinkle the flatbread with 1/2 tsp (2 mL) coarse sea salt.

## Storage Tip

Store the cooled flatbread, wrapped in foil or plastic wrap, in the refrigerator for up to 1 day.

- **Preheat oven to 400°F (200°C)**
- **Coffee or spice grinder or small food processor**
- **Large rimmed baking sheet, oiled (preferably with olive oil)**

### Za'atar

| | | |
|---|---|---|
| 3 tbsp | chopped toasted hazelnuts or almonds | 45 mL |
| 3 tbsp | sesame seeds | 45 mL |
| 1 tsp | cumin seeds | 5 mL |
| 3/4 tsp | dried thyme | 3 mL |
| 1/2 tsp | coarse sea salt | 2 mL |
| 1/2 tsp | whole black peppercorns | 2 mL |

### Dough

| | | |
|---|---|---|
| 1 1/2 cups | quinoa flour | 375 mL |
| 2 tsp | baking powder (GF, if needed) | 10 mL |
| 1/2 tsp | fine sea salt | 2 mL |
| 1 | large egg, beaten | 1 |
| 2/3 cup | water | 150 mL |
| 2 tbsp | olive oil, divided | 30 mL |

1. *Za'atar:* In coffee grinder, combine hazelnuts, sesame seeds, cumin seeds, thyme, salt and peppercorns; pulse until finely ground (but not a paste).

2. *Dough:* In a large bowl, whisk together quinoa flour, baking powder and salt. Using a wooden spoon, stir in egg, water and 1 tbsp (15 mL) of the oil until blended.

3. Turn dough out onto a work surface lightly floured with quinoa flour. Knead for 1 minute.

4. Transfer dough to prepared baking sheet and pat into a 13- by 9-inch (33 by 23 cm) rectangle. (Dough will be very thin.) Brush or drizzle dough with the remaining oil and sprinkle with za'atar.

5. Bake in preheated oven for 22 to 25 minutes or until golden brown. Let cool on pan on a wire rack for 5 minutes, then transfer to a cutting board. Using a sharp, heavy knife, cut into 16 slices. Serve warm or let cool completely.

# Quinoa Tortillas

*An ancient Andean
ingredient shines in this
fantastic take on tortillas.
Don't be intimated about
making them from
scratch: they are really
quite easy to prepare and
come together in minutes.*

## Tip

If you do not have a tortilla press, you can use a rolling pin. Place a 6-inch (15 cm) wide bowl upside down on the sealable plastic bag and trace a circle around it. Cut out the circle into two rounds. Place a round on either side of the dough ball before rolling it out. The plastic rounds help ensure that the tortillas do not stick and are all the same size.

## Storage Tip

Store the cooled tortillas, wrapped in foil or plastic wrap, in the refrigerator for up to 5 days. Alternatively, wrap them in plastic wrap, then foil, completely enclosing bread, and freeze for up to 3 months. Let thaw at room temperature for 4 to 6 hours before serving.

- **Tortilla press (see tip, at left)**
- **Cast-iron or other heavy skillet**

| | | |
|---|---|---|
| 2 cups | quinoa flour | 500 mL |
| 1/3 cup | brown rice flour | 75 mL |
| 1/2 tsp | fine sea salt | 2 mL |
| 2/3 cup | hot (not boiling) water | 150 mL |
| 2 tsp | vegetable oil | 10 mL |

1. Cut two rounds from a heavy-duty sealable plastic bag to fit the shape of the tortilla press. Set aside.
2. In a large bowl, whisk together quinoa flour, brown rice flour and salt. Stir in hot water and oil until mixture comes together into a smooth dough.
3. Turn dough out onto a work surface lightly floured with quinoa flour or brown rice flour. Knead for about 1 minute. Cut dough into 9 equal pieces and shape each into a ball. Cover loosely with plastic wrap.
4. Place a plastic round on the bottom half of the tortilla press. Place a dough ball in the center. Top with the second plastic round. Close press, flattening dough to about 1/8 inch (3 mm) thick and forming a 6-inch (15 cm) round. If thickness of tortilla is uneven, lift dough round, in plastic, and rotate 180 degrees. Press tortilla lightly to even out. Peel off top sheet of plastic.
5. Heat cast-iron skillet over medium-high heat. Cook tortilla, turning once, for about 45 seconds per side, until it looks slightly dry at the edges, starts to release from the surface of the skillet and is lightly browned in spots. Transfer to a plate.
6. Repeat steps 4 and 5 with the remaining dough balls.

# Quinoa Pizza Dough

*Don't wait around for yeast: this baking powder version of pizza dough yields a crisp crust in a fraction of the time. Quinoa flour, with its naturally nutty, faintly sweet flavor, makes the dough a standout.*

## Tip

One of the secrets to great pizza is restraint with the toppings. A smear of sauce, a sprinkle of cheese and a light hand with any additional toppings is all you need.

- **Preheat oven to 400°F (200°C)**
- **Large pizza pan or rimmed baking sheet, oiled (preferably with olive oil)**

| | | |
|---|---|---|
| 1½ cups | quinoa flour | 375 mL |
| 1 tbsp | baking powder (GF, if needed) | 15 mL |
| ½ tsp | fine sea salt | 2 mL |
| ⅔ cup | water | 150 mL |
| 2 tbsp | olive oil | 30 mL |

**Suggested Toppings**

Marinara sauce

Basil pesto

Shredded or grated cheese (such as mozzarella, Parmesan, Gouda or fontina)

Leftover grilled or roasted vegetables, coarsely chopped

Diced cooked lean meat or sausage (such as roasted chicken, Canadian bacon or chicken sausage)

Pitted ripe or brine-cured black olives, sliced or quartered (lengthwise)

1. In a large bowl, whisk together quinoa flour, baking powder and salt. Using a wooden spoon, stir in water and oil until a shaggy dough forms.

2. Turn dough out onto a work surface lightly floured with quinoa flour. Knead for 1 to 2 minutes or until smooth and cohesive. Shape into a ball. Use immediately.

**To Make Pizza**

3. Place ball on prepared pan and pat into a large round (if using a pizza pan) or rectangle (if using a baking sheet). Add any of the suggested toppings, as desired.

4. Bake for 19 to 24 minutes or until crust is golden and cheese is bubbly. Let cool on pan on a wire rack for 5 minutes, then transfer to a cutting board. Cut into 10 wedges or squares.

# Desserts

# Quinoa Pie Crust

*Buttery, nutty and quick — this pie crust has it all. Use it for all of your favorite fillings, from sweet fruit pies and creamy custard to savory quiche.*

## Tip

The pie and tart recipes in this chapter call for either a "parbaked" or a "baked" crust. Make sure to note which is specified and follow the appropriate version of step 4, at right, including letting the crust cool as instructed, before proceeding with the recipe.

- **Preheat oven to 375°F (190°C)**
- **Food processor**
- **9-inch (23 cm) pie plate**

| | | |
|---|---|---|
| ¾ cup | quinoa flour | 175 mL |
| ⅓ cup | almond meal or almond flour | 75 mL |
| 5 tbsp | cornstarch or arrowroot, divided | 75 mL |
| 1 tbsp | natural cane sugar or granulated sugar (optional) | 15 mL |
| ½ tsp | fine sea salt | 2 mL |
| ½ cup | cold unsalted butter, cut into small pieces | 125 mL |
| 1 | large egg, lightly beaten | 1 |

1. In food processor, combine quinoa flour, almond meal, 4 tbsp (60 mL) of the cornstarch, sugar (if using) and salt; pulse to blend. Add butter and pulse until mixture resembles coarse crumbs. Add egg and pulse until a slightly sticky dough forms.

2. Turn dough out onto a large sheet of waxed paper dusted with cornstarch. Sprinkle the remaining cornstarch over dough and knead gently until dough holds together and is no longer sticky but is still very pliable. Using your fingertips, press dough into a 10-inch (25 cm) circle.

3. Invert pie plate on top of dough. Quickly flip both pan and dough over so that the dough rests in the pan. Gently peel away and discard waxed paper. Press dough into pie plate, patching it together, if necessary. Crimp and trim the edges as desired. Using a fork, prick the sides and bottom all over.

### To Parbake

4. Bake in preheated oven for 14 to 18 minutes or until golden. Let cool slightly on a wire rack, then fill and bake as directed in the recipe.

### To Bake Completely

4. Bake in preheated oven for 24 to 28 minutes or until golden brown and set at the edges. Let cool completely on a wire rack. Fill as desired.

# Quinoa Flake Pie or Tart Crust

*This fantastic pie crust
gives graham cracker
crusts a run for their
money. Light and crispy,
it works especially well
with sweet custard- or
fruit-filled pies.*

## Tip

The pie and tart recipes in
this chapter call for either
a "parbaked" or a "baked"
crust. Make sure to note
which is specified and
follow the appropriate
version of step 3, at right,
including letting the
crust cool as instructed,
before proceeding with
the recipe.

- **Preheat oven to 350°F (180°C)**
- **9-inch (23 cm) pie plate or fluted tart pan with removable bottom**

| | | |
|---|---|---|
| 1½ cups | quinoa flakes or quick-cooking rolled oats (certified GF, if needed) | 375 mL |
| ¾ cup | quinoa flour | 175 mL |
| ⅓ cup | natural cane sugar or packed light brown sugar | 75 mL |
| ¼ tsp | fine sea salt | 1 mL |
| 6 tbsp | unsalted butter, melted and cooled slightly | 90 mL |
| 6 tbsp | milk or plain non-dairy milk (such as soy, almond, rice or hemp) | 90 mL |

1. In a large bowl, combine quinoa flakes, quinoa flour, sugar and salt. Stir in butter and milk until blended.
2. Transfer quinoa mixture to pie plate. Using moist fingers, press mixture over bottom and up sides of plate. Place pie plate on a large baking sheet.

### To Parbake

3. Bake in preheated oven for 12 to 15 minutes or until golden. Let cool slightly on a wire rack, then fill and bake as directed in the recipe.

### To Bake Completely

3. Bake in preheated oven for 23 to 27 minutes or until golden brown and set at the edges. Let cool completely on a wire rack. Fill as desired.

# Walnut-Quinoa Pie or Tart Crust

*Have leftover quinoa?
Make this easy crust,
then use it for any sweet
or savory filling.*

## Tips

For best results, spread the
dough somewhat thinner
on the bottom and slightly
thicker on the walls of the
pie plate.

The pie and tart recipes in
this chapter call for either
a "parbaked" or a "baked"
crust. Make sure to note
which is specified and
follow the appropriate
version of step 3, at right,
including letting the
crust cool as instructed,
before proceeding with
the recipe.

- **Preheat oven to 350°F (180°C)**
- **Food processor**
- **9-inch (23 cm) pie plate or fluted tart pan with removable bottom**

| | | |
|---|---|---|
| 1½ cups | chopped walnuts | 375 mL |
| 1 cup | cooked quinoa (see page 10), cooled | 250 mL |
| 1 tsp | baking soda | 5 mL |
| ¼ tsp | fine sea salt | 1 mL |
| 2 tbsp | unsalted butter, melted, or unrefined virgin coconut oil, warmed | 30 mL |

1. In food processor, combine walnuts, quinoa, baking soda and salt; process until finely ground. Add butter and pulse until blended.
2. Transfer walnut mixture to pie plate. Using moist fingers, press mixture over bottom and up sides of plate. Place pie plate on a large baking sheet.

### To Parbake

3. Bake in preheated oven for 14 to 17 minutes or until golden. Let cool slightly on a wire rack, then fill and bake as directed in the recipe.

### To Bake Completely

3. Bake in preheated oven for 23 to 27 minutes or until golden brown and set at the edges. Let cool completely on a wire rack. Fill as desired.

## Variation

*Pecan-Quinoa Pie Crust:* Replace the walnuts with chopped pecans.

# Apple Custard Pie

*Tart-sweet apples and honey-sweetened custard mingle in this updated version of a North American favorite. It's a showstopper when paired with the lightly sweet quinoa flake crust.*

## Storage Tip

Store the cooled pie, loosely wrapped in foil or waxed paper, in the refrigerator for up to 2 days.

- **Preheat oven to 350°F (180°C)**
- **Rimmed baking sheet**

| | | |
|---|---|---|
| 2 | large eggs | 2 |
| ⅓ cup | liquid honey or pure maple syrup | 75 mL |
| 1 tsp | vanilla extract (GF, if needed) | 5 mL |
| ¾ cup | milk or plain non-dairy milk (such as soy, almond, rice or hemp) | 175 mL |
| 6 cups | sliced peeled tart-sweet apples (such as Gala or Braeburn) | 1.5 L |
| 1 | parbaked Quinoa Flake Pie Crust (page 445) | 1 |
| 1 tbsp | turbinado or natural cane sugar | 15 mL |
| ½ tsp | ground cinnamon | 2 mL |

1. In a medium bowl, whisk together eggs, honey and vanilla. Whisk in milk until blended. Arrange apples in prepared crust and pour egg mixture evenly over apples. Place pie plate on baking sheet.
2. Bake in preheated oven for 25 minutes.
3. In a small bowl, combine sugar and cinnamon. Sprinkle over pie and bake for 10 to 15 minutes or until filling is set. Let cool completely on a wire rack.

# Cranberry Orange Tart

*Fresh orange and a toasty quinoa crust balance the tartness in this custardy Southern pie.*

## Tip

An equal amount of brown rice syrup, pure maple syrup or agave nectar may be used in place of the honey.

## Storage Tip

Store the cooled tart, loosely wrapped in foil or waxed paper, in the refrigerator for up to 2 days.

| | | |
|---|---|---|
| 2½ tbsp | cornstarch or arrowroot | 37 mL |
| ¾ cup | liquid honey | 175 mL |
| 1 tbsp | finely grated orange zest | 15 mL |
| ⅓ cup | freshly squeezed orange juice | 75 mL |
| 3 cups | fresh or frozen cranberries | 750 mL |
| ½ cup | chopped toasted walnuts (optional) | 125 mL |
| 1 | parbaked Walnut-Quinoa Tart Crust (page 446) or Quinoa Flake Tart Crust (page 445) | 1 |

1. In a medium saucepan, whisk together cornstarch, honey, orange zest and orange juice. Stir in cranberries. Bring to a boil over medium-high heat, stirring constantly. Reduce heat and simmer, stirring occasionally, for 5 to 7 minutes or until mixture thickens and cranberries begin to pop. Remove from heat and let cool to room temperature.
2. Meanwhile, preheat oven to 350°F (180°C).
3. If desired, stir walnuts into filling. Pour filling into prepared crust.
4. Bake in preheated oven for 25 to 30 minutes or until crust is golden brown at the edges. Let cool completely on a wire rack.

# Toasted Coconut Cream Pie

**Makes
8 servings**

*This tart is all about the coconut. Don't expect an overly sweet, cloying confection, though; this one is a buttery shell filled with creamy egg- and dairy-free custard and topped with nutty toasted coconut.*

## Tip

To toast coconut, preheat oven to 300°F (150°C). Spread coconut in a thin, even layer on an ungreased baking sheet. Bake for 15 to 20 minutes, stirring every 5 minutes, until golden brown and fragrant. Transfer to a plate and let cool completely.

## Storage Tip

Store the cooled pie, loosely wrapped in foil or plastic wrap, in the refrigerator for up to 1 day.

- **Blender or food processor**

| | | |
|---|---|---|
| 8 oz | firm silken tofu, drained | 250 g |
| 1/2 cup | agave nectar, brown rice syrup or liquid honey | 125 mL |
| 6 tbsp | cornstarch or arrowroot | 90 mL |
| 1/8 tsp | fine sea salt | 0.5 mL |
| 2 cups | light coconut milk | 500 mL |
| 1 tsp | vanilla extract (GF, if needed) | 5 mL |
| 1 | baked Quinoa Flake Pie Crust (page 445) | 1 |
| 1 cup | unsweetened flaked coconut, toasted (see tip, at left) | 250 mL |

1. In blender, combine tofu and agave nectar; process for 2 to 3 minutes or until smooth.
2. In a medium saucepan, whisk cornstarch, salt and 1/2 cup (125 mL) of the coconut milk until smooth. Whisk in remaining coconut milk. Bring to a gentle boil over medium-high heat, whisking constantly. Reduce heat and cook, whisking occasionally, for 7 to 10 minutes or until thickened. Remove from heat and whisk in tofu mixture and vanilla until blended.
3. Spread filling in prepared crust and sprinkle with coconut. Loosely cover with plastic wrap or foil and refrigerate for at least 4 hours, until firm, or overnight.

# Pumpkin Pie

*Thanksgiving without
pumpkin pie is almost
unthinkable, but that
doesn't mean you can't
have some fun with
the ingredients. Here,
pumpkin is sweetened
with maple syrup for a
full, autumnal sweetness.
There's a bit of tang, too,
from the yogurt and an
underlying warmth from
the quinoa crust.*

## Storage Tip

Store the cooled pie,
loosely wrapped in foil
or waxed paper, in the
refrigerator for up to
3 days.

**• Preheat oven to 350°F (180°C)**

| | | |
|---|---|---|
| 2 tbsp | quinoa flour | 30 mL |
| 2½ tsp | pumpkin pie spice | 12 mL |
| ¼ tsp | fine sea salt | 1 mL |
| 3 | large eggs | 3 |
| 1 | can (15 oz/425 mL) pumpkin purée (not pie filling) | 1 |
| ¾ cup | pure maple syrup or liquid honey | 175 mL |
| ½ cup | milk or plain non-dairy milk (such as soy, almond, rice or hemp) | 125 mL |
| ⅓ cup | plain Greek yogurt | 75 mL |
| 1 | parbaked Quinoa Pie Crust (page 444) | 1 |

1. In a large bowl, whisk together quinoa flour, pumpkin pie spice, salt, eggs, pumpkin, maple syrup, milk and yogurt until well blended. Spread filling in prepared crust.
2. Bake in preheated oven for 55 to 60 minutes or until center is set. Let cool completely on a wire rack.

# Sweet Potato Whiskey Pie

*In many sweet potato desserts, the other ingredients — especially sugar — overwhelm the potatoes. By contrast, this pie plays to the flavor of the tubers. The result? Southern charm.*

## Tip

To make 2 cups (500 mL) sweet potato purée, you'll need 1½ lbs (750 g) sweet potatoes (about 3 medium-large). Using a fork, prick sweet potatoes all over. Place on a large plate and microwave on High, turning every 5 minutes, for 15 to 20 minutes or until very soft. Immediately cut in half to release steam. When cool enough to handle, scoop flesh into a bowl and mash until smooth. Measure 2 cups (500 mL), reserving any extra for another use.

## Storage Tip

Store the cooled pie, loosely wrapped in foil or waxed paper, in the refrigerator for up to 3 days.

- **Preheat oven to 350°F (180°C)**
- **Rimmed baking sheet**

| | | |
|---|---|---|
| ¾ cup | natural cane sugar or packed light brown sugar | 175 mL |
| ¼ cup | quinoa flour | 60 mL |
| 1 tsp | ground cinnamon | 5 mL |
| ½ tsp | ground nutmeg | 2 mL |
| ¼ tsp | fine sea salt | 1 mL |
| 3 | large eggs | 3 |
| 2 cups | cooked sweet potato purée (see tip, at left) | 500 mL |
| 2 tbsp | whiskey or bourbon | 30 mL |
| 1 | parbaked Pecan-Quinoa Pie Crust (variation, page 446) | 1 |

1. In a large bowl, whisk together sugar, quinoa flour, cinnamon, nutmeg, salt, eggs, sweet potato and whiskey until well blended.
2. Spread filling in prepared crust. Place pie plate on baking sheet.
3. Bake in preheated oven for 45 to 50 minutes or until center is set. Let cool completely on a wire rack.

# Chocolate Cream Pie

*A perfect combination of cocoa, chocolate and espresso powder, this is a dessert experience for those who welcome the true essence of chocolate — with a bit of modern flair from the walnut-quinoa crust.*

## Storage Tip

Store the cooled pie, with the surface covered in plastic wrap, in the refrigerator for up to 1 day.

| | | |
|---|---|---|
| ⅔ cup | natural cane sugar or packed light brown sugar | 150 mL |
| ½ cup | unsweetened cocoa powder (not Dutch process) | 125 mL |
| 3 tbsp | cornstarch or arrowroot | 45 mL |
| 1 tsp | instant espresso powder (optional) | 5 mL |
| ⅛ tsp | fine sea salt | 0.5 mL |
| 1 | large egg | 1 |
| 2 cups | milk or plain non-dairy milk (such as soy, almond, rice or hemp), divided | 500 mL |
| ⅓ cup | semisweet chocolate chips (GF, if needed) | 75 mL |
| 1 tsp | vanilla extract (GF, if needed) | 5 mL |
| 1 | baked Walnut-Quinoa Pie Crust (page 446) or Quinoa Flake Pie Crust (page 445) | 1 |

1. In a large bowl, whisk together sugar, cocoa powder, cornstarch, espresso powder (if using) and salt. Whisk in egg and ½ cup (125 mL) of the milk until blended.

2. In a medium saucepan, bring the remaining milk to a gentle boil over medium-high heat. Remove from heat and slowly whisk hot milk into cocoa mixture. Return milk mixture to pan and add chocolate chips. Cook over medium heat, whisking constantly, for 4 to 5 minutes or until thick and bubbly. Reduce heat and simmer, whisking, for 2 minutes. Remove from heat and whisk in vanilla.

3. Spread filling in prepared crust. Cover surface of filling with plastic wrap and refrigerate for 3 hours or until chilled.

# Chocolate and Cashew Butter Pie

**Tip**

Other natural nut or seed butters, such as peanut, almond, sunflower or sesame, may be used in place of the cashew butter.

**Storage Tip**

Store the cooled pie, with the surface covered in plastic wrap, in the refrigerator for up to 2 days.

- **Food processor or blender**

| | | |
|---|---|---|
| 1 cup | semisweet chocolate chips (GF, if needed) | 250 mL |
| 12 oz | firm silken tofu, drained | 375 g |
| ½ cup | pure maple syrup or brown rice syrup | 125 mL |
| 1 cup | unsweetened natural cashew butter | 250 mL |
| 1 | baked Quinoa Flake Pie Crust (page 445) | 1 |

1. In a small microwave-safe bowl, microwave chocolate chips on Medium (70%) for 30 seconds. Stir. Microwave on Medium (70%) in 15-second intervals, stirring after each, until melted and smooth.
2. In food processor, combine tofu and maple syrup; process until smooth. Add cashew butter and process until smooth. Scrape down sides of bowl. Add melted chocolate and process until smooth.
3. Spread filling in prepared crust. Cover surface of filling with plastic wrap and refrigerate for 3 hours or until filling is set.

# Chocolate Pecan Tart

*This swanky tart, filled with toasted pecans and dark chocolate, is a wonderful take on pecan pie.*

**Storage Tip**

Store the cooled tart, loosely wrapped in foil or waxed paper, in the refrigerator for up to 3 days.

- **Preheat oven to 375°F (190°C)**

| | | |
|---|---|---|
| 1 cup | semisweet chocolate chips (GF, if needed) | 250 mL |
| ¼ cup | unsalted butter, cut into pieces | 60 mL |
| 2 tbsp | quinoa flour | 30 mL |
| ¼ tsp | fine sea salt | 1 mL |
| ½ cup | pure maple syrup or brown rice syrup | 125 mL |
| 2 tsp | vanilla extract (GF, if needed) | 10 mL |
| 3 cups | coarsely chopped toasted pecans | 750 mL |
| 1 | parbaked Quinoa Flake Tart Crust (page 445) | 1 |

1. In a medium saucepan, melt chocolate and butter over low heat, stirring until smooth. Remove from heat and whisk in quinoa flour, salt, maple syrup and vanilla until blended. Stir in pecans.
2. Spread filling in prepared crust.
3. Bake in preheated oven for 22 to 25 minutes or until crust is golden brown at the edges and filling is just set. Let cool completely on a wire rack.

# Mixed Berry Crisp

*The appeal of this simple dessert is unmistakable: it takes lush summer berries and cooks them down so that everything good about them becomes even better. A crisp topping clinches the deal.*

## Tip

For the berries, try blueberries, raspberries and/or blackberries.

## Storage Tip

Store the cooled crisp, loosely wrapped in foil or waxed paper, in the refrigerator for up to 2 days. Serve cold, or warm in the microwave on Medium (70%) for about 1 minute.

- **Preheat oven to 375°F (190°C)**
- **8- or 9-inch (20 or 23 cm) square glass baking dish, sprayed with nonstick cooking spray**

| | | |
|---|---|---|
| 6 cups | assorted fresh or thawed frozen berries | 1.5 L |
| 1 tbsp | cornstarch or arrowroot | 15 mL |
| 2 tbsp | brown rice syrup, liquid honey or pure maple syrup | 30 mL |
| 1 tbsp | freshly squeezed lemon juice | 15 mL |
| 2/3 cup | quinoa flour | 150 mL |
| 1/2 cup | quinoa flakes or large-flake (old-fashioned) rolled oats (certified GF, if needed) | 125 mL |
| 1/2 cup | natural cane sugar or packed light brown sugar | 125 mL |
| 3/4 tsp | ground cinnamon | 3 mL |
| 1/8 tsp | fine sea salt | 0.5 mL |
| 1/3 cup | cold unsalted butter or unrefined virgin coconut oil, cut into small pieces | 75 mL |
| | Honey- or vanilla-flavored Greek yogurt | |

1. In a large bowl, combine berries, cornstarch, brown rice syrup and lemon juice. Transfer to prepared baking dish.
2. In a medium bowl, whisk together quinoa flour, quinoa flakes, sugar, cinnamon and salt. Using a pastry blender or two knives, cut in butter until mixture resembles coarse crumbs. Sprinkle over berry mixture.
3. Bake in preheated oven for 28 to 33 minutes or until berries are bubbling and topping is golden brown. Let cool on a wire rack for 10 minutes before serving.

# Blueberry Crumble

*Fruit crumbles are such happy desserts. Perhaps because they are often made when berries, peaches and other lush fruits are in season — during the summer — fruit crumbles seem to call out for taking it easy and enjoying the day.*

## Tip

Other berries, such as blackberries or raspberries, may be used in place of the blueberries.

## Storage Tip

Store the cooled crumble, loosely wrapped in foil or waxed paper, in the refrigerator for up to 2 days. Serve cold, or warm in the microwave on Medium (70%) for about 1 minute.

- **Preheat oven to 350°F (180°C)**
- **8- or 9-inch (20 or 23 cm) square glass baking dish, sprayed with nonstick cooking spray**

| | | |
|---|---|---|
| 3 cups | fresh or thawed frozen blueberries | 750 mL |
| 2 tbsp | freshly squeezed lemon juice | 30 mL |
| 2 cups | cooked quinoa (see page 10), cooled | 500 mL |
| 2/3 cup | natural cane sugar or packed light brown sugar | 150 mL |
| 1/2 cup | quinoa flour | 125 mL |
| 2 tsp | ground cinnamon | 10 mL |
| 1/4 cup | unsalted butter, melted | 60 mL |
| | Vanilla- or honey-flavored Greek yogurt (optional) | |

1. Place blueberries in prepared baking dish and sprinkle with lemon juice.
2. In a medium bowl, combine quinoa, sugar, quinoa flour, cinnamon and butter. Sprinkle over blueberries.
3. Bake in preheated oven for 25 to 30 minutes or until berries are bubbling and topping is golden brown. Let cool on a wire rack for 15 minutes. Serve warm or at room temperature, topped with a dollop of yogurt, if desired.

# Honey Apple Crumble

**Makes
9 servings**

The combination of honey and apples has been a favorite since Ancient Greek times. But here they are thoroughly modern in a cozy quinoa crumble that is further enhanced with cinnamon and vanilla.

## Tips

You'll need about 6 large apples to make 10 cups (2.5 L) sliced.

Removing the foil halfway through baking allows the topping to become crisp and browned.

## Storage Tip

Store the cooled crumble, loosely wrapped in foil or waxed paper, in the refrigerator for up to 2 days. Serve cold, or warm in the microwave on Medium (70%) for about 1 minute.

- **Preheat oven to 375°F (190°C)**
- **13- by 9-inch (33 by 23 cm) glass baking dish, sprayed with nonstick cooking spray**

| | | |
|---|---|---|
| 1¼ cups | quinoa flakes or large-flake (old-fashioned) oats (certified GF, if needed) | 300 mL |
| ¾ cup | quinoa flour | 175 mL |
| ½ cup | natural cane sugar or packed light brown sugar | 125 mL |
| 1 tsp | ground cinnamon | 5 mL |
| ½ tsp | fine sea salt | 2 mL |
| ½ cup | unsalted butter, melted and cooled slightly | 125 mL |
| 2 tsp | vanilla extract (GF, if needed), divided | 10 mL |
| 1½ tsp | cornstarch | 7 mL |
| ½ cup | unsweetened apple juice | 125 mL |
| 3 tbsp | liquid honey or pure maple syrup | 45 mL |
| 10 cups | sliced peeled tart-sweet apples (such as Braeburn or Gala) | 2.5 L |
| | Vanilla-flavored Greek yogurt (optional) | |

1. In a medium bowl, whisk together quinoa flakes, quinoa flour, sugar, cinnamon and salt. Stir in butter and half the vanilla until moist and crumbly.

2. In a large bowl, whisk together cornstarch, apple juice, honey and the remaining vanilla. Add apples and toss to coat.

3. Spoon apple mixture into baking prepared dish and sprinkle with quinoa flake mixture. Cover with foil.

4. Bake in preheated oven for 30 minutes. Remove foil and bake for 25 to 30 minutes or until browned and bubbling and apples are tender. Let cool on a wire rack for 30 minutes. Serve warm or at room temperature, topped with a dollop of yogurt, if desired.

## Variation

*Honey Peach Crumble:* Replace the apples with an equal amount of sliced peeled peaches (fresh or thawed frozen).

*Rhubarb Crumble:* Replace the apples with an equal amount of fresh or thawed frozen sliced rhubarb (½-inch/1 cm slices). Increase the honey to ⅓ cup (75 mL).

# Pear and Honey Clafouti

*Clafouti is something of a cross between a flan and a fruit-filled pancake. Traditional versions embrace cherries, but any fruit, such as lush, fragrant pears, can be used. The clafouti will puff up dramatically during baking, then collapse. Let it cool slightly before serving, then chill the leftovers for a delicious breakfast treat the next morning.*

## Storage Tip

Store the cooled clafouti, loosely wrapped in foil or waxed paper, in the refrigerator for up to 2 days.

- **Preheat oven to 400°F (200°C)**
- **8- or 9-inch (20 or 23 cm) square glass baking dish, sprayed with nonstick cooking spray**

| | | |
|---|---|---|
| 3 | large pears (about 1½ lbs/750 g), cored and cut into sixths | 3 |
| ¼ cup | liquid honey | 60 mL |
| 4 | large eggs | 4 |
| ¾ cup | quinoa flour | 175 mL |
| 3 tbsp | natural cane sugar or granulated sugar, divided | 45 mL |
| ¼ tsp | ground nutmeg | 1 mL |
| ¼ tsp | fine sea salt | 1 mL |
| 1 cup + 1 tbsp | milk | 265 mL |
| 3 tbsp | unsalted butter, melted and cooled | 45 mL |

1. Arrange pears in prepared baking dish and drizzle with honey.
2. Separate 3 of the eggs.
3. In a large bowl, whisk together quinoa flour, 2 tbsp (30 mL) of the sugar, nutmeg and salt. Whisk in egg yolks, the remaining whole egg and milk until blended. Whisk in butter.
4. In a medium bowl, using an electric mixer on low speed, beat egg whites until foamy. Add the remaining sugar and beat on medium-high speed until soft peaks form. Fold egg whites into batter. Pour batter over pears.
5. Bake in preheated oven for 25 to 30 minutes or until puffed and golden. Let cool completely on a wire rack.

## Variation

Use an equal amount of pure maple syrup in place of the honey.

# Baked Apples with Quinoa and Dried Cherry Filling

*After a rich main course in the colder months, you'll love the minimalist sensibility of these baked apples. Leftovers are fabulous for breakfast, served cold or warm.*

## Tip

Other varieties of dried fruit, such as blueberries, raisins or chopped apricots, may be used in place of the cherries

## Storage Tip

Store the cooled apples, loosely covered in foil or plastic wrap, in the refrigerator for up to 1 day. Serve cold, or warm in the microwave on Medium (70%) for about 1 minute.

- **Preheat oven to 350°F (180°C)**
- **8- or 9-inch (20 or 23 cm) square glass baking dish or glass pie plate**

| 4 | tart-sweet apples (such as Braeburn, Gala or Fuji), cored | 4 |
|---|---|---|
| ½ cup | cooked quinoa (see page 10), cooled | 125 mL |
| ⅓ cup | dried cherries or cranberries | 75 mL |
| ⅓ cup | chopped toasted pecans | 75 mL |
| ½ tsp | ground cinnamon | 2 mL |
| 6 tbsp | pure maple syrup or liquid honey, divided | 90 mL |
| 4 tbsp | plain Greek yogurt | 60 mL |

1. Using a vegetable peeler, peel top 1 inch (2.5 cm) of apples. Place apples, top side up, in baking dish.
2. In a small bowl, combine quinoa, cherries, pecans, cinnamon and 2 tbsp (30 mL) of the maple syrup. Stuff quinoa mixture into apple cavities. Drizzle 1 tbsp (15 mL) of the remaining maple syrup over each apple.
3. Bake in preheated oven for 45 to 55 minutes, brushing occasionally with accumulated juices, until apples are tender.
4. Transfer apples to a plate and pour pan juices over top. Serve each apple dolloped with 1 tbsp (15 mL) yogurt.

# Cocoa, Quinoa and Cashew Truffles

**Makes 2 dozen truffles**

*Cocoa powder is nothing if not versatile: you can transform it into a quick chocolate sauce, make it into hot cocoa in minutes or use it as the base for cookies. But if you're feeling even mildly industrious, use it to make these truffles. The combination of cashews, quinoa, dates and cocoa powder produces a deeply flavored, not-too-sweet confection.*

## Tip

Dutch process cocoa powder may be used in place of the natural cocoa in this recipe, but I prefer the latter for its deep, true chocolate flavor and minimal processing.

## Storage Tip

Store the truffles in an airtight container in the refrigerator for up to 1 week.

- **Food processor**

| 1 cup | raw cashews | 250 mL |
| | Cold water | |
| 1 cup | cooked quinoa (see page 10), cooled | 250 mL |
| 2 cups | packed chopped pitted dates | 500 mL |
| ⅔ cup | unsweetened cocoa powder (preferably natural cocoa) | 150 mL |
| ¼ tsp | fine sea salt | 1 mL |
| 1 tbsp | vanilla extract (GF, if needed) | 15 mL |
| | Additional unsweetened cocoa powder (optional) | |

1. Place cashews in a medium bowl and add enough cold water to cover. Let soak for 4 to 6 hours to soften. Drain well.

2. In food processor, pulse softened cashews and quinoa until mixture becomes a paste. Add dates, cocoa powder, salt and vanilla; process until almost smooth, stopping once or twice to scrape sides of bowl. Transfer to a medium bowl, cover and refrigerate for at least 2 hours or until firm enough to roll.

3. Roll quinoa mixture into 1-inch (2.5 cm) balls. If desired, roll in cocoa powder to coat.

# Basic Quinoa Thumbprints

*For their sheer cuteness alone, these jam-filled cookies are irresistible. Quinoa flour gives the shortbread bases a nutty flavor that perfectly complements the jam centers. Any flavor of jam or preserves will work for the filling; for a colorful variety, fill a batch with a few different types.*

## Tip

If the edges crack too much when you're pressing your thumb into the dough, reroll the dough and try again.

## Storage Tip

Store the cooled cookies in an airtight container in the refrigerator for up to 5 days.

- **Preheat oven to 350°F (180°C)**
- **Small baking sheet, lined with parchment paper**

| | | |
|---|---|---|
| 7 tbsp | natural cane sugar or granulated sugar, divided | 105 mL |
| ⅓ cup | unsalted butter, at room temperature | 75 mL |
| 1 tsp | vanilla extract (GF, if needed) | 5 mL |
| ¾ cup | quinoa flour | 175 mL |
| ¼ cup | jam, preserves or marmalade | 60 mL |

**1.** In a medium bowl, using an electric mixer on medium speed, beat 5 tbsp (75 mL) of the sugar and the butter until light and fluffy. Beat in vanilla until blended. Using a wooden spoon, stir in quinoa flour until blended.

**2.** Roll dough into twelve 1-inch (2.5 cm) balls. Place the remaining sugar in a shallow dish and roll balls in sugar to coat. Place balls 2 inches (5 cm) apart on prepared baking sheet. Using your thumb, make a small indentation in the center of each ball.

**3.** Bake in preheated oven for 11 to 13 minutes or until puffed and just set at the edges. Let cool on pan on a wire rack for 2 minutes, then transfer to the rack to cool. Just before serving, spoon about ¼ tsp (1 mL) jam into each indentation.

# No-Bake Jam Thumbprints

**Makes
18 cookies**

*A hearty dose of quinoa flakes and natural nut butter balances the mild sweetness of these no-bake charmers. Consider the recipe a blueprint for countless variations: change the nut butter, juice and jam according to your whims or what's on hand.*

## Tips

You can use any unsweetened natural nut or seed butter, such as peanut, cashew or sunflower, in place of the almond butter.

There's no need to clean the food processor bowl between steps 2 and 3.

## Storage Tip

Store the chilled cookies in an airtight container in the refrigerator for up to 1 week.

- **Food processor**
- **Small baking sheet, lined with parchment paper or foil**

| | | |
|---|---|---|
| ½ cup | chopped pitted dates | 125 mL |
| | Hot water | |
| 1½ cups | quinoa flakes | 375 mL |
| ⅓ cup | unsweetened flaked coconut | 75 mL |
| ½ tsp | ground cinnamon | 2 mL |
| ¼ tsp | fine sea salt | 1 mL |
| 1 tsp | finely grated orange zest | 5 mL |
| ¼ cup | freshly squeezed orange juice | 60 mL |
| ¾ cup | unsweetened natural almond butter | 175 mL |
| ¼ cup | raspberry or other fruit jam sweetened with fruit juice | 60 mL |

1. Place dates in a medium bowl and add enough hot water to cover. Let soak for 15 minutes. Drain, reserving ½ cup (125 mL) soaking liquid.

2. Meanwhile, in food processor, combine quinoa flakes, coconut, cinnamon and salt; pulse until coarsely ground. Transfer to a large bowl.

3. In food processor, combine soaked dates, the reserved soaking liquid, orange zest and orange juice; purée until smooth.

4. Add the date mixture and almond butter to the quinoa mixture, mixing with a wooden spoon or your hands to make a cohesive dough.

5. Roll dough into eighteen 1-inch (2.5 cm) balls. Place on prepared baking sheet. Using your thumb, make a small indentation in the center of each ball. Loosely cover with foil or plastic wrap and refrigerate for 1 hour or until chilled. Just before serving, spoon ¼ tsp (1 mL) jam into each indentation.

# Oatmeal Quinoa Cookies

*It's likely you've nibbled one too many cookies whose sweetness overpowers the other ingredients. These oatmeal cookies couldn't be more of a contrast. The restrained, mellow sweetness from the dates and brown rice syrup still allows the toasty flavor of the oats and walnuts to come through.*

## Storage Tip

Store the cooled cookies in an airtight container in the refrigerator for up to 5 days.

- **Preheat oven to 350°F (180°C)**
- **Food processor**
- **Large baking sheet, lined with parchment paper**

| | | |
|---|---|---|
| 1 cup | chopped pitted dates | 250 mL |
| 1 cup | chopped walnuts or pecans | 250 mL |
| 1 cup | large-flake (old-fashioned) rolled oats (certified GF, if needed) | 250 mL |
| ¾ cup | quinoa flour | 175 mL |
| ½ tsp | ground cinnamon | 2 mL |
| ½ tsp | fine sea salt | 2 mL |
| ¼ tsp | baking soda | 1 mL |
| 1 | large egg, at room temperature | 1 |
| ¼ cup | brown rice syrup, pure maple syrup or liquid honey | 60 mL |
| ¼ cup | unsweetened applesauce | 60 mL |
| ¼ cup | vegetable oil | 60 mL |
| 1 tsp | vanilla extract (GF, if needed) | 5 mL |

1. In food processor, combine dates and walnuts; pulse until finely chopped.
2. In a large bowl, whisk together oats, quinoa flour, cinnamon, salt and baking soda. Stir in date mixture, egg, brown rice syrup, applesauce, oil and vanilla until just blended.
3. Drop dough by tablespoonfuls (15 mL) onto prepared baking sheet, spacing them 2 inches (5 cm) apart. Flatten slightly with your fingertips.
4. Bake in preheated oven for 20 to 25 minutes or until just set at the center. Let cool on pan on a wire rack for 2 minutes, then transfer to the rack to cool.
5. Repeat steps 3 and 4 with the remaining dough.

## Variations

Substitute pumpkin purée (not pie filling) for the applesauce.

Use quinoa flakes in place of the oats.

# Maple Cinnamon Cookies

*These aromatic cookies
may bring to mind winter
holidays, but they are
worth baking — and
eating — throughout
the year.*

## Storage Tip

Store the cooled cookies
in an airtight container in
the refrigerator for up to
5 days.

- **Preheat oven to 350°F (180°C)**
- **Large baking sheet, lined with parchment paper**

| | | |
|---|---|---|
| 2 cups | quinoa flakes | 500 mL |
| 1 cup | quinoa flour | 250 mL |
| 1½ tsp | ground cinnamon | 7 mL |
| ¼ tsp | fine sea salt | 1 mL |
| ¼ tsp | baking soda | 1 mL |
| ½ cup | vegetable oil | 125 mL |
| ½ cup | pure maple syrup | 125 mL |
| 2 tsp | vanilla extract (GF, if needed) | 10 mL |

1. In a large bowl, whisk together quinoa flakes, quinoa flour, cinnamon, salt and baking soda. Stir in oil, maple syrup and vanilla until just blended.
2. Drop dough by tablespoonfuls (15 mL) onto prepared baking sheet, spacing them 2 inches (5 cm) apart. Flatten slightly with your fingertips.
3. Bake in preheated oven for 12 to 15 minutes or until just set at the center. Let cool on pan on a wire rack for 5 minutes, then transfer to the rack to cool.
4. Repeat steps 2 and 3 with the remaining dough.

## Variation

*Honey Cardamom Cookies:* Replace the maple syrup with liquid honey and replace the cinnamon with 1 tsp (5 mL) ground cardamom.

# Ginger Quinoa Crinkles

**Makes
30 cookies**

*Turbinado sugar
(sometimes called
raw sugar) adds a
sophisticated sparkle
and crunch to these spicy
favorites. The nutty-sweet
flavor of quinoa flour
boosts the deep flavor of
the molasses and spices.*

## Storage Tip

Store the cooled cookies
in an airtight container in
the refrigerator for up to
5 days.

• **2 large baking sheets, lined with parchment paper**

| | | |
|---|---|---|
| 1⅓ cups | quinoa flour | 325 mL |
| 2½ tsp | ground ginger | 12 mL |
| 2 tsp | baking soda | 10 mL |
| 1 tsp | ground cinnamon | 5 mL |
| ¼ tsp | ground cloves | 1 mL |
| ¼ tsp | fine sea salt | 1 mL |
| ⅔ cup | natural cane sugar or packed dark brown sugar | 150 mL |
| ⅓ cup | unsalted butter, softened | 75 mL |
| 1 | large egg | 1 |
| ¼ cup | dark (cooking) molasses | 60 mL |
| ¾ cup | cooked quinoa (see page 10), cooled | 175 mL |
| 3 tbsp | turbinado sugar | 45 mL |

1. In a small bowl, whisk together quinoa flour, ginger, baking soda, cinnamon, cloves and salt.

2. In a large bowl, using an electric mixer on medium speed, beat cane sugar and butter until light and fluffy. Beat in egg and molasses until blended. Using a wooden spoon, stir in quinoa. Stir in flour mixture until just blended. Cover and refrigerate for 1 hour.

3. Preheat oven to 350°F (180°C).

4. Roll dough into thirty 1-inch (2.5 cm) balls. Place turbinado sugar in a shallow dish and roll balls in sugar to coat. Place balls 2 inches (5 cm) apart on prepared baking sheets.

5. Bake, one sheet at a time, for 9 to 12 minutes or until puffed and set at the edges. Let cool on pan on a wire rack for 3 minutes, then transfer to the rack to cool.

# Peanut Butter and Jam Cookies

*A vibrant dab of jam in the center of salty-nutty peanut butter dough creates a time-honored flavor combination with a subtle quinoa twist.*

## Tip

Other natural nut or seed butters, such as cashew, almond, sunflower or sesame, may be used in place of the peanut butter.

## Storage Tip

Store the cooled cookies in an airtight container in the refrigerator for up to 5 days.

- **2 large baking sheets, lined with parchment paper**

| | | |
|---|---|---|
| ¾ cup | natural cane sugar or granulated sugar | 175 mL |
| ¾ cup | unsweetened natural peanut butter | 175 mL |
| 1 | large egg, beaten | 1 |
| ⅓ cup | quinoa flour | 75 mL |
| 6 tbsp | raspberry jam or preserves sweetened with fruit juice | 90 mL |

1. In a medium bowl, using an electric mixer on medium speed, beat sugar and peanut butter until smooth. Add egg, beating on low speed until blended. Using a wooden spoon, stir in quinoa flour until just blended.
2. Roll dough into thirty-six 1-inch (2.5 cm) balls. Place balls 1 inch (2.5 cm) apart on prepared baking sheets. Using your thumb, make a small indentation in the center of each ball. Cover and refrigerate for 3 hours.
3. Preheat oven to 375°F (190°C).
4. Bake, one sheet at a time, for 10 to 12 minutes or until just set. Let cool on pan on a wire rack for 2 minutes, then transfer to the rack to cool. Just before serving, spoon about ½ tsp (2 mL) jam into each indentation.

# Cinnamon Raisin Cookies

*Your subconscious will
register "cozy comfort"
with this nostalgic
combination of cinnamon,
raisins and vanilla.
Cooked quinoa in the
dough gives the cookies
a unique and incredibly
appealing texture
reminiscent of oatmeal
and a flavor hinting of
toasted nuts and sesame.*

## Tip

Other dried fruits, such as
cranberries, blueberries or
chopped apricots, may be
used in place of the raisins.

## Storage Tip

Store the cooled cookies
in an airtight container in
the refrigerator for up to
5 days.

- **Preheat oven to 350°F (180°C)**
- **Large baking sheet, lined with parchment paper**

| | | |
|---|---|---|
| 1¼ cups | quinoa flour | 300 mL |
| 1 tbsp | cornstarch or arrowroot | 15 mL |
| ½ tsp | baking soda | 2 mL |
| 1½ tsp | ground cinnamon | 7 mL |
| ½ tsp | fine sea salt | 2 mL |
| 1 cup | natural cane sugar or packed dark brown sugar | 250 mL |
| 1 | large egg | 1 |
| ½ cup | unrefined virgin coconut oil, warmed slightly, or unsalted butter, softened | 125 mL |
| 1 tsp | vanilla extract (GF, if needed) | 5 mL |
| 1½ cups | cooked quinoa (see page 10), cooled | 375 mL |
| ¾ cup | raisins | 175 mL |
| ½ cup | chopped toasted pecans or walnuts (optional) | 125 mL |

1. In a small bowl, whisk together quinoa flour, cornstarch, baking soda, cinnamon and salt.
2. In a large bowl, using an electric mixer on medium speed, beat sugar, egg, oil and vanilla until blended. Using a wooden spoon, stir in flour mixture until just blended. Stir in quinoa, raisins and pecans (if using).
3. Drop dough by tablespoonfuls (15 mL) onto prepared baking sheet, spacing them 2 inches (5 cm) apart.
4. Bake in preheated oven for 9 to 12 minutes or until golden brown. Let cool on pan on a wire rack for 2 minutes, then transfer to the rack to cool.
5. Repeat steps 3 and 4 with the remaining dough.

# Soft Apple Cookies

*These tender spiced cookies are reminiscent of apple pie. A double dose of apple in the batter — applesauce and chopped fresh apples — keeps them exceptionally moist.*

## Storage Tip

Store the cooled cookies in an airtight container in the refrigerator for up to 3 days.

- **Preheat oven to 325°F (160°C)**
- **Large baking sheet, lined with parchment paper**

| | | |
|---|---|---|
| 1½ cups | quinoa flour | 375 mL |
| 1 cup | large-flake (old-fashioned) rolled oats (certified GF, if needed) | 250 mL |
| ¾ cup | natural cane sugar or granulated sugar | 175 mL |
| 2 tsp | ground cinnamon | 10 mL |
| 1½ tsp | baking powder (GF, if needed) | 7 mL |
| 1 tsp | baking soda | 5 mL |
| ¼ tsp | ground nutmeg | 1 mL |
| ¼ tsp | fine sea salt | 1 mL |
| 1 | large egg, lightly beaten | 1 |
| ¼ cup | unsweetened applesauce | 60 mL |
| 3 tbsp | vegetable oil | 45 mL |
| 3 tbsp | pure maple syrup or liquid honey | 45 mL |
| 1 cup | finely chopped peeled tart-sweet apples (such as Braeburn, Gala or Pippin) | 250 mL |

1. In a large bowl, whisk together quinoa flour, oats, sugar, cinnamon, baking powder, baking soda, nutmeg and salt. Stir in egg, applesauce, oil and maple syrup until just blended. Gently fold in apples.

2. Drop dough by tablespoonfuls (15 mL) onto prepared baking sheet, spacing them 2 inches (5 cm) apart.

3. Bake in preheated oven for 12 to 15 minutes or until just set at the center. Let cool on pan on a wire rack for 5 minutes, then transfer to the rack to cool.

4. Repeat steps 2 and 3 with the remaining dough.

# Coconut and Cranberry Macaroons

*I'm a bit of a snob about macaroons — I like the kind that strikes a good balance between chewy and crisp, with just a slight nuance of almond flavor. This recipe fits the bill. Better still, you can bang out a batch in well under an hour.*

## Tips

Natural cane confectioners' (icing) sugar is made using the same process as regular confectioners' sugar (granulated sugar is crushed to a fine white powder), but is made with less processed natural cane sugar. Regular confectioners' sugar may be used in its place.

If you like, you can moisten your fingertips and shape the drops into rounded or peaked mounds before baking.

## Storage Tip

Store the cooled cookies in an airtight container at room temperature for up to 5 days.

- **Preheat oven to 300°F (150°C)**
- **Food processor**
- **Large baking sheet, lined with parchment paper**

| | | |
|---|---|---|
| 2½ cups | unsweetened flaked coconut | 625 mL |
| 3 | large egg whites, at room temperature | 3 |
| ⅛ tsp | fine sea salt | 0.5 mL |
| ½ cup + 2 tbsp | natural cane confectioners' (icing) sugar | 155 mL |
| 1 tsp | almond extract (GF, if needed) | 5 mL |
| ⅔ cup | quinoa flakes | 150 mL |
| ½ cup | dried cranberries, finely chopped | 125 mL |

1. In food processor, process coconut until very finely chopped.
2. In a large bowl, using an electric mixer on medium-high speed, beat egg whites and salt until soft peaks form. Reduce speed to medium and gradually beat in confectioners' sugar. Beat in almond extract. Using a rubber spatula, gently fold in coconut, quinoa flakes and cranberries.
3. Drop dough by rounded tablespoonfuls (15 mL) onto prepared baking sheet, spacing them 2 inches (5 cm) apart.
4. Bake in preheated oven for 20 to 25 minutes or until tops and bottoms are golden brown and slightly crisped. Let cool on pan on a wire rack for 5 minutes, then transfer to the rack to cool.
5. Repeat steps 3 and 4 with the remaining dough.

# Coconut Pecan Cookies

*Newfangled has never been better. Crunchy pecans, chewy coconut and nutty quinoa? Hooray for innovation!*

## Storage Tip

Store the cooled cookies in an airtight container in the refrigerator for up to 5 days.

- **Preheat oven to 350°F (180°C)**
- **Large baking sheet, lined with parchment paper**

| | | |
|---|---|---|
| 1 cup | quinoa flour | 250 mL |
| 1½ tsp | baking powder (GF, if needed) | 7 mL |
| ¼ tsp | fine sea salt | 1 mL |
| ¾ cup | natural cane sugar or packed dark brown sugar | 175 mL |
| ½ cup | unrefined virgin coconut oil, warmed slightly, or unsalted butter, softened | 125 mL |
| 1 | large egg | 1 |
| 1 tsp | vanilla extract (GF, if needed) | 5 mL |
| 1¾ cups | cooked quinoa (see page 10), cooled | 425 mL |
| 1 cup | unsweetened flaked coconut | 250 mL |
| ¾ cup | chopped toasted pecans | 175 mL |

1. In a small bowl, whisk together quinoa flour, baking powder and salt.

2. In a large bowl, using an electric mixer on medium speed, beat sugar and oil until blended. Beat in egg and vanilla until blended. Using a wooden spoon, stir in quinoa. Stir in flour mixture until just blended. Gently fold in coconut and pecans.

3. Drop dough by tablespoonfuls (15 mL) onto prepared baking sheet, spacing them 2 inches (5 cm) apart. Flatten slightly with your fingertips.

4. Bake in preheated oven for 11 to 13 minutes or until golden brown and just set at the center. Let cool on pan on a wire rack for 2 minutes, then transfer to the rack to cool.

5. Repeat steps 3 and 4 with the remaining dough.

# Island Banana Cookies

*The inspiration for these cookies comes from the Caribbean, where bananas and coconut are popular ingredients in a wide range of both sweet and savory dishes. Here, the two ingredients converge in sweet, petite quinoa cookie harmony.*

## Tip

To toast coconut, preheat oven to 300°F (150°C). Spread coconut in a thin, even layer on an ungreased baking sheet. Bake for 15 to 20 minutes, stirring every 5 minutes, until golden brown and fragrant. Transfer to a plate and let cool completely.

## Storage Tip

Store the cooled cookies in an airtight container in the refrigerator for up to 3 days.

- **Preheat oven to 350°F (180°C)**
- **Large baking sheet, lined with parchment paper**

| | | |
|---|---|---|
| 1¾ cups | large-flake (old-fashioned) rolled oats (certified GF, if needed) | 425 mL |
| 1¼ cups | quinoa flour | 300 mL |
| 1½ tsp | ground allspice | 7 mL |
| 1 tsp | baking soda | 5 mL |
| ½ tsp | fine sea salt | 2 mL |
| ¾ cup | natural cane sugar or packed light brown sugar | 175 mL |
| 1 | large egg | 1 |
| ⅔ cup | mashed ripe banana | 150 mL |
| ¼ cup | unrefined virgin coconut oil, warmed slightly, or unsalted butter, softened | 60 mL |
| 1 tsp | vanilla extract (GF, if needed) | 5 mL |
| 1 cup | unsweetened flaked coconut, toasted (see tip, at left) | 250 mL |

1. In a medium bowl, whisk together oats, quinoa flour, allspice, baking soda and salt.
2. In a large bowl, using an electric mixer on medium speed, beat sugar, egg, banana, oil and vanilla until blended. Using a wooden spoon, stir in oat mixture and coconut until blended.
3. Drop dough by tablespoonfuls (15 mL) onto prepared baking sheet, spacing them 2 inches (5 cm) apart.
4. Bake in preheated oven for 15 to 18 minutes or until just set at the center. Let cool on pan on a wire rack for 2 minutes, then transfer to the rack to cool.
5. Repeat steps 3 and 4 with the remaining dough.

## Variation

Add ½ cup (125 mL) miniature semisweet chocolate chips (GF, if needed) with the coconut.

# Pumpkin Quinoa Cookies

*Be the hit of the party
when you arrive with a
platter of these crowd-
pleasing pumpkin
cookies. They'll satisfy
guests far beyond
taste alone.*

## Storage Tip

Store the cooled cookies
in an airtight container in
the refrigerator for up to
3 days.

- **Preheat oven to 350°F (180°C)**
- **Large baking sheet, lined with parchment paper**

| | | |
|---|---|---|
| 1⅓ cups | quinoa flour | 325 mL |
| 1 tsp | baking powder (GF, if needed) | 5 mL |
| 1 tsp | ground cinnamon | 5 mL |
| ¾ tsp | ground ginger | 3 mL |
| ½ tsp | baking soda | 2 mL |
| ½ tsp | fine sea salt | 2 mL |
| ¼ tsp | ground nutmeg | 1 mL |
| ¾ cup | natural cane sugar or packed light brown sugar | 175 mL |
| 2 | large eggs, at room temperature | 2 |
| ¾ cup | pumpkin purée (not pie filling) | 175 mL |
| ¼ cup | vegetable oil | 60 mL |
| ¼ cup | dark (cooking) molasses or liquid honey | 60 mL |
| 1 cup | dried cranberries or raisins | 250 mL |

1. In a large bowl, whisk together quinoa flour, baking powder, cinnamon, ginger, baking soda, salt and nutmeg.

2. In a medium bowl, whisk together sugar, eggs, pumpkin, oil and molasses until blended.

3. Add the pumpkin mixture to the flour mixture and stir until just blended. Gently fold in cranberries.

4. Drop dough by tablespoonfuls (15 mL) onto prepared baking sheet, spacing them 2 inches (5 cm) apart.

5. Bake in preheated oven for 10 to 12 minutes or until just set at the center. Let cool on pan on a wire rack for 5 minutes, then transfer to the rack to cool.

6. Repeat steps 4 and 5 with the remaining dough.

# Chocolate Quinoa Flake No-Bakes

*So easy and so good, variations of this great chocolate no-bake cookie — typically made with oats — abound. But traditional versions have up to an entire stick of butter per batch. My enlightened version slashes the butter without any sacrifice of chocolate goodness.*

## Storage Tip

Store the cookies in an airtight container in the refrigerator for up to 1 week.

- **Large plate or platter, lined with waxed paper or foil**

| | | |
|---|---|---|
| 1 cup | natural cane sugar or packed light brown sugar | 250 mL |
| ½ cup | milk or plain non-dairy milk (such as soy, almond, rice or hemp) | 125 mL |
| 2 tbsp | unsalted butter or unrefined virgin coconut oil | 30 mL |
| 1¼ cups | quinoa flakes | 300 mL |
| ½ cup | chopped toasted pecans | 125 mL |
| ½ cup | unsweetened cocoa powder (not Dutch process), divided | 125 mL |
| 1 tsp | vanilla extract (GF, if needed) | 5 mL |

1. In a medium saucepan, combine sugar, milk and butter. Bring to a boil over medium-high heat. Reduce heat and simmer, stirring constantly, for 3 minutes. Remove from heat and stir in quinoa flakes, pecans, ⅓ cup (75 mL) of the cocoa powder and vanilla until blended. Transfer to a medium bowl, cover and refrigerate for 1 hour or until firm.

2. Roll dough into eighteen 1-inch (2.5 cm) balls. Sift the remaining cocoa powder into a shallow dish and roll balls in cocoa powder to coat. Place balls on prepared plate.

# Multigrain Chocolate Chip Cookies

*Classic chocolate chippers get several new-fashioned, whole-grain twists — quinoa flour, flaxseed meal and oats — that add as much flavor as they do good health. Chilling the dough for an hour before baking allows the flour and oats to better absorb the liquid, yielding tender cookies.*

## Storage Tip

Store the cooled cookies in an airtight container in the refrigerator for up to 5 days.

- **Large baking sheet, lined with parchment paper**

| | | |
|---|---|---|
| 1¼ cups | quinoa flour | 300 mL |
| 1 cup | large-flake (old-fashioned) rolled oats (certified GF, if needed) | 250 mL |
| 3 tbsp | ground flax seeds (flaxseed meal) | 45 mL |
| ½ tsp | baking powder (GF, if needed) | 2 mL |
| ¼ tsp | baking soda | 1 mL |
| ¼ tsp | fine sea salt | 1 mL |
| ¾ cup | natural cane sugar or packed dark brown sugar | 175 mL |
| ⅓ cup | unsalted butter, softened | 75 mL |
| 2 | large eggs | 2 |
| 3 tbsp | liquid honey or brown rice syrup | 45 mL |
| 1½ tsp | vanilla extract (GF, if needed) | 7 mL |
| ¾ cup | miniature semisweet chocolate chips (GF, if needed) | 175 mL |

1. In a medium bowl, whisk together quinoa flour, oats, flax seeds, baking powder, baking soda and salt.
2. In a large bowl, using an electric mixer on medium speed, beat sugar and butter until light and fluffy. Beat in eggs, honey and vanilla until blended. Using a wooden spoon, stir in flour mixture until just blended. Gently stir in chocolate chips. Cover and refrigerate for at least 1 hour, until firm, or overnight.
3. Preheat oven to 350°F (180°C).
4. Drop dough by tablespoonfuls (15 mL) onto prepared baking sheet, spacing them 2 inches (5 cm) apart.
5. Bake for 10 to 12 minutes or until golden brown and just set at the edges. Let cool on pan on a wire rack for 2 minutes, then transfer to the rack to cool.
6. Repeat steps 4 and 5 with the remaining dough.

# Toasted Walnut Chocolate Chip Cookies

*Despite being loaded with superfood ingredients — walnuts, double quinoa and dark chocolate — these cookies are designed to thrill with their decadent flavor.*

## Storage Tip

Store the cooled cookies in an airtight container in the refrigerator for up to 5 days.

- **Preheat oven to 350°F (180°C)**
- **Food processor**
- **2 large baking sheets, lined with parchment paper**

| | | |
|---|---|---|
| 2 cups | toasted walnut or pecan halves | 500 mL |
| 1/3 cup | walnut or vegetable oil | 75 mL |
| 1 cup | brown rice syrup or pure maple syrup | 250 mL |
| 2 tsp | vanilla extract (GF, if needed) | 10 mL |
| 1 1/3 cups | quinoa flour | 325 mL |
| 1 tsp | baking soda | 5 mL |
| 1 tsp | fine sea salt | 5 mL |
| 2 cups | quinoa flakes or large-flake (old-fashioned) rolled oats (certified GF, if needed) | 500 mL |
| 1 1/2 cups | semisweet chocolate chips (GF, if needed) | 375 mL |

1. In food processor, process walnuts and oil for 3 to 5 minutes, stopping to scrape down sides of bowl several times, until mixture has the consistency of natural peanut butter. Add brown rice syrup and vanilla; process for 1 minute or until blended.

2. In a large bowl, whisk together quinoa flour, baking soda and salt. Stir in walnut mixture until blended. Stir in quinoa flakes and chocolate chips.

3. Roll dough into thirty 2-inch (5 cm) balls. Place balls 2 inches (5 cm) apart on prepared baking sheets and flatten with the bottom of a drinking glass dipped in water.

4. Bake, one sheet at a time, in preheated oven for 9 to 12 minutes or until golden brown and just set at the center. Let cool on pan on a wire rack for 3 minutes, then transfer to the rack to cool.

# Crisp Quinoa Chocolate Chunkers

**Makes about 30 cookies**

*If any cookie can make you feel like a kid again, it's a chocolate chipper still warm from the oven. You'll make this double quinoa version again and again, not because the cookies are packed with good-for-you ingredients, but because they're so darn good.*

## Storage Tip

Store the cooled cookies in an airtight container in the refrigerator for up to 5 days.

- **Preheat oven to 350°F (180°C)**
- **Large baking sheet, lined with parchment paper**

| | | |
|---|---|---|
| 1½ cups | quinoa flakes or quick-cooking rolled oats (certified GF, if needed) | 375 mL |
| ⅔ cup | quinoa flour | 150 mL |
| ¾ tsp | baking soda | 3 mL |
| ½ tsp | fine sea salt | 2 mL |
| ¾ cup | natural cane sugar or packed light brown sugar | 175 mL |
| 6 tbsp | unrefined virgin coconut oil, warmed, or unsalted butter, melted | 90 mL |
| 1 | large egg, lightly beaten | 1 |
| 1 tsp | vanilla extract (GF, if needed) | 5 mL |
| 4 oz | bittersweet (dark) or semisweet chocolate (GF, if needed), coarsely chopped | 125 g |
| ½ cup | chopped toasted pecans or walnuts (optional) | 125 mL |

1. In a large bowl, whisk together quinoa flakes, quinoa flour, baking soda and salt.
2. In a small bowl, whisk together sugar and oil until blended. Whisk in egg and vanilla until blended.
3. Add the egg mixture to the flour mixture and stir until just blended. Gently fold in chocolate and pecans (if using).
4. Drop dough by tablespoonfuls (15 mL) onto prepared baking sheet, spacing them 2 inches (5 cm) apart.
5. Bake in preheated oven for 11 to 13 minutes or until golden brown. Let cool on pan on a wire rack for 2 minutes, then transfer to the rack to cool.
6. Repeat steps 4 and 5 with the remaining dough.

# Chocolate Quinoa Crackles

*It's a good idea to have a napkin handy when eating these crackle-top chocolate cookies — the powdered sugar coating can get all over the place. But they are so very worth the mess!*

## Tip

Natural cane confectioners' (icing) sugar is made using the same process as regular confectioners' sugar (granulated sugar is crushed to a fine white powder), but is made with less processed natural cane sugar. Regular confectioners' sugar may be used in its place.

## Storage Tip

Store the cooled cookies in an airtight container in the refrigerator for up to 5 days.

- **Preheat oven to 350°F (180°C)**
- **Large baking sheet, lined with parchment paper**

| | | |
|---|---|---|
| 1⅓ cups | quinoa flour | 325 mL |
| ½ cup | unsweetened cocoa powder (not Dutch process) | 125 mL |
| ⅓ cup | natural cane sugar or packed light brown sugar | 75 mL |
| 1 tsp | baking powder (GF, if needed) | 5 mL |
| ¼ tsp | fine sea salt | 1 mL |
| ⅛ tsp | baking soda | 0.5 mL |
| ¼ cup | cold unsalted butter or unrefined virgin coconut oil, cut into small pieces | 60 mL |
| 3 | large egg whites | 3 |
| 1 tsp | vanilla extract (GF, if needed) | 5 mL |
| ½ cup | natural cane confectioners' (icing) sugar | 125 mL |

1. In a medium bowl, whisk together quinoa flour, cocoa powder, cane sugar, baking powder, salt and baking soda. Using a pastry blender or two knives, cut in butter until mixture resembles coarse crumbs. Using a wooden spoon, stir in egg whites and vanilla until just blended.

2. Roll dough into eighteen 1-inch (2.5 cm) balls. Place confectioners' sugar in a shallow dish and roll balls in sugar to coat. Place balls 2 inches (5 cm) apart on prepared baking sheet.

3. Bake in preheated oven for 11 to 13 minutes or until puffed and just set at the edges. Let cool on pan on a wire rack for 1 minute, then transfer to the rack to cool.

# Quinoa Anzac Biscuits

*Anzac biscuits were popularized by World War I care packages to soldiers of the Australian and New Zealand Army Corps (ANZAC), since they kept well on the overseas voyage to Europe. I've refashioned the cookies with quinoa flakes and quinoa flour, as they, too, are excellent travelers!*

## Storage Tip

Store the cooled biscuits in an airtight container in the refrigerator for up to 1 week.

- **Preheat oven to 325°F (160°C)**
- **Large baking sheet, lined with parchment paper**

| | | |
|---|---|---|
| 1 cup | quinoa flakes or quick-cooking rolled oats (certified GF, if needed) | 250 mL |
| 1 cup | quinoa flour | 250 mL |
| 1 cup | natural cane sugar or packed light brown sugar | 250 mL |
| ½ cup | unsweetened flaked coconut | 125 mL |
| ½ tsp | baking soda | 2 mL |
| ¼ tsp | fine sea salt | 1 mL |
| ¼ cup | unrefined virgin coconut oil, warmed, or unsalted butter, melted and cooled slightly | 60 mL |
| 3 tbsp | water | 45 mL |
| 2 tbsp | brown rice syrup, pure maple syrup or liquid honey | 30 mL |

1. In a large bowl, whisk together quinoa flakes, quinoa flour, sugar, coconut, baking soda and salt. Stir in oil, water and brown rice syrup until well blended.

2. Drop dough by tablespoonfuls (15 mL) onto prepared baking sheet, spacing them 2 inches (5 cm) apart.

3. Bake in preheated oven for 11 to 13 minutes or until golden brown. Let cool on pan on a wire rack for 2 minutes, then transfer to the rack to cool.

4. Repeat steps 2 and 3 with the remaining dough.

## Variation

*Tropical Anzac Biscuits:* Add ⅓ cup (75 mL) golden raisins, ¼ cup (60 mL) chopped macadamia nuts and ¾ tsp (3 mL) ground allspice with the coconut.

# Olive Oil Quinoa Biscotti

*Olive oil may sound like an unusual ingredient for biscotti, but it's actually quite traditional in many regions of Italy. The flavor can range from bold to nuanced to indistinguishable, depending on the olive oil you choose.*

## Tips

For the nuts, try walnuts, pecans, hazelnuts, pistachios or almonds. For the dried fruit, try raisins, cherries or chopped apricots.

The biscotti will continue to harden after the second bake, as they cool.

## Storage Tip

Store the cooled biscotti in an airtight container at room temperature for up to 5 days.

- **Preheat oven to 300°F (150°C)**
- **Large baking sheet, lined with parchment paper**

| | | |
|---|---|---|
| 1²⁄₃ cups | quinoa flour | 400 mL |
| 1 tsp | baking powder (GF, if needed) | 5 mL |
| ¼ tsp | fine sea salt | 1 mL |
| 1¼ cups | coarsely chopped nuts (see tip, at left) | 300 mL |
| ¾ cup | chopped dried fruit | 175 mL |
| ¾ cup | natural cane sugar or granulated sugar | 175 mL |
| 2 | large eggs, at room temperature | 2 |
| ⅓ cup | extra virgin olive oil | 75 mL |
| 2 tsp | vanilla extract (GF, if needed) | 10 mL |

1. In a medium bowl, whisk together quinoa flour, baking powder and salt. Stir in nuts and dried fruit.

2. In a large bowl, whisk together sugar, eggs, oil and vanilla until blended. Gradually add the flour mixture, stirring until just blended. Divide dough in half.

3. Place dough halves on prepared baking sheet and, using moistened hands, shape into two parallel 12- by 2-inch (30 by 5 cm) rectangles, spaced about 3 inches (7.5 cm) apart.

4. Bake in preheated oven for 30 to 35 minutes or until golden and center is set. Let cool on pan on a wire rack for 15 minutes.

5. Cut rectangles crosswise into ¹⁄₂-inch (1 cm) slices. Place slices, cut side down, on baking sheet. Bake for 8 to 10 minutes or until edges are dark golden. Let cool on pan for 1 minute, then transfer to wire racks to cool completely.

# Chocolate Almond Biscotti

*Combining two classic dessert flavors — chocolate and almond — these biscotti are always in fashion.*

## Tip

The biscotti will continue to harden after the second bake, as they cool.

## Storage Tip

Store the cooled biscotti in an airtight container at room temperature for up to 5 days.

- **Preheat oven to 325°F (160°C)**
- **Large baking sheet, lined with parchment paper**

| | | |
|---|---|---|
| 1½ cups | quinoa flour | 375 mL |
| ⅓ cup | unsweetened cocoa powder (not Dutch process) | 75 mL |
| ¾ tsp | baking soda | 3 mL |
| ¼ tsp | fine sea salt | 1 mL |
| ½ cup | unsweetened natural almond butter | 125 mL |
| ⅔ cup | brown rice syrup or liquid honey | 150 mL |
| 2 | large eggs, at room temperature | 2 |
| ¾ tsp | almond extract (GF, if needed) | 3 mL |
| ½ cup | slivered almonds | 125 mL |

1. In a medium bowl, whisk together quinoa flour, cocoa powder, baking soda and salt.

2. In a large bowl, using an electric mixer on medium speed, beat almond butter and brown rice syrup until blended. Add eggs and almond extract, beating on low speed until just blended.

3. Add the flour mixture to the egg mixture, stirring until just blended. Gently fold in almonds. Divide dough in half.

4. Place dough halves on prepared baking sheet and, using moistened hands, shape into two parallel 12- by 2-inch (30 by 5 cm) rectangles, spaced about 3 inches (7.5 cm) apart.

5. Bake in preheated oven for 30 to 35 minutes or until center is set. Let cool on pan on a wire rack for 15 minutes.

6. Cut rectangles crosswise into ½-inch (1 cm) slices. Place slices, cut side down, on baking sheet. Bake for 8 to 10 minutes or until centers are set. Let cool on pan for 1 minute, then transfer to wire racks to cool completely.

# Quinoa Fekkas

**Makes 3 dozen cookies**

*Akin to biscotti, these Moroccan tea biscuits have an exotic scent — orange, anise, almonds and sesame — that is nothing short of intoxicating as they bake.*

## Tips

To toast sesame seeds, place up to 3 tbsp (45 mL) seeds in a medium skillet set over medium heat. Cook, shaking the skillet, for 3 to 5 minutes or until seeds are golden brown and fragrant. Let cool completely before use.

The biscuits will continue to harden after the second bake, as they cool.

## Storage Tip

Store the cooled biscuits in an airtight container at room temperature for up to 5 days.

- **Preheat oven to 300°F (150°C)**
- **Large baking sheet, lined with parchment paper**

| | | |
|---|---|---|
| 1¾ cups | quinoa flour | 425 mL |
| 2 tsp | anise seeds, crushed | 10 mL |
| 1 tsp | baking powder (GF, if needed) | 5 mL |
| ¼ tsp | fine sea salt | 1 mL |
| 1 cup | coarsely chopped toasted almonds | 250 mL |
| ⅓ cup | sesame seeds, toasted (see tip, at left) | 75 mL |
| ¾ cup | natural cane sugar or granulated sugar | 175 mL |
| 3 | large eggs, at room temperature | 3 |
| ¼ cup | unsalted butter, melted, or unrefined virgin coconut oil, warmed | 60 mL |
| 1 tbsp | finely grated orange zest | 15 mL |
| 1 tsp | almond extract (GF, if needed) | 5 mL |

1. In a medium bowl, whisk together quinoa flour, anise seeds, baking powder and salt. Stir in almonds and sesame seeds.

2. In a large bowl, whisk together sugar, eggs, butter, orange zest and almond extract until blended. Gradually add the flour mixture, stirring until just blended. Divide dough in half.

3. Place dough halves on prepared baking sheet and, using moistened hands, shape into two parallel 12- by 2-inch (30 by 5 cm) rectangles, spaced about 3 inches (7.5 cm) apart.

4. Bake in preheated oven for 30 to 35 minutes or until golden and center is set. Let cool on pan on a wire rack for 15 minutes.

5. Cut rectangles crosswise into ½-inch (1 cm) slices. Place slices, cut side down, on baking sheet. Bake for 8 to 10 minutes or until edges are dark golden. Let cool on pan for 1 minute, then transfer to wire racks to cool completely.

# Tahini Quinoa Shortbread

*Tahini and quinoa flour unexpectedly embolden basic buttery shortbread with their sesame flavors and earthy richness. Watch everyone (yourself included) go back for seconds and thirds.*

## Tips

Lining a pan with foil is easy. Begin by turning the pan upside down. Tear off a piece of foil longer than the pan, then mold the foil over the pan. Remove the foil and set it aside. Flip the pan over and gently fit the shaped foil into the pan, allowing the foil to hang over the sides (the overhang ends will work as "handles" when the contents of the pan are removed).

Be sure to cut the shortbread while it is still warm; if left to cool completely, it will crumble when cut. To cut 18 bars, cut three horizontal rows, then six vertical rows.

## Storage Tip

Store the cooled bars in an airtight container in the refrigerator for up to 5 days.

- **Preheat oven to 350°F (180°C)**
- **Food processor**
- **9-inch (23 cm) square metal baking pan, lined with foil (see tip, at left)**

| | | |
|---|---|---|
| 1¼ cups | natural cane sugar or packed light brown sugar | 300 mL |
| ¼ tsp | fine sea salt | 1 mL |
| ¾ cup | unsalted butter, softened | 175 mL |
| ½ cup | tahini | 125 mL |
| 2 cups | quinoa flour | 500 mL |
| ⅔ cup | chopped toasted walnuts, pecans or almonds | 150 mL |

1. In food processor, combine sugar, salt, butter and tahini; pulse until well blended. Add quinoa flour and walnuts; pulse until just blended (dough will be stiff).

2. Transfer dough to prepared pan and, using your fingertips or a large square of waxed paper, press into an even thickness, smoothing top.

3. Bake in preheated oven for 20 to 25 minutes or until edges are golden brown. Let cool in pan on a wire rack for 5 minutes. Using foil liner, lift mixture from pan and invert onto a cutting board. Peel off foil and cut into 18 bars. Transfer bars to rack and let cool completely.

# Quinoa Almond Butter Blondies

**Makes
16 blondies**

*The brownie has legions
of loyal fans, but the
blondie has equally
steadfast enthusiasts. The
reasons are clearer than
ever with this quinoa
interpretation: a chewy,
nutty butterscotch bar,
enriched with cashew
butter and highly
transportable to boot.*

## Tip

Other natural nut or seed
butters, such as peanut,
almond or sunflower, or
tahini, may be used in
place of the cashew butter.

## Storage Tip

Store the cooled blondies
in an airtight container in
the refrigerator for up to
5 days.

- **Preheat oven to 350°F (180°C)**
- **8-inch (20 cm) square metal baking pan, sprayed with nonstick cooking spray**

| | | |
|---|---|---|
| 1¼ cups | quinoa flour | 300 mL |
| 1 tsp | baking powder (GF, if needed) | 5 mL |
| ½ tsp | fine sea salt | 2 mL |
| ½ cup | unsweetened natural almond butter | 125 mL |
| ¼ cup | unsalted butter, softened | 60 mL |
| 1 cup | natural cane sugar or packed light brown sugar | 250 mL |
| ½ cup | brown rice syrup or pure maple syrup | 125 mL |
| 2 | large eggs | 2 |
| 1 tsp | vanilla extract (GF, if needed) | 5 mL |

1. In a medium bowl, whisk together quinoa flour, baking powder and salt.

2. In a large bowl, using an electric mixer on medium speed, beat almond butter and butter until fluffy. Beat in sugar and brown rice syrup until blended. Add eggs, one at a time, beating well after each addition. Beat in vanilla until smooth. Using a wooden spoon, stir in flour mixture until just blended.

3. Spread batter evenly in prepared pan.

4. Bake in preheated oven for 28 to 32 minutes or until a toothpick inserted in the center comes out with a few moist crumbs attached. Let cool completely in pan on a wire rack. Cut into 16 squares.

# Quinoa Brownies

*These have all the
qualities you want in a
brownie: they're dense,
chewy and rich with
chocolate flavor. Using
brown rice syrup as part
of the sweetener keeps
them moist and fudgy.*

## Storage Tip

Store the cooled brownies
in an airtight container in
the refrigerator for up to
5 days.

- **Preheat oven to 350°F (180°C)**
- **9-inch (23 cm) square metal baking pan, sprayed with nonstick cooking spray**

| | | |
|---|---|---|
| 1 cup | natural cane sugar or packed dark brown sugar | 250 mL |
| ¾ cup | quinoa flour | 175 mL |
| ¾ cup | unsweetened cocoa powder (not Dutch process) | 175 mL |
| ½ tsp | baking powder (GF, if needed) | 2 mL |
| ¼ tsp | fine sea salt | 1 mL |
| 1 cup | semisweet chocolate chips (GF, if needed), divided | 250 mL |
| 6 tbsp | unsalted butter | 90 mL |
| ½ cup | brown rice syrup, pure maple syrup or liquid honey | 125 mL |
| ⅓ cup | milk or plain non-dairy milk (such as soy, almond, rice or hemp) | 75 mL |
| 2 | large eggs | 2 |
| 1 tsp | vanilla extract (GF, if needed) | 15 mL |
| ½ cup | chopped toasted walnuts or pecans (optional) | 125 mL |

1. In a large bowl, whisk together sugar, quinoa flour, cocoa powder, baking powder and salt.
2. In a medium microwave-safe bowl, microwave ⅔ cup (150 mL) of the chocolate chips and the butter on Medium (70%) for 30 seconds. Stir. Microwave on Medium (70%) in 15-second intervals, stirring after each, until melted and smooth. Whisk in brown rice syrup and milk until blended. Whisk in eggs and vanilla until blended.
3. Add the egg mixture to the flour mixture, stirring until just blended. Gently fold in walnuts (if using) and the remaining chocolate chips.
4. Spread batter evenly in prepared pan.
5. Bake in preheated oven for 16 to 19 minutes or until a toothpick inserted in center comes out with a few moist crumbs attached. Let cool completely in pan on a wire rack. Cut into 16 squares.

# Chocolate Hazelnut Brownie Bites

*These decadent morsels have a bit of European flair thanks to the hazelnut chocolate spread in the batter. One taste makes it abundantly clear why the chocolate-hazelnut combination is a classic.*

## Storage Tip

Store the cooled brownies in an airtight container in the refrigerator for up to 5 days.

- **Preheat oven to 350°F (180°C)**
- **12-cup mini muffin pan, lined with paper liners**

| | | |
|---|---|---|
| ⅓ cup | quinoa flour | 75 mL |
| ¼ tsp | baking powder (GF, if needed) | 1 mL |
| 1 | large egg | 1 |
| ½ cup | hazelnut chocolate spread (such as Nutella) | 125 mL |
| 2 tbsp | milk or plain non-dairy milk (such as soy, almond, rice or hemp) | 30 mL |
| ⅓ cup | chopped toasted hazelnuts | 75 mL |

1. In a small bowl, whisk together quinoa flour and baking powder.
2. In a medium bowl, whisk together egg, hazelnut chocolate spread and milk until blended. Stir in flour mixture until blended. Gently fold in hazelnuts.
3. Divide batter equally among prepared muffin cups.
4. Bake in preheated oven for 10 to 13 minutes or until a toothpick inserted in the center comes out with moist (but not wet) crumbs attached. Let cool in pan on a wire rack for 1 minute, then transfer to the rack to cool.

# Date Bars

*Date bars have long been a favorite curl-up-with-a-cup-of-tea option, and this version is no different.*

## Tip

For the best results, use whole pitted dates and chop them yourself. Pre-chopped dates are typically tossed with oat flour (to prevent sticking) and sugar. In addition, they tend to be fairly hard. If pre-chopped dates are the only option available, give them a quick rinse in hot (not boiling) water to remove any coatings and soften them slightly.

## Storage Tip

Store the cooled bars in an airtight container in the refrigerator for up to 5 days.

- **Preheat oven to 375°F (190°C)**
- **Blender or food processor**
- **8-inch (20 cm) square metal baking pan, sprayed with nonstick cooking spray**

| | | |
|---|---|---|
| 1¼ cups | quinoa flakes or quick-cooking rolled oats (certified GF, if needed) | 300 mL |
| ½ cup | quinoa flour | 125 mL |
| ½ tsp | ground cinnamon | 2 mL |
| ½ tsp | baking powder (GF, if needed) | 2 mL |
| ¼ tsp | fine sea salt | 1 mL |
| ⅔ cup | chopped pitted dates, divided | 150 mL |
| 1 tsp | finely grated orange zest | 5 mL |
| ¼ cup | freshly squeezed orange juice | 60 mL |
| ¼ cup | vegetable oil | 60 mL |
| 1 | large egg, at room temperature | 1 |

1. In a medium bowl, whisk together quinoa flakes, quinoa flour, cinnamon, baking powder and salt.
2. In blender, combine half the dates, orange zest, orange juice and oil; purée until very smooth. Add egg and blend until just combined.
3. Add the date mixture to the flour mixture, stirring until just blended. Gently fold in the remaining dates.
4. Spread batter evenly in prepared pan.
5. Bake in preheated oven for 15 to 20 minutes or until golden brown and set at the center. Let cool completely in pan on a wire rack. Cut into 16 bars.

# Apricot Crumb Squares

*A distinctive double-apricot filling nestles between layers of nutmeg-spiced quinoa crumble in these delicious squares. The combination of flavors and textures is extremely appealing.*

## Tip

Lining a pan with foil is easy. Begin by turning the pan upside down. Tear off a piece of foil longer than the pan, then mold the foil over the pan. Remove the foil and set it aside. Flip the pan over and gently fit the shaped foil into the pan, allowing the foil to hang over the sides (the overhang ends will work as "handles" when the contents of the pan are removed).

## Storage Tip

Store the cooled squares in an airtight container in the refrigerator for up to 5 days.

- **Preheat oven to 350°F (180°C)**
- **Food processor**
- **8-inch (20 cm) square metal baking pan, lined with foil (see tip, at left) and sprayed with nonstick cooking spray**

| | | |
|---|---|---|
| 1½ cups | large-flake (old-fashioned) rolled oats (certified GF, if needed) | 375 mL |
| 1 cup | quinoa flour | 250 mL |
| ⅓ cup | natural cane sugar or packed light brown sugar | 75 mL |
| ¼ tsp | ground nutmeg | 1 mL |
| 6 tbsp | cold unsalted butter or unrefined virgin coconut oil | 90 mL |
| ¾ cup | apricot preserves sweetened with fruit juice | 175 mL |
| ½ cup | finely chopped dried apricots | 125 mL |

1. In food processor, combine oats, quinoa flour, sugar, nutmeg and butter; pulse until mixture resembles coarse crumbs.
2. Firmly press two-thirds of the oat mixture into prepared pan. Bake in preheated oven for 10 minutes.
3. In a small bowl, combine preserves and apricots. Spread over warm crust. Sprinkle with the remaining oat mixture, gently pressing it into the preserves.
4. Bake for 20 to 25 minutes or until lightly browned and bubbling. Let cool completely in pan on a wire rack. Using foil liner, lift mixture from pan and invert onto a cutting board. Peel off foil and cut into 16 squares.

## Variation

Other flavors of preserves, such as raspberry, strawberry or peach, may be used in place of the apricot preserves, and other varieties of dried fruit, such as cherries, cranberries or blueberries, may be used in place of the apricots.

# Quinoa Gingerbread

*Even if you're not a
ginger lover, you'll
love this quinoa
gingerbread. Freshly
grated gingerroot and
the rounded complexity
of dark molasses lend
it a rich flavor and an
intoxicating scent.*

## Tips

For a milder-flavored
cake, use pure maple
syrup, brown rice syrup or
liquid honey in place of
the molasses.

Natural cane confectioners'
(icing) sugar is made
using the same process
as regular confectioners'
sugar (granulated sugar
is crushed to a fine white
powder), but is made with
less processed natural
cane sugar. Regular
confectioners' sugar may
be used in its place.

## Storage Tip

Store the cooled cake,
loosely wrapped in foil
or plastic wrap, in the
refrigerator for up to
5 days. Alternatively, wrap
it in plastic wrap, then
foil, completely enclosing
cake, and freeze for up
to 6 months. Let thaw at
room temperature for 4 to
6 hours before serving.

- **Preheat oven to 350°F (180°C)**
- **8-inch (20 cm) square metal baking pan, sprayed with nonstick cooking spray**

| | | |
|---|---|---:|
| 1¼ cups | quinoa flour | 300 mL |
| 1 tsp | ground cinnamon | 5 mL |
| ½ tsp | baking soda | 2 mL |
| ⅛ tsp | fine sea salt | 0.5 mL |
| ⅛ tsp | ground cloves | 0.5 mL |
| ⅓ cup | natural cane sugar or packed dark brown sugar | 75 mL |
| 2 tbsp | grated gingerroot | 30 mL |
| 1 | large egg, at room temperature | 1 |
| ½ cup | buttermilk | 125 mL |
| ½ cup | dark (cooking) molasses | 125 mL |
| ⅓ cup | vegetable oil | 75 mL |
| 1 tbsp | natural cane confectioners' (icing) sugar (optional) | 15 mL |

1. In a large bowl, whisk together quinoa flour, cinnamon, baking soda, salt and cloves.
2. Add sugar, ginger, egg, buttermilk, molasses and oil to flour mixture. Using an electric mixer on medium-low speed, beat for 1 minute, until blended. Scrape sides and bottom of bowl with a spatula. Beat on medium speed for 1 minute.
3. Spread batter evenly in prepared pan.
4. Bake in preheated oven for 25 to 30 minutes or until a toothpick inserted in the center comes out with a few moist crumbs attached. Let cool in pan on a wire rack for 10 minutes, then invert cake onto rack to cool completely. If desired, sprinkle confectioners' sugar over top of cooled cake.

# Cinnamon Streusel Snack Cake

| | |
|---|---|
| **Makes**<br>**9 servings** | |

*For cozy comfort, this cinnamon-scented cake is hard to beat. Wonderfully homey, it's equally good with afternoon tea, after a meal or for breakfast with a cup of dark-roast coffee.*

## Tip

An equal amount of unrefined virgin coconut oil may be used in place of the butter.

## Storage Tip

Store the cooled cake, loosely wrapped in foil or plastic wrap, in the refrigerator for up to 5 days. Alternatively, wrap it in plastic wrap, then foil, completely enclosing cake and freeze for up to 6 months. Let thaw at room temperature for 4 to 6 hours before serving.

- **Preheat oven to 350°F (180°C)**
- **8-inch (20 cm) square metal baking pan, sprayed with nonstick cooking spray**

| | | |
|---|---|---|
| 1¼ cups | quinoa flour | 300 mL |
| ⅔ cup | natural cane sugar or packed dark brown sugar | 150 mL |
| 1½ tsp | ground cinnamon, divided | 7 mL |
| ¼ tsp | fine sea salt | 1 mL |
| ¼ cup | cold unsalted butter, cut into small pieces | 60 mL |
| ½ tsp | baking powder (GF, if needed) | 2 mL |
| ½ tsp | baking soda | 2 mL |
| 2 | large eggs | 2 |
| ⅓ cup | buttermilk | 75 mL |
| 1 tsp | vanilla extract (GF, if needed) | 5 mL |

1. In a medium bowl, whisk together quinoa flour, sugar, 1 tsp (5 mL) of the cinnamon and salt. Using a pastry blender or two knives, cut in butter until mixture resembles coarse crumbs. Transfer ½ cup (125 mL) flour mixture to a small bowl and stir in the remaining cinnamon.

2. To the remaining flour mixture, stir in baking powder and baking soda. Add eggs, buttermilk and vanilla. Using an electric mixer on medium speed, beat for 1 to 2 minutes or until blended.

3. Spread batter evenly in prepared pan. Sprinkle the reserved flour mixture over top.

4. Bake in preheated oven for 27 to 30 minutes or until a toothpick inserted in the center comes out with a few moist crumbs attached. Let cool completely in pan on a wire rack.

# Quinoa Angel Food Cake

*Angel food cake — which is surprisingly simple to assemble — owes its ethereal lightness and fine texture to whipped egg whites. The volume of the cake continues to expand in the oven as a result of steam, which evaporates from the liquid in the egg whites. Savor it on its own or with berries and cream, or use it as the base for trifles or tiramisu.*

## Tip

The leftover egg yolks can be stored in an airtight container in the refrigerator for up to 1 day or in the freezer for up to 2 months. They can be used in a wide range of recipes, from cookies to ice cream to lemon curd.

## Storage Tip

Store the cooled cake in a cake keeper, or loosely wrapped in foil or plastic wrap, at room temperature for up to 5 days. Alternatively, wrap it in plastic wrap, then foil, completely enclosing cake, and freeze for up to 6 months. Let thaw at room temperature for 2 to 3 hours before serving.

- **Preheat oven to 350°F (180°C)**
- **10-inch (25 cm) tube pan (angel food cake pan)**

| | | |
|---|---|---|
| 1 cup | quinoa flour | 250 mL |
| 1½ cups | natural cane sugar or granulated sugar, divided | 375 mL |
| 2 cups | large egg whites (about 15 large eggs), at room temperature | 500 mL |
| 2 tsp | cream of tartar | 10 mL |
| ¾ tsp | fine sea salt | 3 mL |
| 2 tsp | vanilla extract (GF, if needed) | 10 mL |

1. In a medium bowl, whisk together quinoa flour and ½ cup (125 mL) of the sugar.

2. In a large bowl, using an electric mixer on low speed, beat egg whites, cream of tartar and salt for 1 minute, until blended and frothy. Increase speed to medium and gradually beat in the remaining sugar, a few tablespoons at a time. Continue beating until medium peaks form. Beat in vanilla. Using a rubber spatula, fold in flour mixture, ⅓ cup (75 mL) at a time.

3. Spread batter evenly in pan.

4. Bake in preheated oven for 35 to 40 minutes or until cake is brown and crusty on top and a piece of uncooked spaghetti inserted in the center comes out clean. Turn pan upside down and fit center onto a slender bottle neck. Let cool completely. Slide a knife around pan sides to loosen cake and turn cake out onto a platter or cake plate.

## Variation

*Chocolate Quinoa Angel Food Cake:* Reduce the flour by 2 tbsp (30 mL). Sift ⅓ cup (75 mL) unsweetened cocoa powder (not Dutch process) and add to the flour mixture in step 1.

# Maple Sugar Chiffon Cake

*At once rich and light, this delicate maple cake is a big bite of nostalgia. Think pancakes and syrup, all dressed up. A sweet maple glaze and toasty pecans team up on top for a crunchy, tasty embellishment.*

## Tip

Natural cane confectioners' (icing) sugar is made using the same process as regular confectioners' sugar (granulated sugar is crushed to a fine white powder), but is made with less processed natural cane sugar. Regular confectioners' sugar may be used in its place.

## Storage Tip

Store the cooled cake in a cake keeper, or loosely wrapped in foil or plastic wrap, at room temperature for up to 5 days. Alternatively, wrap it in plastic wrap, then foil, completely enclosing cake, and freeze for up to 6 months. Let thaw at room temperature for 2 to 3 hours before serving.

- **Preheat oven to 350°F (180°C)**
- **10-inch (25 cm) tube pan (angel food cake pan)**

| | | |
|---|---|---|
| 1 cup | quinoa flour | 250 mL |
| ½ cup | natural cane sugar or packed light brown sugar | 125 mL |
| 1 tsp | baking powder (GF, if needed) | 5 mL |
| ½ tsp | ground cinnamon | 2 mL |
| ¼ tsp | fine sea salt | 1 mL |
| 2 | large egg yolks, at room temperature | 2 |
| ¼ cup | milk or plain non-dairy milk (such as soy, almond, rice or hemp) | 60 mL |
| 1 tbsp | vegetable oil | 15 mL |
| 1 tbsp | natural maple extract | 15 mL |
| 6 | large egg whites, at room temperature | 6 |
| ¼ tsp | cream of tartar | 1 mL |
| 6 tbsp | natural cane confectioners' (icing) sugar | 90 mL |
| 3 tbsp | pure maple syrup | 45 mL |
| ⅔ cup | chopped toasted pecans (optional) | 150 mL |

1. In a large bowl, whisk together quinoa flour, cane sugar, baking powder, cinnamon and salt.
2. Add egg yolks, milk, oil and maple extract to flour mixture. Using an electric mixer on medium speed, beat until smooth, stopping once or twice to scrape sides and bottom of bowl. Set bowl aside. Clean and dry beaters.
3. In another large bowl, using electric mixer on high speed, beat egg whites and cream of tartar until stiff (but not dry) peaks form. Gently stir one-quarter of the egg whites into batter. Fold in the remaining egg whites.
4. Spread batter evenly in pan.
5. Bake in preheated oven for 23 to 26 minutes or until cake springs back when lightly touched. Let cool in pan on a wire rack for 5 minutes, then invert cake onto rack to cool completely.
6. In a small bowl, whisk together confectioners' sugar and maple syrup until smooth. Drizzle over top of cooled cake. If desired, sprinkle with pecans.

# Swedish Honey and Spice Cake

*This crowd-pleasing cake takes its cue from a Swedish blend of spices: cinnamon, cardamom and cloves. It's great to have on hand all through the holiday season. The honey glaze keeps the cake moist while accentuating the earthy nuances of the quinoa flour.*

## Storage Tip

Store the cooled cake, loosely wrapped in foil or waxed paper, in the refrigerator for up to 3 days. Alternatively, wrap it in plastic wrap, then foil, completely enclosing cake, and freeze for up to 6 months. Let thaw at room temperature for 4 to 6 hours before serving.

- **Preheat oven to 325°F (160°C)**
- **9-inch (23 cm) square metal baking pan, sprayed with nonstick cooking spray**

| | | |
|---|---|---|
| 1½ cups | quinoa flour | 375 mL |
| ⅓ cup | natural cane sugar or packed light brown sugar | 75 mL |
| 2 tsp | ground ginger | 10 mL |
| 1 tsp | ground cinnamon | 5 mL |
| ¾ tsp | baking powder (GF, if needed) | 3 mL |
| ¾ tsp | ground cardamom | 3 mL |
| ½ tsp | baking soda | 2 mL |
| ½ tsp | fine sea salt | 2 mL |
| 2 | large eggs, at room temperature | 2 |
| ⅓ cup | vegetable oil | 75 mL |
| ⅔ cup | liquid honey | 150 mL |
| ⅓ cup | milk | 75 mL |

1. In a large bowl, whisk together quinoa flour, sugar, ginger, cinnamon, baking powder, cardamom, baking soda and salt.

2. Add eggs, oil, honey and milk to flour mixture. Using an electric mixer on medium-low speed, beat for 1 minute, until blended. Scrape sides and bottom of bowl with a spatula. Beat on medium speed for 1 minute.

3. Spread batter evenly in prepared pan.

4. Bake in preheated oven for 25 to 30 minutes or until a toothpick inserted in the center comes out with a few moist crumbs attached. Let cool completely in pan on a wire rack.

# Dark and Damp Molasses Cake

*This dark, damp and deliciously spiced cake captures the fragrant earthiness of quinoa flour. Best of all, it's a breeze to make.*

## Storage Tip

Store the cooled cake, loosely wrapped in foil or plastic wrap, in the refrigerator for up to 5 days. Alternatively, wrap it in plastic wrap, then foil, completely enclosing cake, and freeze for up to 6 months. Let thaw at room temperature for 4 to 6 hours before serving.

- **Preheat oven to 350°F (180°C)**
- **9-inch (23 cm) square metal baking pan, sprayed with nonstick cooking spray**

| | | |
|---|---|---|
| 2 cups | quinoa flour | 500 mL |
| 2 tsp | instant espresso powder (optional) | 10 mL |
| 1½ tsp | ground cinnamon | 7 mL |
| ½ tsp | ground ginger | 2 mL |
| 1 tsp | baking soda | 5 mL |
| ½ tsp | fine sea salt | 2 mL |
| 2 | large eggs, at room temperature | 2 |
| 1 cup | unsweetened applesauce | 250 mL |
| ¼ cup | vegetable oil | 60 mL |
| ¾ cup | dark (cooking) molasses | 175 mL |
| 1 tsp | vanilla extract (GF, if needed) | 5 mL |

1. In a large bowl, whisk together quinoa flour, espresso powder (if using), cinnamon, ginger, baking soda and salt.
2. Add eggs, applesauce, oil, molasses and vanilla to flour mixture. Using an electric mixer on medium-low speed, beat for 1 minute, until blended. Scrape sides and bottom of bowl with a spatula. Beat on medium speed for 1 minute.
3. Spread batter evenly in prepared pan.
4. Bake in preheated oven for 32 to 38 minutes or until a toothpick inserted in the center comes out with a few moist crumbs attached. Let cool completely in pan on a wire rack.

# Easy Applesauce Cake

*Whether you use store-bought applesauce or make your own, this humble cake will please one and all.*

## Storage Tip

Store the cooled cake, loosely wrapped in foil or plastic wrap, in the refrigerator for up to 5 days. Alternatively, wrap it in plastic wrap, then foil, completely enclosing cake, and freeze for up to 6 months. Let thaw at room temperature for 4 to 6 hours before serving.

- Preheat oven to 350°F (180°C)
- 9-inch (23 cm) square metal baking pan, sprayed with nonstick cooking spray

| | | |
|---|---|---|
| 1 cup | quinoa flour | 250 mL |
| 1 tsp | ground cinnamon | 5 mL |
| ¾ tsp | baking soda | 3 mL |
| ½ tsp | baking powder (GF, if needed) | 2 mL |
| ½ tsp | fine sea salt | 2 mL |
| 1 | large egg, at room temperature | 1 |
| ¾ cup | unsweetened applesauce | 175 mL |
| ¾ cup | brown rice syrup, pure maple syrup or liquid honey | 175 mL |
| ¼ cup | unsalted butter, melted and cooled slightly | 60 mL |
| 1 tsp | vanilla extract (GF, if needed) | 5 mL |
| ½ cup | raisins or dried cranberries | 125 mL |

1. In a large bowl, whisk together quinoa flour, cinnamon, baking soda, baking powder and salt.
2. Add egg, applesauce, brown rice syrup, butter and vanilla to flour mixture. Using an electric mixer on medium-low speed, beat for 1 minute, until blended. Scrape sides and bottom of bowl with a spatula. Beat on medium speed for 1 minute. Gently stir in raisins.
3. Spread batter evenly in prepared pan.
4. Bake in preheated oven for 23 to 28 minutes or until a toothpick inserted in the center comes out with a few moist crumbs attached. Let cool completely in pan on a wire rack.

# Maple Apple Cake

*Though it's quite irresistible when still warm from the oven, this moist apple cake is perfect potluck or picnic food, since it's also terrific cold or at room temperature.*

## Tip

Liquid honey may be used in place of the maple syrup.

## Storage Tip

Store the cooled cake, loosely wrapped in foil or plastic wrap, in the refrigerator for up to 5 days. Alternatively, wrap it in plastic wrap, then foil, completely enclosing cake, and freeze for up to 6 months. Let thaw at room temperature for 4 to 6 hours before serving.

- **Preheat oven to 350°F (180°C)**
- **Food processor**
- **9-inch (23 cm) square metal baking pan, sprayed with nonstick cooking spray**

| | | |
|---|---|---|
| 1 cup | large-flake (old-fashioned) rolled oats (certified GF, if needed) | 250 mL |
| 1½ cups | quinoa flour | 375 mL |
| 2 tsp | baking powder (GF, if needed) | 10 mL |
| 2 tsp | ground cinnamon | 10 mL |
| ½ tsp | fine sea salt | 2 mL |
| ½ tsp | baking soda | 2 mL |
| 2 | large eggs, at room temperature | 2 |
| 1 cup | buttermilk | 250 mL |
| ¼ cup | vegetable oil | 60 mL |
| ¾ cup | pure maple syrup | 175 mL |
| 2 tsp | vanilla extract (GF, if needed) | 10 mL |
| 2 cups | chopped peeled tart-sweet apples (such as Braeburn or Gala) | 500 mL |

1. In food processor, process oats until powdery.
2. In a large bowl, whisk together oats, quinoa flour, baking powder, cinnamon, salt and baking soda.
3. In a medium bowl, whisk together eggs, buttermilk, oil, maple syrup and vanilla until well blended.
4. Add the egg mixture to the flour mixture and stir until just blended. Gently fold in apples.
5. Spread batter evenly in prepared pan.
6. Bake in preheated oven for 45 to 50 minutes or until a toothpick inserted in the center comes out with a few moist crumbs attached. Let cool in pan on a wire rack for 10 minutes, then invert cake onto rack to cool slightly. Serve warm or let cool completely.

# Summer Berry Spoon Cake

*A jumble of summer berries and delicate cake creates quite a picture, and there is flavor to match. Although spoon cake sounds unusual, it's familiar: part cake, part cobbler, it's a dessert made for serving in bowls and gobbling up with a spoon. Better still, it's a breeze to whip together. Serve with ice cream, if desired.*

## Tips

Frozen berries may be substituted for the fresh berries. Let thaw for 10 minutes before using.

Natural cane confectioners' (icing) sugar is made using the same process as regular confectioners' sugar (granulated sugar is crushed to a fine white powder), but is made with less processed natural cane sugar. Regular confectioners' sugar may be used in its place.

## Storage Tip

Store the cooled cake, loosely wrapped in foil or waxed paper, in the refrigerator for up to 2 days.

- **Preheat oven to 350°F (180°C)**
- **13- by 9-inch (33 by 23 cm) metal baking pan, sprayed with nonstick cooking spray**

| | | |
|---|---|---|
| 2 cups | blueberries | 500 mL |
| 2 cups | raspberries | 500 mL |
| ¼ cup | agave nectar, liquid honey or pure maple syrup | 60 mL |
| 1 cup | quinoa flour | 250 mL |
| ¾ cup | natural cane sugar or granulated sugar | 175 mL |
| 1 tsp | baking powder (GF, if needed) | 5 mL |
| ¼ tsp | fine sea salt | 1 mL |
| 4 | large eggs, at room temperature | 4 |
| 1 tbsp | finely grated orange zest | 15 mL |
| 1 tbsp | olive oil | 15 mL |
| 1 tsp | vanilla extract (GF, if needed) | 5 mL |
| 2 tbsp | natural cane confectioners' (icing) sugar | 30 mL |

1. In prepared pan, combine blueberries, raspberries and agave nectar. Spread evenly in pan.
2. In a large bowl, whisk together quinoa flour, cane sugar, baking powder and salt. Whisk in eggs, orange zest, oil and vanilla until smooth. Carefully spoon batter over berries, spreading evenly.
3. Bake in preheated oven for 27 to 32 minutes or until top is golden and springs back when touched. Let cool in pan on a wire rack for 1 hour. Sprinkle with confectioners' sugar, then scoop into bowls.

# Banana Quinoa Cake

**Makes
9 servings**

*I love banana cake for its homespun flavor and lack of pretense. This version gets a double dose of banana. It's perfect for picnics and packing in lunch bags.*

## Storage Tip

Store the cooled cake, loosely wrapped in foil or plastic wrap, in the refrigerator for up to 5 days. Alternatively, wrap it in plastic wrap, then foil, completely enclosing cake, and freeze for up to 6 months. Let thaw at room temperature for 4 to 6 hours before serving.

- **Preheat oven to 350°F (180°C)**
- **9-inch (23 cm) square metal baking pan, sprayed with nonstick cooking spray**

| | | |
|---|---|---|
| 2 cups | quinoa flour | 500 mL |
| 1½ tsp | baking soda | 7 mL |
| ½ tsp | ground nutmeg | 2 mL |
| ¾ cup | natural cane sugar or packed light brown sugar | 175 mL |
| ¼ cup | unsalted butter, softened, or unrefined virgin coconut oil, warmed slightly | 60 mL |
| 3 | large eggs | 3 |
| ½ cup | buttermilk | 125 mL |
| 1 cup | mashed ripe bananas | 250 mL |
| ½ cup | diced firm-ripe banana | 125 mL |
| 2 tbsp | freshly squeezed lemon juice | 30 mL |

1. In a medium bowl, whisk together quinoa flour, baking soda and nutmeg. Set aside.
2. In a large bowl, using an electric mixer on medium speed, beat sugar and butter for 2 to 3 minutes or until light and fluffy. Beat in eggs until well blended. Add buttermilk and beat on low speed until blended.
3. In a medium bowl, combine mashed bananas, diced bananas and lemon juice.
4. Gently stir banana mixture into egg mixture. Stir in flour mixture until just blended.
5. Spread batter evenly in prepared pan.
6. Bake in preheated oven for 30 to 34 minutes or until or until a toothpick inserted in the center comes out with a few moist crumbs attached. Let cool completely in pan on a wire rack.

# Plum Crumble Cake

This delectable dessert is reminiscent of a cake my friend Louisa used to make. The recipe was passed down from her mother, who hailed from Bühl, in southwestern Germany. According to Louisa, the cake was traditionally made each year during festival time to celebrate the plum harvest. The one-bowl batter is covered with wedges of fall plums; a sprinkling of hazelnut streusel bakes into a crunchy topping.

## Tip

An equal amount of unrefined virgin coconut oil may be used in place of the butter.

## Storage Tip

Store the cooled cake, loosely wrapped in foil or plastic wrap, in the refrigerator for up to 3 days. Alternatively, wrap it in plastic wrap, then foil, completely enclosing cake, and freeze for up to 6 months. Let thaw at room temperature for 4 to 6 hours before serving.

- **Preheat oven to 350°F (180°C)**
- **8-inch (20 cm) square metal baking pan, sprayed with nonstick cooking spray**

| | | |
|---|---|---|
| 1 cup | quinoa flour | 250 mL |
| ⅓ cup | natural cane sugar or packed light brown sugar | 75 mL |
| ¼ tsp | fine sea salt | 1 mL |
| ¼ cup | cold unsalted butter, cut into small pieces | 60 mL |
| ⅓ cup | chopped toasted hazelnuts | 75 mL |
| ½ tsp | baking powder (GF, if needed) | 2 mL |
| ¼ tsp | baking soda | 1 mL |
| 1 | large egg, lightly beaten | 1 |
| ½ cup | plain yogurt | 125 mL |
| 1 tsp | vanilla extract (GF, if needed) | 5 mL |
| ½ tsp | almond extract (GF, if needed) | 2 mL |
| 2 tbsp | natural cane sugar or granulated sugar | 30 mL |
| 1 | large egg white | 1 |
| ½ cup | ricotta cheese (reduced-fat or regular) | 125 mL |
| ¼ cup | plum jam or preserves | 60 mL |
| 6 | purple or red plums, pitted and quartered | 6 |

1. In a medium bowl, whisk together quinoa flour, ⅓ cup (75 mL) sugar and salt. Using a pastry blender or two knives, cut in butter until mixture resembles coarse crumbs. Transfer ½ cup (125 mL) flour mixture to a small bowl and stir in hazelnuts.
2. To the remaining flour mixture, stir in baking powder and baking soda. Stir in egg, yogurt, vanilla and almond extract until blended.
3. Spread batter evenly in prepared pan.
4. In a small bowl, whisk together 2 tbsp (30 mL) sugar, egg white and cheese until blended. Spread evenly over batter. Dot with jam. Top with plums and sprinkle with hazelnut mixture.
5. Bake in preheated oven for 27 to 30 minutes or until a toothpick inserted in the center comes out with a few moist crumbs attached. Let cool completely in pan on a wire rack.

# Dried Fruit and Toasted Nut Fruitcake

Not all fruitcakes are super-sweet, dense and dark. This golden version — rich with roasted nuts and dried fruits but spare on sugar and flour — almost qualifies as health food (I have very broad standards). There's no chance of this fruitcake hanging around unnoticed; it will undoubtedly be eaten sooner rather than later.

## Storage Tip

Store the cooled cake, loosely wrapped in foil or plastic wrap, in the refrigerator for up to 1 week. Alternatively, wrap it in plastic wrap, then foil, completely enclosing cake, and freeze for up to 6 months. Let thaw at room temperature for 4 to 6 hours before serving.

- **Preheat oven to 300°F (150°C)**
- **9- by 5-inch (23 by 12.5 cm) metal loaf pan, sprayed with nonstick cooking spray**

| | | |
|---|---|---|
| ¾ cup | quinoa flour | 175 mL |
| ⅔ cup | natural cane sugar or granulated sugar | 150 mL |
| 1 tsp | pumpkin pie spice | 5 mL |
| ½ tsp | baking powder (GF, if needed) | 2 mL |
| ½ tsp | fine sea salt | 2 mL |
| 3 | large eggs, at room temperature | 3 |
| 2 tsp | vanilla extract (GF, if needed) | 10 mL |
| 3 cups | coarsely chopped roasted salted deluxe mixed nuts (such as pecans, almonds, cashews and Brazil nuts) | 750 mL |
| 8 oz | pitted dates, chopped | 250 g |
| 1½ cups | dried cranberries, coarsely chopped | 375 mL |
| 1½ cups | coarsely chopped dried apricots | 375 mL |

1. In a large bowl, whisk together quinoa flour, sugar, pumpkin pie spice, baking powder and salt.
2. Add eggs and vanilla to flour mixture and stir with a wooden spoon until just blended. Stir in nuts, dates, cranberries and apricots (batter will be very stiff).
3. Spread batter evenly in prepared pan.
4. Bake in preheated oven for 90 to 100 minutes or until top is deep golden brown and a piece of uncooked spaghetti inserted in the center comes out with a few moist crumbs attached. Let cool in pan on a wire rack for 10 minutes, then invert cake onto rack to cool completely.

# Pumpkin Cranberry Cake

**Makes
10 servings**

*This easy cake, fragrant
with traditional
pumpkin pie spices, is
an innovative yet still
comforting way to make
pumpkin brand new.*

## Tips

To make your own
pumpkin pie spice,
combine 2 tbsp (30 mL)
ground cinnamon, 1 tbsp
(15 mL) ground ginger,
2 tsp (10 mL) ground
nutmeg, ½ tsp (2 mL)
ground allspice and
½ tsp (2 mL) ground
cloves. Store in an airtight
container. Makes ¼ cup
(60 mL).

Be sure to use pumpkin
purée, not the sweetened,
spiced pie filling.

## Storage Tip

Store the cooled cake,
loosely wrapped in foil
or waxed paper, in the
refrigerator for up to
3 days. Alternatively, wrap
it in plastic wrap, then
foil, completely enclosing
cake, and freeze for up
to 6 months. Let thaw at
room temperature for 4 to
6 hours before serving.

- **Preheat oven to 350°F (180°C)**
- **9-inch (23 cm) square metal baking pan, sprayed with
  nonstick cooking spray**

| | | |
|---|---|---|
| 1¼ cups | quinoa flour | 300 mL |
| ¾ cup | natural cane sugar or granulated sugar | 175 mL |
| 2½ tsp | pumpkin pie spice (see tip, at left) | 12 mL |
| 1 tsp | baking powder (GF, if needed) | 5 mL |
| ½ tsp | baking soda | 2 mL |
| ½ tsp | fine sea salt | 2 mL |
| 2 | large eggs, at room temperature | 2 |
| 1 cup | canned pumpkin purée (not pie filling) | 250 mL |
| ½ cup | vegetable oil | 125 mL |
| 1 tsp | vanilla extract (GF, if needed) | 5 mL |
| ⅔ cup | dried cranberries, chopped | 150 mL |
| ½ cup | chopped toasted pecans (optional) | 125 mL |
| | Natural cane confectioners' sugar (optional) | |

1. In a large bowl, whisk together quinoa flour, cane
   sugar, pumpkin pie spice, baking powder, baking soda
   and salt.
2. Add eggs, pumpkin, oil and vanilla to flour mixture and
   stir with a wooden spoon until blended. Gently stir in
   cranberries and pecans (if using).
3. Spread batter evenly in prepared pan.
4. Bake in preheated oven for 28 to 33 minutes or until a
   toothpick inserted in the center comes out with a few
   moist crumbs attached. Let cool completely in pan on
   a wire rack. If desired, sprinkle top of cooled cake with
   confectioners' sugar.

## Variation

*Sweet Potato Cranberry Cake:* Use cooled mashed sweet
potatoes in place of the pumpkin and packed light
brown sugar in place of the cane sugar.

# Spiced Carrot Cake

*A classic cake takes a
healthy turn with quinoa
flour, oats and honey. Of
course, you could gild
it with cream cheese
frosting, but why bother?
It's delicious as is.*

## Storage Tip

Store the cooled cake
in a cake keeper, or
loosely wrapped in foil
or plastic wrap, at room
temperature for up to
3 days. Alternatively, wrap
it in plastic wrap, then
foil, completely enclosing
cake, and freeze for up
to 6 months. Let thaw at
room temperature for 4 to
6 hours before serving.

- **Preheat oven to 325°F (160°C)**
- **Food processor**
- **9-inch (23 cm) square metal baking pan, sprayed with nonstick cooking spray**

| | | |
|---|---|---|
| 1 cup | quick-cooking rolled oats (certified GF, if needed) or quinoa flakes | 250 mL |
| 1 cup | chopped walnuts or pecans | 250 mL |
| 1 cup | quinoa flour | 250 mL |
| 2 tsp | baking powder (GF, if needed) | 10 mL |
| 1 tsp | baking soda | 5 mL |
| 1 tsp | ground cinnamon | 5 mL |
| ½ tsp | ground ginger | 2 mL |
| ½ tsp | fine sea salt | 2 mL |
| 2 cups | shredded carrots | 500 mL |
| ⅔ cup | dried currants | 150 mL |
| ½ cup | unsweetened flaked coconut | 125 mL |
| 1 cup | liquid honey, pure maple syrup or brown rice syrup | 250 mL |
| 2 tsp | vanilla extract (GF, if needed) | 10 mL |

1. In food processor, combine oats and walnuts; pulse until coarsely ground.
2. In a large bowl, whisk together oat mixture, quinoa flour, baking powder, baking soda, cinnamon, ginger and salt.
3. In a medium bowl, combine carrots, currants, coconut, honey and vanilla.
4. Add the carrot mixture to the flour mixture and stir with a wooden spoon until blended.
5. Spread batter evenly in prepared pan.
6. Bake in preheated oven for 50 to 60 minutes or until a toothpick inserted in the center comes out with a few moist crumbs attached. Let cool completely in pan on a wire rack.

# Zucchini Quinoa Cake

*Even diehard vegetable dodgers love this zucchini quinoa cake. The vanilla and spices likely influence matters, but the cake itself is so incredibly moist and delicious, it can stand alone.*

## Storage Tip

Store the cooled cake, loosely wrapped in foil or waxed paper, in the refrigerator for up to 3 days. Alternatively, wrap it in plastic wrap, then foil, completely enclosing cake, and freeze for up to 6 months. Let thaw at room temperature for 4 to 6 hours before serving.

- **Preheat oven to 350°F (180°C)**
- **9-inch (23 cm) square metal baking pan, sprayed with nonstick cooking spray**

| | | |
|---|---|---|
| 1¼ cups | quinoa flour | 300 mL |
| ⅔ cup | natural cane sugar or packed light brown sugar | 150 mL |
| 1 tsp | ground cinnamon | 5 mL |
| 1 tsp | baking powder (GF, if needed) | 5 mL |
| ½ tsp | baking soda | 2 mL |
| ½ tsp | fine sea salt | 2 mL |
| ¼ tsp | ground cloves | 1 mL |
| 2 | large eggs, at room temperature | 2 |
| ¼ cup | milk or plain non-dairy milk (such as soy, almond, rice or hemp) | 60 mL |
| 3 tbsp | vegetable oil | 45 mL |
| 1 tsp | vanilla extract (GF, if needed) | 5 mL |
| ¾ cup | shredded zucchini | 175 mL |

1. In a large bowl, whisk together quinoa flour, sugar, cinnamon, baking powder, baking soda, salt and cloves.
2. Add eggs, milk, oil and vanilla to flour mixture and stir with a wooden spoon until blended. Gently stir in zucchini.
3. Spread batter evenly in prepared pan.
4. Bake in preheated oven for 30 to 35 minutes or until a toothpick inserted in the center comes out with a few moist crumbs attached. Let cool completely in pan on a wire rack.

# Anytime Chocolate Quinoa Cake

*This old-fashioned, deeply chocolate pantry cake (no eggs or dairy required) always gets rave reviews from kids and adults alike. It keeps particularly well, too — perfect for late-night refrigerator raids.*

## Tip

Unsweetened carob powder may be used in place of the cocoa powder.

## Storage Tip

Store the cooled cake, loosely wrapped in foil or plastic wrap, in the refrigerator for up to 1 week. Alternatively, wrap it in plastic wrap, then foil, completely enclosing cake, and freeze for up to 6 months. Let thaw at room temperature for 4 to 6 hours before serving.

- **Preheat oven to 350°F (180°C)**
- **8-inch (20 cm) square metal baking pan, sprayed with nonstick cooking spray**

| | | |
|---|---|---|
| 1⅓ cups | quinoa flour | 325 mL |
| ⅓ cup | unsweetened cocoa powder (not Dutch process) | 75 mL |
| ¾ tsp | baking soda | 3 mL |
| ½ tsp | fine sea salt | 2 mL |
| ½ cup | vegetable oil | 125 mL |
| 2 tsp | cider vinegar or white vinegar | 10 mL |
| 1½ tsp | vanilla extract (GF, if needed) | 7 mL |
| 1 cup | water | 250 mL |
| ¾ cup | brown rice syrup or liquid honey | 175 mL |

1. In a large bowl, whisk together quinoa flour, cocoa powder, baking soda and salt.

2. Using the end of a wooden spoon, make one large and two small holes in flour mixture. Add oil to large hole, vinegar to one of the small holes and vanilla to the other small hole. Pour water and brown rice syrup over top and stir until just blended.

3. Immediately pour batter into prepared pan.

4. Bake in preheated oven for 27 to 32 minutes or until a toothpick inserted in the center comes out with a few moist crumbs attached. Let cool completely in pan on a wire rack.

# Chocolate Fudge Brownie Cake

*Suitable for any occasion, this fudgy, dense, delicious treat — part cake, part brownie — falls into the "most requested" category.*

## Tip

To line and spray the springform pan, begin by placing the cake pan on a square of parchment paper that is slightly larger than the pan. Trace around the edge of the pan with a pencil, then set the pan aside. Cut out the circle and place it inside the pan. Spray the paper and the sides of the pan with nonstick cooking spray.

## Storage Tip

Store the cooled cake, loosely wrapped in foil or plastic wrap, in the refrigerator for up to 5 days. Alternatively, wrap it in plastic wrap, then foil, completely enclosing cake, and freeze for up to 6 months. Let thaw at room temperature for 4 to 6 hours before serving.

- **Preheat oven to 350°F (180°C)**
- **9-inch (20 cm) springform pan, lined and sprayed (see tip, at left)**

| | | |
|---|---|---|
| ⅓ cup | semisweet chocolate chips (GF, if needed) | 75 mL |
| 1 cup | quinoa flour | 250 mL |
| 1 cup | natural cane sugar or packed light brown sugar | 250 mL |
| ½ cup | unsweetened cocoa powder (not Dutch process) | 125 mL |
| 1 tsp | baking powder (GF, if needed) | 5 mL |
| ½ tsp | fine sea salt | 2 mL |
| 2 tsp | instant espresso powder | 10 mL |
| 2 | large eggs | 2 |
| 2 | large egg whites | 2 |
| ¾ cup | unsweetened applesauce | 175 mL |
| ½ cup | unrefined virgin coconut oil, warmed, or vegetable oil | 125 mL |
| 2 tsp | vanilla extract (GF, if needed) | 10 mL |
| 1 tbsp | natural cane confectioners' (icing) sugar (optional) | 15 mL |

1. In a small microwave-safe bowl, microwave chocolate chips on Medium (70%) for 30 seconds. Stir. Microwave on Medium (70%) in 15-second intervals, stirring after each, until melted and smooth.

2. In a medium bowl, whisk together quinoa flour, cane sugar, cocoa powder, baking powder and salt.

3. In a large bowl, whisk together espresso powder, eggs, egg whites, applesauce, oil, vanilla and melted chocolate until blended. Stir in flour mixture until just blended.

4. Spread batter evenly in prepared pan.

5. Bake in preheated oven for 30 to 35 minutes or until a toothpick inserted in the center comes out with a few moist crumbs attached. Let cool in pan on a wire rack for 30 minutes.

6. Run a knife around edge of pan, then remove sides of pan. Using parchment paper, lift cake off pan bottom and invert onto rack. Gently peel off parchment, carefully turn cake right side up on rack and let cool completely. If desired, sprinkle confectioners' sugar over cooled cake.

# Chocolate Zucchini Cake

*Rich, moist and
decadently chocolatey,
this cake ranks as one
of my favorite ways
to eat my vegetables.
It's delicious to the
last crumb.*

## Storage Tip

Store the cooled cake,
loosely wrapped in foil
or waxed paper, in the
refrigerator for up to
1 week. Alternatively, wrap
it in plastic wrap, then
foil, completely enclosing
cake, and freeze for up
to 6 months. Let thaw at
room temperature for 4 to
6 hours before serving.

- **Preheat oven to 350°F (180°C)**
- **8-inch (20 cm) square metal baking pan, sprayed with nonstick cooking spray**

| | | |
|---|---|---:|
| 1¼ cups | quinoa flour | 300 mL |
| ¾ cup | natural cane sugar or granulated sugar | 175 mL |
| ⅓ cup | unsweetened cocoa powder (not Dutch process) | 75 mL |
| ¾ tsp | baking soda | 3 mL |
| ½ tsp | fine sea salt | 2 mL |
| 1 | large egg, at room temperature, lightly beaten | 1 |
| ⅓ cup | unsweetened applesauce | 75 mL |
| ¼ cup | buttermilk | 60 mL |
| ¼ cup | vegetable oil | 60 mL |
| 1 tsp | vanilla extract (GF, if needed) | 5 mL |
| 1 cup | shredded zucchini | 250 mL |
| ½ cup | miniature semisweet chocolate chips (GF, if needed) | 125 mL |

1. In a medium bowl, whisk together quinoa flour, sugar, cocoa powder, baking soda and salt.
2. Add egg, applesauce, buttermilk, oil and vanilla to flour mixture. Using an electric mixer on medium-low speed, beat for 1 minute, until blended. Scrape sides and bottom of bowl with a spatula. Beat on medium speed for 1 minute. Gently stir in zucchini.
3. Spread batter evenly in prepared pan.
4. Bake in preheated oven for 15 minutes. Sprinkle with chocolate chips. Bake for 7 to 11 minutes or until a toothpick inserted in the center comes out with a few moist crumbs attached. Let cool completely in pan on a wire rack.

# Raspberry and Toasted Quinoa Cranachan

*There are many versions
of this traditional Scottish
pudding, the simplest
being a stir-up of toasted
oats, whiskey, honey
and cream. Modern
versions make the
most of raspberries by
folding them in at the
last minute.*

## • Medium glass trifle dish or 4 parfait glasses

| | | |
|---|---|---:|
| 1 tbsp | unsalted butter | 15 mL |
| 1 cup | quinoa flakes | 250 mL |
| 3 tsp | natural cane sugar or granulated sugar, divided | 15 mL |
| 2 cups | raspberries, divided | 500 mL |
| 2 cups | plain Greek yogurt | 500 mL |
| 3 tbsp | liquid honey | 45 mL |
| 1 tbsp | whiskey | 15 mL |

**1.** In a large nonstick skillet, melt butter over medium heat. Add quinoa flakes and cook, stirring, for 2 to 3 minutes or until fragrant and golden. Sprinkle with 1 tsp (5 mL) of the sugar and cook, stirring, for 1 minute. Transfer to a plate and let cool completely.

**2.** In a medium bowl, crush 1 cup (250 mL) of the raspberries with a fork. Gently stir in the remaining raspberries and the remaining sugar.

**3.** In another medium bowl, whisk together yogurt, honey and whiskey until blended.

**4.** In trifle dish, layer half the raspberry mixture, half the yogurt mixture and half the quinoa flakes. Repeat layers. Serve immediately.

# Minted Fruit and Quinoa Salad

*With tones of jewel red and blue-black, plus yellows and greens that pop, this salad is both pretty as a painting and utterly delicious.*

## Storage Tip

This salad is best served within 1 to 2 hours of being prepared, but can be stored in an airtight container in the refrigerator for up to 1 day.

| | | |
|---|---|---|
| 1½ cups | quartered hulled strawberries | 375 mL |
| 1½ cups | blackberries | 375 mL |
| 1¼ cups | cooked quinoa (see page 10), cooled | 300 mL |
| 1 cup | fresh pineapple chunks | 250 mL |
| 1 cup | diced kiwifruit | 250 mL |
| 1 cup | loosely packed mint leaves, chopped | 250 mL |
| 2 tbsp | freshly squeezed lime juice | 30 mL |
| 2 tbsp | agave nectar or liquid honey | 30 mL |

1. In a large bowl, gently combine strawberries, blackberries, quinoa, pineapple, kiwi, mint, lime juice and agave nectar.

## Variations

Serve the salad atop lightly sweetened Greek yogurt.

Use an equal amount of fresh basil leaves in place of the mint.

# Creamy Quinoa Millet Butterscotch Pudding

*The true flavor of butterscotch is captured in this easy, creamy, whole-grain pudding. Millet becomes velvety, rich and smooth with a long simmer; quinoa adds a delicate complementary texture and subtle undercurrent of earthy flavor.*

| | | |
|---|---|---|
| ½ cup | quinoa, rinsed | 125 mL |
| ½ cup | millet | 125 mL |
| ⅓ cup | natural cane sugar or packed dark brown sugar | 75 mL |
| ⅛ tsp | fine sea salt | 0.5 mL |
| 3¾ cups | milk or plain non-dairy milk (such as soy, almond, rice or hemp) | 925 mL |
| 2 tsp | vanilla extract (GF, if needed) | 10 mL |

1. In a medium saucepan, combine quinoa, millet, sugar, salt and milk. Bring to a gentle boil over medium heat. Reduce heat to medium-low, cover, leaving lid ajar, and simmer, stirring occasionally, for about 35 minutes or until thickened and creamy. Remove from heat and stir in vanilla.

2. Transfer quinoa mixture to a medium heatproof bowl and let cool to room temperature. Serve at room temperature or cover and refrigerate until cold.

# Quintessential Quinoa Pudding

*The unique texture
of quinoa makes an
incredible pudding. This
polka-dotted dessert is
akin to tapioca, but more
delicate, with the bonus of
a nuanced nutty-sesame
flavor. The possibilities
for variation are vast, but
vanilla, along with a faint
touch of cinnamon, is
always a winner.*

| | | |
|---|---|---|
| 1 cup | quinoa, rinsed | 250 mL |
| 1/4 cup | natural cane sugar or granulated sugar | 60 mL |
| 1/4 tsp | ground cinnamon | 1 mL |
| 1/8 tsp | fine sea salt | 0.5 mL |
| 3 cups | milk or plain non-dairy milk (such as soy, almond, rice or hemp) | 750 mL |
| 2/3 cup | water | 150 mL |
| 2 tsp | vanilla extract (GF, if needed) | 10 mL |

1. In a medium saucepan, combine quinoa, sugar, cinnamon, salt, milk and water. Bring to a gentle boil over medium heat. Reduce heat to medium-low, cover, leaving lid ajar, and simmer, stirring occasionally, for 30 to 35 minutes or until quinoa is very soft and mixture is thickened. Remove from heat and stir in vanilla.

2. Transfer quinoa mixture to a medium heatproof bowl and let cool to room temperature. Serve at room temperature or cover and refrigerate until cold.

## Variations

Add 1/2 cup (125 mL) dried fruit (such as raisins, cherries, blueberries, currants or chopped apricots) with the quinoa in step 1.

Use an equal amount of ground cardamom, allspice or ginger in place of the cinnamon.

Omit the cinnamon and replace the vanilla with 1/2 tsp (2 mL) almond extract (GF, if needed). If desired, sprinkle the pudding with toasted sliced almonds before serving.

# Chocolate Quinoa Pudding

<table>
<tr><td>Makes<br>6 servings</td></tr>
</table>

*Rich and decadent chocolate pudding is always in fashion. This superfood version, however — flush with quinoa, cocoa powder and almond milk — will invoke glee, not guilt.*

## Tip

Milk or another plain non-dairy milk (such as soy, rice or hemp) may be used in place of the almond milk.

• **Six ³⁄₄-cup (175 mL) ramekins or dessert glasses**

| | | |
|---|---|---|
| ³⁄₄ cup | quinoa, rinsed | 175 mL |
| ¹⁄₃ cup | natural cane sugar or packed light brown sugar | 75 mL |
| ¹⁄₃ cup | unsweetened cocoa powder (not Dutch process) | 75 mL |
| 2 tsp | instant espresso powder (optional) | 10 mL |
| ¹⁄₄ tsp | fine sea salt | 1 mL |
| 3¹⁄₂ cups | almond milk | 875 mL |
| 1 | large egg | 1 |
| ¹⁄₃ cup | semisweet chocolate chips (GF, if needed) | 75 mL |
| 1 tbsp | unsalted butter or unrefined virgin coconut oil | 15 mL |
| 1 tsp | vanilla extract (GF, if needed) | 5 mL |

1. In a medium saucepan, combine quinoa, sugar, cocoa powder, espresso power (if using), salt and almond milk. Bring to a gentle boil over medium-high heat. Reduce heat and simmer, stirring often, for 15 minutes.

2. In a small bowl, whisk egg until well blended. Gradually whisk in about 1 cup (250 mL) hot quinoa mixture. Gradually whisk egg mixture into the pan and simmer, stirring constantly, for 10 to 12 minutes or until thickened. Remove from heat and whisk in chocolate chips, butter and vanilla until chocolate and butter are melted.

3. Spoon pudding into ramekins and cover tops with plastic wrap, allowing wrap to touch the surface of the pudding. Let cool to room temperature. Serve at room temperature or refrigerate for 2 to 3 hours, until chilled.

# Baked Quinoa Raisin Pudding

*There are few better
desserts to cozy up with
on a chilly autumn
evening than this
creamy baked pudding,
sweetened with maple
syrup and fragrant
with vanilla, cinnamon
and nutmeg. Quinoa
makes a fantastic and
unexpected foundation.*

## Tip

Other dried fruits, such as
dried cranberries, dried
blueberries, chopped dried
apricots or dried cherries,
may be used in place of
the raisins.

- **Preheat oven to 325°F (160°C)**
- **8-cup (2 L) baking dish, sprayed with nonstick cooking spray**
- **16-cup (4 L) baking dish or roasting pan**
- **Large rimmed baking sheet**

| | | |
|---|---|---|
| ¾ tsp | ground cinnamon | 3 mL |
| ½ tsp | fine sea salt | 2 mL |
| ¼ tsp | ground nutmeg | 1 mL |
| 3 | large eggs | 3 |
| ⅓ cup | pure maple syrup or liquid honey | 75 mL |
| 2 tsp | vanilla extract (GF, if needed) | 10 mL |
| 2 cups | milk or plain non-dairy milk (such as soy, almond, rice or hemp) | 500 mL |
| 3 cups | cooked quinoa (see page 10), cooled | 750 mL |
| 1 cup | raisins | 250 mL |
| | Boiling water | |

1. In a large bowl, whisk together cinnamon, salt, nutmeg, eggs, maple syrup and vanilla until blended. Whisk in milk. Stir in quinoa and raisins.

2. Pour quinoa mixture into prepared 8-cup (2 L) baking dish. Place 16-cup (4 L) baking dish on baking sheet. Set filled baking dish inside larger dish. Transfer baking sheet to the oven and carefully add enough boiling water to the larger dish to reach halfway up the sides of the smaller dish.

3. Bake for 23 to 28 minutes or until golden and set at the center. Transfer filled baking dish to a wire rack and let cool for 20 minutes. Serve warm or let cool completely, cover and refrigerate until cold.

# Maple Quinoa Pudding with Dried Cherries

*Comfort food at its best, this easy quinoa pudding gets loads of flavor and natural sweetness from pure maple syrup and dried cherries.*

## Storage Tip

Store leftover pudding in an airtight container in the refrigerator for up to 2 days.

| | | |
|---|---|---|
| 2 cups | cooked quinoa (see page 10), cooled | 500 mL |
| ¾ cup | dried cherries or cranberries | 175 mL |
| ½ tsp | ground cinnamon | 2 mL |
| ⅛ tsp | fine sea salt | 0.5 mL |
| 1½ cups | milk or plain non-dairy milk (such as soy, almond, rice or hemp) | 375 mL |
| ¼ cup | pure maple syrup | 60 mL |
| 1 tsp | vanilla extract (GF, if needed) | 5 mL |
| ½ cup | chopped toasted pecans | 125 mL |

1. In a medium saucepan, combine quinoa, cherries, cinnamon, salt, milk and maple syrup. Bring to a simmer over medium-high heat. Reduce heat and simmer, stirring constantly, for 20 to 25 minutes or until thickened. Remove from heat and stir in vanilla. Let cool to room temperature. Serve at room temperature or cover and refrigerate until cold.

## Variation

The pudding is also delicious made with liquid honey or brown rice syrup instead of maple syrup.

# Ricotta Quinoa Pudding with Crushed Blackberry Sauce

*Sure, it's great in lasagna, but ricotta makes equally dazzling appearances in desserts. Here, it combines with subtly sweet quinoa to create an innovative baked pudding. A super-easy blackberry sauce — fragrant and floral, sweet and tart — brings out the pudding's best.*

| | | |
|---|---|---|
| 1 cup | ricotta cheese (reduced-fat or regular) | 250 mL |
| 1 cup | milk or plain non-dairy milk (such as soy, almond, rice or hemp) | 250 mL |
| 5 tbsp | liquid honey, divided | 75 mL |
| 1¼ cups | cooked quinoa (see page 10), cooled | 300 mL |
| 1 | large egg | 1 |
| 1 tsp | vanilla extract (GF, if needed) | 5 mL |
| 1¼ cups | fresh or thawed frozen blackberries | 300 mL |
| 2 tsp | freshly squeezed lemon juice | 10 mL |

1. In a medium saucepan, whisk together cheese, milk and 4 tbsp (60 mL) of the honey until smooth. Stir in quinoa. Cook over medium-low heat, stirring, for 15 to 20 minutes or until thickened and creamy. Remove from heat.

2. In a small bowl, whisk egg until well blended. Gradually whisk in ¼ cup (60 mL) hot quinoa mixture. Gradually whisk egg mixture into the pan and cook over medium-low heat, stirring constantly, for 5 minutes. Remove from heat and stir in vanilla. Let cool to room temperature. Serve at room temperature or cover and refrigerate until cold.

3. In a small bowl, coarsely crush blackberries with a fork. Stir in lemon juice and the remaining honey.

4. Divide pudding among four dessert dishes and top with blackberry sauce.

# Blackberry Quinoa Pudding with Cinnamon Walnut Topping

*A cross between a
pudding and a crumble,
this spoonable dessert
takes a summery
turn with glorious
blackberries heightened
by a cinnamon-spiced
walnut topping.*

- **Preheat oven to 375°F (190°C)**
- **8- or 9-inch (20 or 23 cm) square glass baking dish,
  sprayed with nonstick cooking spray**

| | | |
|---|---|---|
| ¼ cup | quinoa flour | 60 mL |
| ¼ cup | natural cane sugar or packed dark brown sugar | 60 mL |
| ¼ cup | chopped walnuts or pecans | 60 mL |
| 1 tsp | ground cinnamon | 5 mL |
| ¼ tsp | fine sea salt, divided | 1 mL |
| 3 tbsp | cold unsalted butter or unrefined virgin coconut oil | 45 mL |
| 1 | large egg | 1 |
| ¾ cup | milk or plain non-dairy milk (such as soy, almond, rice or hemp) | 175 mL |
| ¼ cup | liquid honey, brown rice syrup or agave nectar | 60 mL |
| 3 cups | cooked quinoa (see page 10), cooled | 750 mL |
| 3 cups | fresh or thawed frozen blackberries | 750 mL |

1. In a small bowl, whisk together quinoa flour, sugar, walnuts, cinnamon and ⅛ tsp (0.5 mL) of the salt. Using a pastry blender or two knives, cut in butter until mixture resembles coarse crumbs. Set aside.

2. In a large bowl, whisk together egg, milk, honey and the remaining salt. Stir in quinoa. Gently stir in blackberries.

3. Spoon quinoa mixture into prepared baking dish. Sprinkle with walnut mixture.

4. Bake in preheated oven for 25 to 30 minutes or until berries are bubbling and topping is golden brown. Let cool on a wire rack for 10 minutes. Serve warm or let cool to room temperature.

# Cardamom Quinoa Pudding with Roasted Plums

*The classic pairing of cardamom and honey invites fresh plums, roasted until their sweetness intensifies, to make this simple dish a symphony of flavor.*

- **Preheat oven to 400°F (200°C)**
- **Large rimmed baking sheet, sprayed with nonstick cooking spray**

| | | |
|---|---|---|
| 8 | large red or purple plums, each cut into 8 wedges | 8 |
| 6 tbsp | liquid honey, divided | 90 mL |
| 1 tsp | ground cardamom | 5 mL |
| 1/8 tsp | fine sea salt | 0.5 mL |
| 2 cups | milk or plain non-dairy milk (such as soy, almond, rice or hemp) | 500 mL |
| 2 cups | cooked quinoa (see page 10), cooled | 500 mL |
| 1 | large egg | 1 |
| 1/2 cup | plain Greek yogurt | 125 mL |
| 1 tsp | vanilla extract (GF, if needed) | 5 mL |

1. In a medium bowl, gently toss plums and 2 tbsp (30 mL) of the honey. Spread in a single layer on prepared baking sheet. Roast in preheated oven for 15 to 20 minutes or until browned at the edges. Let cool completely on pan.

2. Meanwhile, in a medium saucepan, whisk together cardamom, salt, milk and the remaining honey. Stir in quinoa. Bring to a boil over medium heat, stirring constantly. Reduce heat and simmer, stirring occasionally, for 12 to 15 minutes or until thickened.

3. In a small bowl, whisk together egg, yogurt and vanilla until blended. Gradually whisk in 1/2 cup (125 mL) quinoa mixture. Gradually whisk egg mixture into the pan and cook, stirring constantly, for 5 minutes.

4. Transfer pudding to a medium bowl and let cool to room temperature. Serve at room temperature or cover surface of pudding with plastic wrap and refrigerate until cold. Serve topped with roasted plums.

# Toasted Coconut Banana Quinoa Pudding

**Makes 6 servings**

*Coconut, quinoa and banana have a natural affinity for each other, so it's no surprise that they make a wonderful pudding.*

## Tip

To toast coconut, preheat oven to 300°F (150°C). Spread coconut in a thin, even layer on an ungreased baking sheet. Bake for 15 to 20 minutes, stirring every 5 minutes, until golden brown and fragrant. Transfer to a plate and let cool completely.

- **Blender or food processor**

| | | |
|---|---|---|
| 1 cup | quinoa, rinsed | 250 mL |
| 2 cups | water | 500 mL |
| 2 cups | light coconut milk | 500 mL |
| 1 cup | mashed ripe bananas | 250 mL |
| 3 tbsp | liquid honey or agave nectar | 45 mL |
| $\frac{1}{2}$ tsp | ground ginger | 1 mL |
| $\frac{1}{8}$ tsp | fine sea salt | 0.5 mL |
| 2 tsp | vanilla extract (GF, if needed) | 10 mL |
| $\frac{1}{2}$ cup | unsweetened flaked coconut, toasted (see tip, at left) | 125 mL |

1. In a medium saucepan, combine quinoa and water. Bring to a boil over medium-high heat. Reduce heat to low, cover and simmer for 12 to 15 minutes or until liquid is absorbed.

2. Meanwhile, in blender, combine coconut milk, bananas, honey, ginger and salt; purée until smooth.

3. Stir banana mixture into quinoa and cook over medium heat, stirring constantly, for 10 to 12 minutes or until thickened. Remove from heat and stir in vanilla.

4. Transfer quinoa mixture to a medium heatproof bowl and let cool to room temperature. Serve at room temperature or cover and refrigerate until cold. Serve sprinkled with toasted coconut.

# Mango Sticky Quinoa

*Mangos are a typical
dessert offering in
Thailand, served
unadorned or
incorporated into a
sweetened coconut sticky
rice. Here, the latter is
recast with quinoa as
the co-star, with sticky-
scrumptious success.*

| | | |
|---|---|---:|
| 2½ tbsp | cornstarch or arrowroot | 37 mL |
| 1½ cups | light coconut milk, divided | 375 mL |
| 2 tsp | finely grated lime zest | 10 mL |
| 2 tbsp | freshly squeezed lime juice | 30 mL |
| ¼ tsp | fine sea salt | 1 mL |
| ¼ cup | liquid honey or agave nectar | 60 mL |
| 3 cups | cooked quinoa (see page 10), cooled | 750 mL |
| 2 cups | diced fresh or thawed frozen mango | 500 mL |

1. In a medium saucepan, whisk together cornstarch, ¼ cup (60 mL) of the coconut milk, lime zest and lime juice until smooth. Whisk in salt, honey and the remaining coconut milk. Bring to a boil over medium heat, whisking constantly. Reduce heat and simmer, whisking, for 2 to 3 minutes or until thickened. Remove from heat and stir in quinoa and mango.

2. Transfer to a medium bowl or serving dish and let cool completely. Cover and refrigerate for 2 to 3 hours or until chilled.

# Sweet Almond Quinoa with Cardamom and Apricots

*This easily assembled
dessert, scented with
cardamom and sweetened
with honey and apricots,
is inspired by the
aromatic sweets found
in Persian, Turkish and
Indian confections.*

| | | |
|---|---|---:|
| 1 cup | quinoa, rinsed | 250 mL |
| 1 tsp | ground cardamom | 5 mL |
| ⅛ tsp | fine sea salt | 0.5 mL |
| 2 cups | almond milk | 500 mL |
| 3 tbsp | liquid honey or agave nectar | 45 mL |
| ½ tsp | rose water (optional) | 2 mL |
| 1 cup | chopped dried apricots | 250 mL |
| ½ cup | toasted sliced almonds | 125 mL |

1. In a medium saucepan, combine quinoa, cardamom, salt, almond milk and honey. Bring to a boil over medium-high heat. Reduce heat to low, cover and simmer for 12 to 15 minutes or until liquid is absorbed. Remove from heat and stir in rose water (if using). Sprinkle with apricots. Cover and let stand for 5 minutes, then fluff with a fork. Serve sprinkled with almonds.

# Index

**Library and Archives Canada Cataloguing in Publication**

Saulsbury, Camilla V
     500 best quinoa recipes : 100% gluten-free : super-easy superfood / Camilla V. Saulsbury.

Includes index.
ISBN 978-0-7788-0414-7

     1. Cooking (Quinoa) 2. Cookbooks. I. Title. II. Title: Five hundred best quinoa recipes.

TX809.Q55S38 2012          641.6'31          C2012-902808-8